D0044038

Clinical Epidemiology: A Basic Science for Clinical Medicine

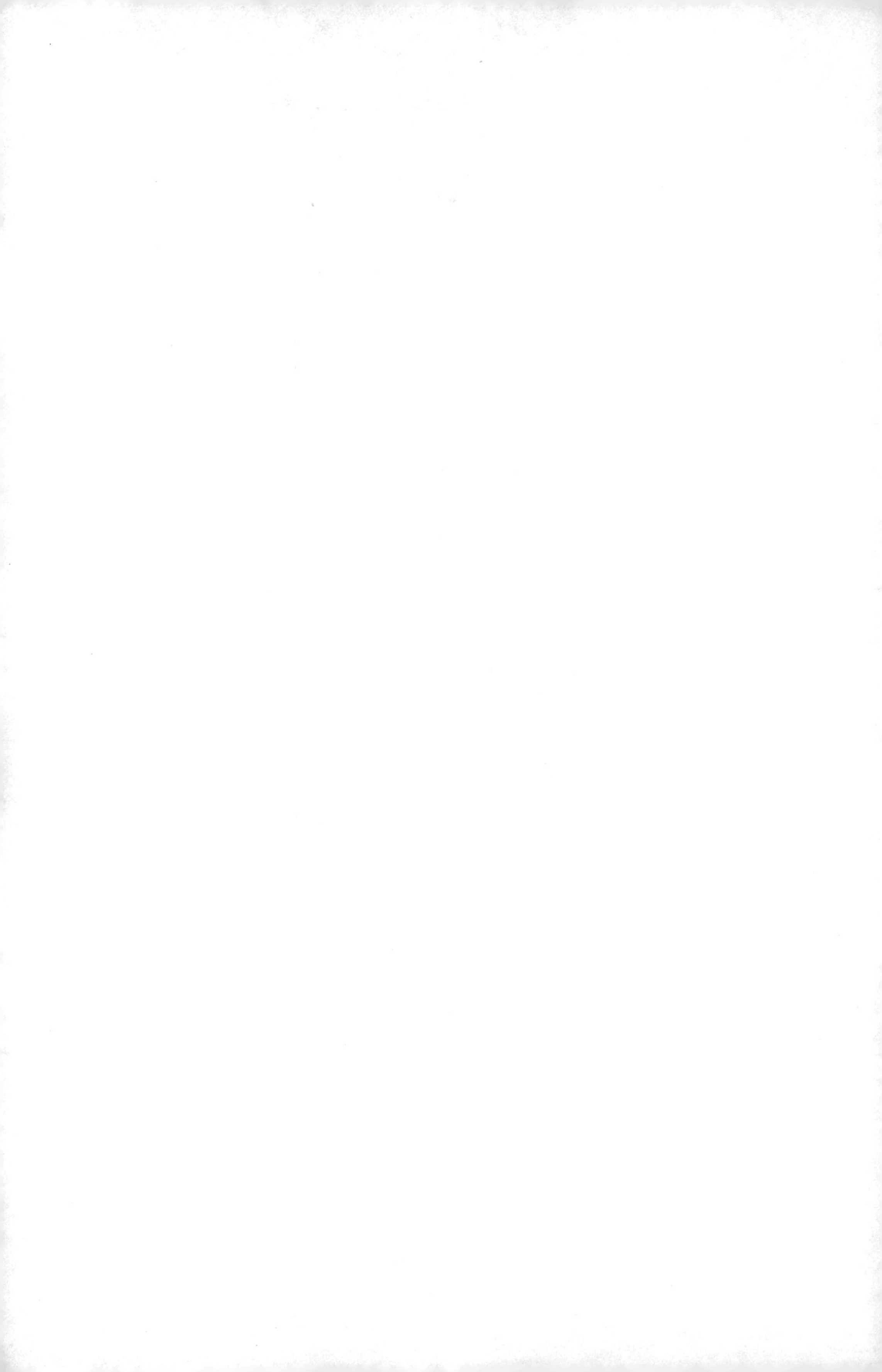

Clinical Epidemiology

A Basic Science for Clinical Medicine

Second Edition

David L. Sackett, M.D., M.Sc.

Professor of Clinical Epidemiology and Biostatistics, and Medicine, McMaster University Faculty of Health Sciences; Attending Physician, Chedoke-McMaster Hospitals, Hamilton, Ontario

R. Brian Haynes, M.D., Ph.D.

Professor of Clinical Epidemiology and Biostatistics, and Medicine, McMaster University Faculty of Health Sciences; Active Staff, Section of Medicine, Chedoke-McMaster Hospitals, Hamilton, Ontario

Gordon H. Guyatt, M.D.

Associate Professor of Clinical Epidemiolo **M.Sc.**
Biostatistics, and Medicine, McMaster University Faculty of Health Sciences; Attending Physician, Chedoke-McMaster Hospitals, Hamilton, Ontario

Peter Tugwell, M.D., M.Sc.

Professor and Chairman, Department of Medicine, University of Ottawa School of Medicine, Ottawa, Ontario

Little, Brown and Company
Boston/Toronto/London

Second Edition
Fifth Printing

Library of Congress Catalog Card No. 91-61705

ISBN 0-316-76599-6

Printed in the United States of America
RRD-VA

This book is dedicated to
Kilgore Trout, J.G.L., Francois Marie Arouet, and
the Emperor's new clothes

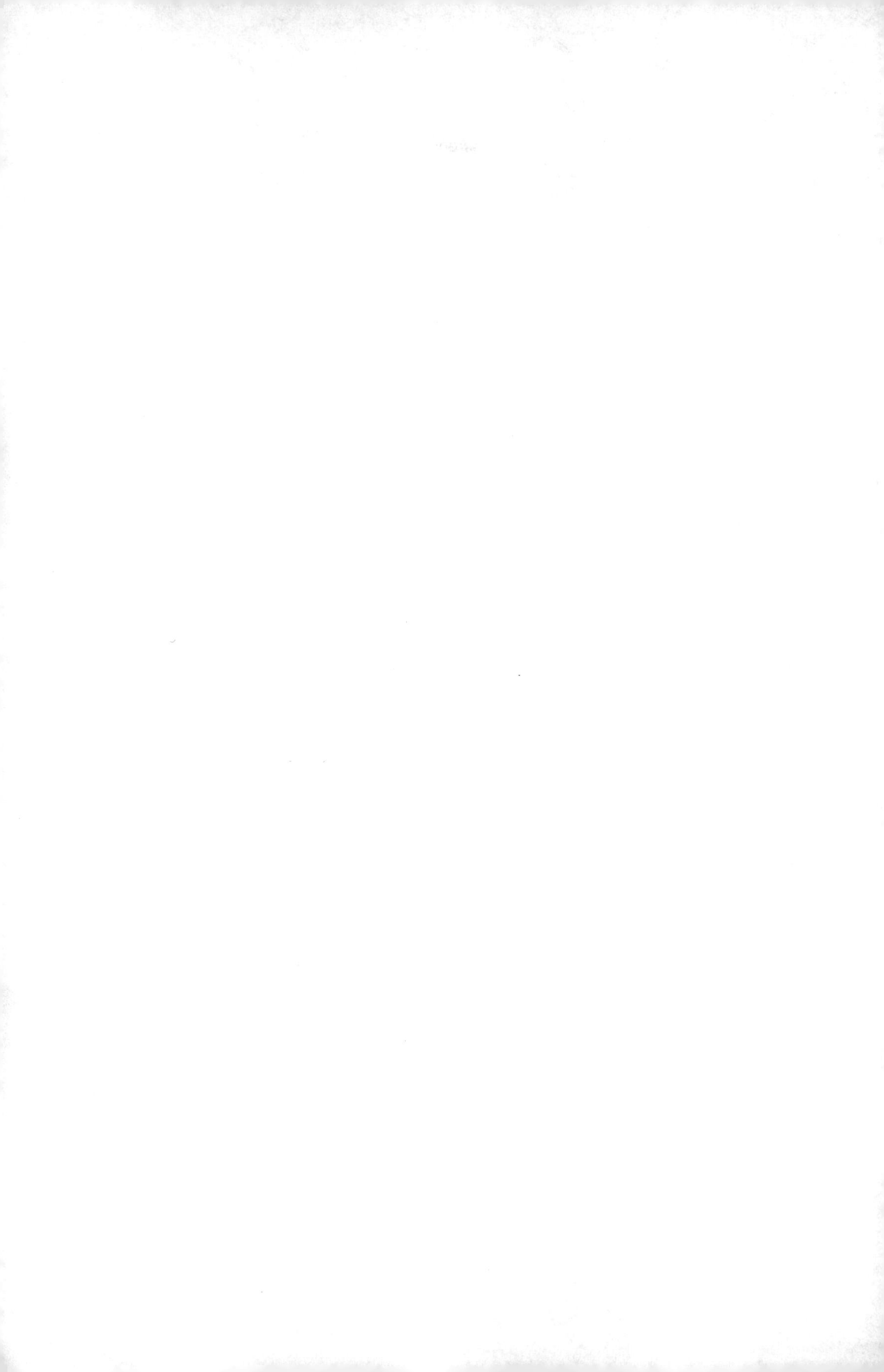

Contents

Preface

Origins

Clinical Epidemiology had its origins in clinical practice, as we struggled with the diagnosis and management of our patients and fell slowly behind in our clinical reading. All of us had been trained in internal medicine, and all of us believed that we were practicing the Art (derived from the beliefs, judgments, and intuitions we could not explain), as well as the Science (derived from the knowledge, logic, and prior experience we could explain), of clinical medicine.

At different times, and in different situations, it dawned on each of us that there was, in fact, a science to the art of medicine. For D.L.S., this realization came when the Cuban missile crisis transformed him, a tenderfoot nephrologist and renal tubular physiologist, into a reluctant field epidemiologist in the U.S. Public Health Service. Although obligated to learn epidemiology (most of it for the first time), he remained a clinician at heart and was repeatedly surprised by the extent to which his growing knowledge of epidemiologic principles could shed light both on the illnesses of patients and on the diagnostic and management behavior of their clinicians. Moreover, it dawned on him that applying these epidemiologic principles (plus a few more from biostatistics) to the beliefs, judgments, and intuitions that comprise the art of medicine might substantially improve the accuracy and efficiency of diagnosis and prognosis, the effectiveness of management, the efficiency of trying to keep up to date, and, of special importance, the ability to teach others how to do these things. The opportunity to explore this science of the art of medicine burgeoned with the creation of a new medical school at McMaster University, which D.L.S. joined in 1967 and where he later teamed up with the other authors to write the first edition of this book.

For R.B.H., the need for an additional basic science for clinical medicine entered his consciousness during a preclerkship lecture on Freudian concepts of psychiatric illness. When he meekly requested the evidence for one of these concepts, the speaker expostulated that the purpose of the lecture was to transmit content, not defend it (and then admitted that he didn't believe it himself). This need for a more systematic approach to gathering and interpreting clinical evidence was reinforced repeatedly during R.B.H.'s early postgraduate training in eastern Canada, most noisily in a running battle between two of his senior attendings as to how he was to measure blood pressures of their patients. These experiences impelled R.B.H. to combine his postgraduate training in internal medicine with graduate work in clinical epidemiology so that he could apply this latter, additional basic science to the interpretation of clinical phenomena. The resulting combined career in clinical epidemiology and clinical practice has led to many things, including the collaboration that produced the first edition.

As a medical student in England, P.T. was attracted to clinical epidemiology by the challenges of trying to apply the principles of population epidemiology to the care of individual patients. However, when he sought career guidance from a world-renowned London epidemiologist, he was informed that it was "amoral" to combine epidemiology with clinical practice! Discouraged from his initial career plan, he entered traditional postgraduate training in internal medicine, spent an exciting three years in Africa, and wound up as Chief Resident in Medicine at McMaster. Encouraged by the attempts to combine clinically oriented epidemiology and clinical medicine that were underway there, P.T. satisfied his rekindled interest by completing training in both clinical epidemiology and rheumatology. He then chaired the Department of Clinical Epidemiology and Biostatistics at McMaster. P.T. practices as an academic rheumatologist, and collaborates with D.L.S. and R.B.H. in projects such as the first edition.

Our common conviction was stated as follows: The important acts we carry out as clinicians require the particularization, to the individual patient, of our prior experiences (both as individual clinicians and collectively) with groups of similar patients. Thus, the rational evaluation of a symptom, sign, or laboratory test result in today's patient demands our critical appraisal of how this clinical finding has behaved previously among groups of patients with the same differential diagnosis. Similarly, the rational selection of a treatment for today's patient requires our appraisal of how similar patients have fared with various treatments in the past. If, on average, they enjoyed better clinical outcomes and fewer side effects on one treatment rather than on others, we will likely prescribe that regimen to today's patient.

If rational clinical practice requires the projection of diagnostic findings, prognoses, and therapeutic responses from groups of patients to the individual patient, then the strategies and tactics used to understand groups of patients (that is, the strategies and tactics of epidemiology and biostatistics) ought to be useful to the clinician. Moreover, it should be possible to take a set of epidemiologic and biostatistical strategies developed to study the distribution and determinants of disease in groups and populations, recast them in a clinical perspective, and use them to improve our clinical performance. The first edition summarized our initial attempts to do so.

In it, we addressed the three challenges that face every clinician every day: reaching the correct diagnosis, selecting the management that does more good than harm, and keeping up to date with useful advances in medicine. In each case, we proposed some practical applications of clinically oriented epidemiology and biostatistics that might help readers improve the accuracy, efficiency, and enjoyment of their clinical efforts.

We begged the readers of the first edition to recognize that it was not a book for the "doers" of research. It contained no discussions on how to pose scientific hypotheses, draw random samples, conduct blind outcome measurements, or perform actuarial analyses. Rather, it was presented as a book for the "users" of research done by others. Moreover, it was organized in terms of clinical actions (diagnosis, management, keeping up to date), not epidemiologic topics. As a result, issues such as statistical significance arose only when they could help in reaching a better clinical decision, and then only within the context of the clinical problem to be solved.

Clinical examples appeared abundantly in those pages, and usually represented actual patients whom we were trying to help when we discovered the usefulness of the particular application of a general strategy of epidemiology or biostatistics. Given the heterogeneity of our intended audience, we anticipated that our readers would be bound to find some of our examples arcane and others oversimplified (and still others managed with approaches unique to southern Ontario) and would risk learning more than they really wanted to know about some of our favorite patients.

Moreover, we emphasized that we all were still pretty new at this game of trying to link group approaches used in epidemiology and biostatistics to individual patients and clinicians and predicted that history (as well as book reviewers) would reveal some spectacular errors in our initial attempts. We hoped, nonetheless, that our mistakes would not prevent our readers from enjoying as well as mastering the lessons to be learned.

Why a Second Edition?

The response to the first edition surprised and delighted us. We made thousands of new friends, received hundreds of letters from students and practitioners who enjoyed both the content and style of the book, and were gratified by the numbers of both young and mid-career clinicians who wrote to tell us how their careers and attitudes toward medicine changed from reading it.

A lot has happened both to us and to the field since we wrote the first edition. D.L.S. decided to put his career where his mouth was and repeated his residency in internal medicine; in addition to being highly educational, this two-year "re-treading" in acute, in-patient referral practice was edifying, terrifying, and hilarious. He then became a full-time clinician on the Chedoke-McMaster medical service, where, surrounded by colleagues whose opinion of his competence was higher than his own, he was made Chief of Medicine. Thus, he has had plenty of recent opportunities to apply the ideas in this book to patient care, to teaching, and to running an ever-busier medical service with ever-fewer resources. Bedside discussions and debates with brilliant clinical clerks, conscientious house staff, and imaginative colleagues have led to the development of some new ways of thinking about and making diagnostic and management decisions, and the ones that have appeared useful are in this edition.

Since the first edition, R.B.H. has become preoccupied with understanding and tightening the connection between the evidence obtained from sound health-care research and what actually happens to patients. Among his activities has been a series of studies on how to find and organize the best clinical evidence right in the emergency room, ICU, ward, or clinic, an effort that has been enriched by always interesting and often productive liaisons with scientists, professional societies, librarians, and colleagues. One of these liaisons found him wearing a penguin suit as he joined several editors of clinical journals in the shadow of Big Ben to celebrate the history of past and present clinical journals. Another has led to his appointment as editor of a new clinical journal, sponsored by the American College of Physicians, the *ACP Journal Club,* which uses the principles of critical appraisal of medical evidence described in this book to identify and present important new findings in internal medicine soon after their primary publication.

P.T. finished his ten years as Chairman of the Department of Clinical Epidemiology and Biostatistics at McMaster, took on a combination of clinical, academic, and administrative responsibilities as director of a new Centre for Arthritic Diseases and Chief of Medicine for the Chedoke Division of Chedoke McMaster Hospitals, and helped form a collaborative group of colleagues at Rheumatic Diseases Units across the country who are combining methodological and clinical questions in their studies. His career as a clinical epidemiologist has been enormously enriched and broadened through involvement in the International Clinical Epidemiology Network (INCLEN) program [4]. Watching and helping the INCLEN fellows and alumni (56 so far at McMaster and more than 150 worldwide) successfully implement locally relevant studies of high quality under extraordinarily difficult circumstances has been a source of inspiration and wonder. As this second edition was going to press, he was named Chairman of the Department of Medicine at the University of Ottawa.

A fourth author has joined us. When G.H.G. was in his final year of postgraduate training and aiming toward a career as a general internist and clinical teacher at a university-affiliated community hospital, he stumbled into the McMaster clinical epidemiology graduate program and decided that it might make that year more interesting. Exhortations from senior colleagues led to an exploratory foray into clinical research. One of the sparks caught and has led to a career at the boundary between research methods and clinical practice. Thus, G.H.G.'s areas of interest are best defined in terms of methods for understanding and solving clinical problems: the measurement of the health-related quality of life, the assessment of health technologies, the application of single-subject (N-of-1) designs to research and clinical practice, the performance and interpretation of scientific overviews, and the practice and teaching of evidence-based medicine.

But, of course, ours has been a small contribution to the total development of the field of clinical epidemiology. Departments and divisions of clinical epidemiology have been created in health science faculties all over the world, and the fastest growing specialty sections of several research societies are devoted to this area. Under the leadership of Alvan Feinstein and Walter Spitzer, a revitalized *Journal of Chronic Disease* has been renamed the *Journal of Clinical Epidemiology.* Clinical epidemiologists have been selected for chairs and chairmanships of departments of medicine and for senior editorships of major clinical journals. Moreover, there has been a salutary critical appraisal of critical appraisal, and we are learning more about when and where it works and doesn't work [1, 3, 5, 6, 7]. A plenitude of new ideas and approaches have come from these developments, and we decided that it was time for us to develop a second edition that would incorporate them.

To our surprise, when we solicited suggestions for how to revise the first edition from about a hundred colleagues here and there, the most common advice we received was "don't fix it if it ain't broke." We were strongly cautioned not to tart up the book or change examples that were already effective in getting our points across. Accordingly, the rules that we applied in revising the book follow.

1. *New examples of the ways of thinking, executing, or learning already presented in the first edition would replace the originals only if they had been shown to be more effective in getting the related principles, strategies, and tactics across to readers.* Thus, the creatine kinase example (based on data from the Edinburgh Royal Infirmary in the 1960s) has yet to be bettered as a means of learning how to interpret diagnostic data, as have the old-fashioned approaches to evaluating exertional chest pain. Our resolve not to bow to calendar time in this matter was strengthened by a reviewer of the first edition who opined: "Less topical examples would have been preferable" [2].

On the other hand, newer or otherwise better examples do appear at several spots in the second edition, especially in Chapters 4, 7, and 9–14.

2. *New ways of thinking about, executing, or learning about diagnosis, management, and keeping up to date would be included if we had been using them for at least a year and their evaluation to date had led us to conclude that they were useful.* This led to the inclusion of 15 new elements or major changes in this edition. Thus, in the section on diagnosis, we've added discussions on the utility of diagnostic tests (page 62), their use in defining the severity of disease (page 54), how to select them when no gold standard is available (page 53), and how to become a faster (as well as more accurate) diagnostician through the application of SpPin and SnNout (page 83).

In the part on management, Chapters 6 (on making a prognosis) and 7 (on deciding on the best therapy) now include sections on how to interpret confidence limits (pages 174 and 217), and the latter has new sections on how to understand utilities (page 209) when they appear in clinical articles about the efficacy of therapy and how to use the number-needed-to-treat as a measure of clinical significance (page 204), and a major, new section on how to conduct your own N-of-1 trials of therapy in your own patients (page 223).

In Part III, Keeping Up to Date, Chapter 10 drops an occasional approach to assessing your own performance that we never faithfully carried out and documents some additional ones that have been shown to improve performance. Breakthroughs in our ability to track down, retrieve, and catalog clinically useful information have led us to rewrite virtually all of Chapter 11 on tracking down the solutions to clinical problems and Chapter 12 on surveying the medical literature in order to keep up to date.

Since our own libraries continue their rapid change, and because we didn't much like the first edition's chapter on creating and running your own library, we dropped it. Moreover, since our earlier chapter on how to read a clinical journal was highly repetitious of information provided elsewhere in the book, we dropped that one, too.

The growing interest in meta-analysis as a means of deciding how to manage patients led us to write a new chapter, which combines guides for reading reviews, overviews, and meta-analyses with our earlier guides for reading economic analyses. Finally, new strategies and tactics for teaching and learning clinical epidemiology at the bedside continue to emerge, and we have revised Chapter 14 accordingly.

On Definitions and Traditions

The first edition lacked a formal definition of clinical epidemiology. So does this one. The reasons are two. First, those readers who don't already know us will soon discover that we are pretty short on formality. Second, we agree with Peter Medawar that: "The innocent belief that words have an essential or inward meaning can lead to appalling confusion and waste of time" [8]. It seems to us that the "essentialist" approach (which invokes ontology and insists that every word has a single, formally correct definition) is simply not up to the tasks that must be carried out in clinical and health care.

Rather, we are forced by both logic and necessity to behave as "nominalists" if we are to cope successfully with the multiple definitions for real-world situations like coronary heart disease (which can be defined in terms of signs and symptoms, or electrocardiograms, or serum enzymes, or gross and microscopic anatomy, or ventricular wall motion, or radioisotopic perfusion, or even symptomless predictors). Again, of course, Medawar said it better: "Let us take it that our business is to attach words to ideas and definitions, not to attach definitions to words." Thus, in order to be helpful to our patients and each other we have lived by the conviction that "clinical epidemiology is what clinical epidemiologists do."* Those who really want to ponder the definition of clinical epidemiology can do it on their own time.†

We also won't attempt to chronicle the development of clinical epidemiology as a basic science for ancient and modern medicine and will leave to others debates about whether Thomas Sydenham, John Snow, or Eve was the first clinical epidemiologist. One thing is clear in 1990, however, and that is that all of us currently working in this field are indebted to Alvan Feinstein for his success in making it scientifically rigorous, academically legitimate, and rollicking fun.

And Finally

If, in the final analysis, the practice of this "science of the art of medicine" is to do more good than harm to patients and clinicians, five additional ingredients must be added to the study of this book. First, its elements must be integrated with those of the other basic sciences, such as morphology, physiology, and biochemistry, as they are applied; were the approaches presented here to consti-

*Actually, we lifted this flagrantly nominalist definition from a "big-E" epidemiologist named Reuel Stallones who, in turn, attributed it to Sandy Gilliam [10].

†The best current starting point is probably the paper from C. David Naylor and his colleagues in the *Journal of Clinical Epidemiology* [9].

tute the sole scientific basis for clinical action, we would simply be substituting a new tyranny of unachievable methodologic rigor for the old tyranny of unteachable clinical art. Second, this approach to diagnosis, management, and keeping up to date must be fed by an increasing body of valid and clinically useful new knowledge, generated from sound, relevant clinical research; without this new knowledge, the approach described in this book could rapidly degenerate into nihilism and therapeutic paralysis. Third, clinical epidemiology must continue to generate new strategies and tactics for identifying and solving problems in diagnosis, management, and keeping up to date; otherwise, this basic science will risk subservience to clinical and information technology. Fourth, this additional basic science for clinical medicine must be applied with abundant humility, recognizing that much of its justification stems from its ability to explain and to teach, not replace, the art of medicine.

Finally, we hope that as you use the strategies and tactics of clinical epidemiology we present in this book, you will add sufficient enthusiasm, irreverence, and merriment to have as much fun in their application as we have had in their development!

D.L.S.
R.B.H.
G.H.G.
P.T.

References

1. Bennett, K. J., Sackett, D. L., Haynes, R. B., et al. A controlled trial of teaching critical appraisal of the literature to medical students. *J.A.M.A.* 257: 2451, 1987.
2. Faergeman, O. Clinical epidemiology: A basic science for clinical medicine (book review). *Int. J. Technol. Assess.* 3: 630, 1987.
3. Frasca, M.A., Dorsch, J. L., Aldag, J. C., et al. A controlled study of a multidisciplinary approach to information management and critical appraisal instruction. *Clin. Res.* 38: 727A, 1990.
4. Halstead, S. B., Tugwell, P., and Bennett, K. J. INCLEN. *J. Clin. Epidemiol.* In press.
5. Hayward, R., Bass, E., Grace, D., et al. Learning critical appraisal in a medical house staff clinic. *Clin. Res.* 38: 728A, 1990.
6. Kitchens, J. M., and Pfeifer, M. P. Teaching residents to read the medical literature: A controlled trial of a curriculum in critical appraisal/clinical epidemiology. *J. Gen. Intern. Med.* 4: 384, 1989.
7. Linzer, M., Brown, J. T., Frazier, L. M., et al. Impact of a medical journal club on house-staff reading habits, knowledge, and critical appraisal skills. *J.A.M.A.* 260: 2537, 1988.
8. Medawar, P. B. The phenomenon of man. In *The Art of the Soluble*. London: Methuen, 1958.
9. Naylor, C. D., Basinski, A., Abrams, H. B., and Detsky, A. S. Clinical and population epidemiology: Beyond sibling rivalry? *J. Clin. Epidemiol.* 43: 607, 1990.
10. Stallones, R. A. Epidemi(olog)^{2}y. *Amer. J. Pub. Health* 53: 82, 1963.

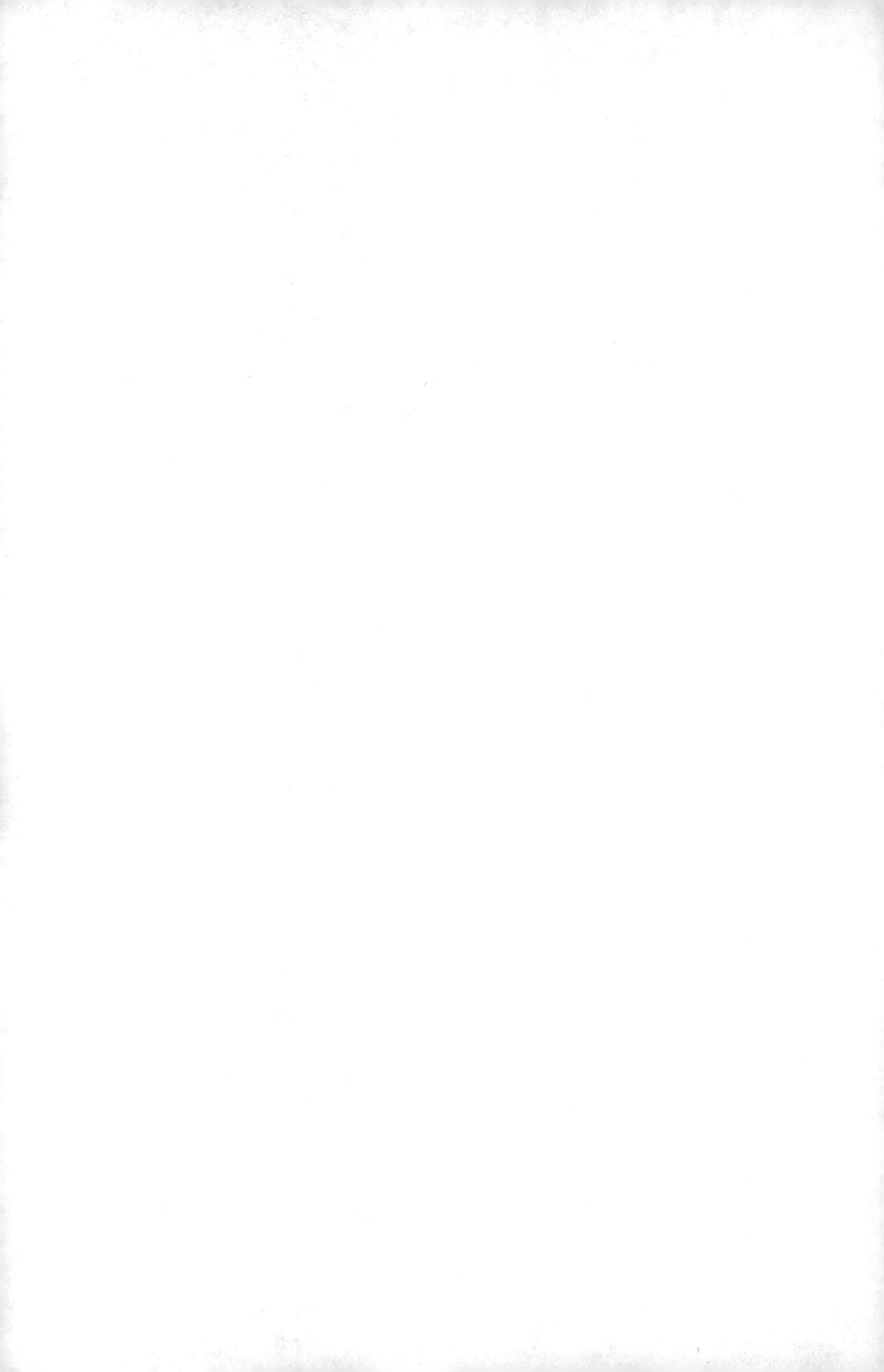

Acknowledgments

This second edition never would have been accomplished without the wonderously effective and tirelessly good-humored Barbara Montesanto, who orchestrated the review of the previous edition by colleagues all over the world, organized and edited the new and revised elements of the manuscript, and kept the unruly authors to their words.

In our first edition, we acknowledged that the book would never have been started without the commitment and support of five men who championed the development of clinical epidemiology at McMaster: John Evans, Jack Hirsh, Bill Spaulding, Jack Laidlaw, and Fraser Mustard. In the interval to the second edition, George Browman and John Cairns have continued this commitment and support, and we thank them for it. Special thanks to Bill Spaulding for serving as D.L.S.'s mentor during his "retreading" as a general internist.

The second edition of this book was written while D.L.S. was on sabbatical at Oxford University, where he received both sanctuary and stimulation from Iain Chalmers, Richard Peto, Richard Doll, and all the McPhersons, as well as generous support from the Anna Grisafi Memorial Fund, the Canadian Heart and Stroke Foundation, the Medical Research Council of Canada, the National Health Research and Development Programme of Canada, the Canadian Society for Clinical Investigation, the Royal College of Physicians and Surgeons of Canada, and the Sir Arthur Sims Travelling Professorship of the Royal College of Surgeons of London.

We thank our loved ones for inspiring our efforts and forgiving our preoccupations.

Don Rosenthal, David Cadman, Irene Uchida, Jack Laidlaw, Bob Volpe, and their patients contributed the color plates that appear in Chapter 1, and we thank them for this. Thanks, too, to Wayne Taylor for Tables 7-15 and 7-16, and to Charlie Goldsmith and Eric Duku for Figure 7-1.

Laurie Anello is the most recent member of a series of editors at Little, Brown who have encouraged and supported our efforts, and Herbert Nolan starred in editing our manuscript in a fashion that corrected its glaring errors, but not its irreverence.

Finally, as with the first edition, our colleagues were wonderfully helpful by proposing changes in the second edition, reading drafts of the resultant revisions, gently pointing out the passages that were obtuse, irrelevant, dead wrong, or really dopey, and offering affectionate advice on how to make them better: Steve Birch, Andrew Brunskill, John Clemens, Deb Cook, Bob Fletcher, John Gately, Dick Heller, Jack Hirsh, Walter Holland, Tom Inui, Len Kurland, Roberta LaBelle, Bob Lachance, Eric Larson, Mitch Levine, Wendy Levinson, Joel Lexchin, Sjef van der Linden, Barb Mueller, Andy Oxman, Akbar Panju, Saul Rosen, Rob Strack van Schijndel, Greg Stoddart, Jan Vandenbroucke, and Kerr White. To them should go the credit for those portions of the book that are lucid, useful, and effective. The authors bear the sole responsibility for the rest.

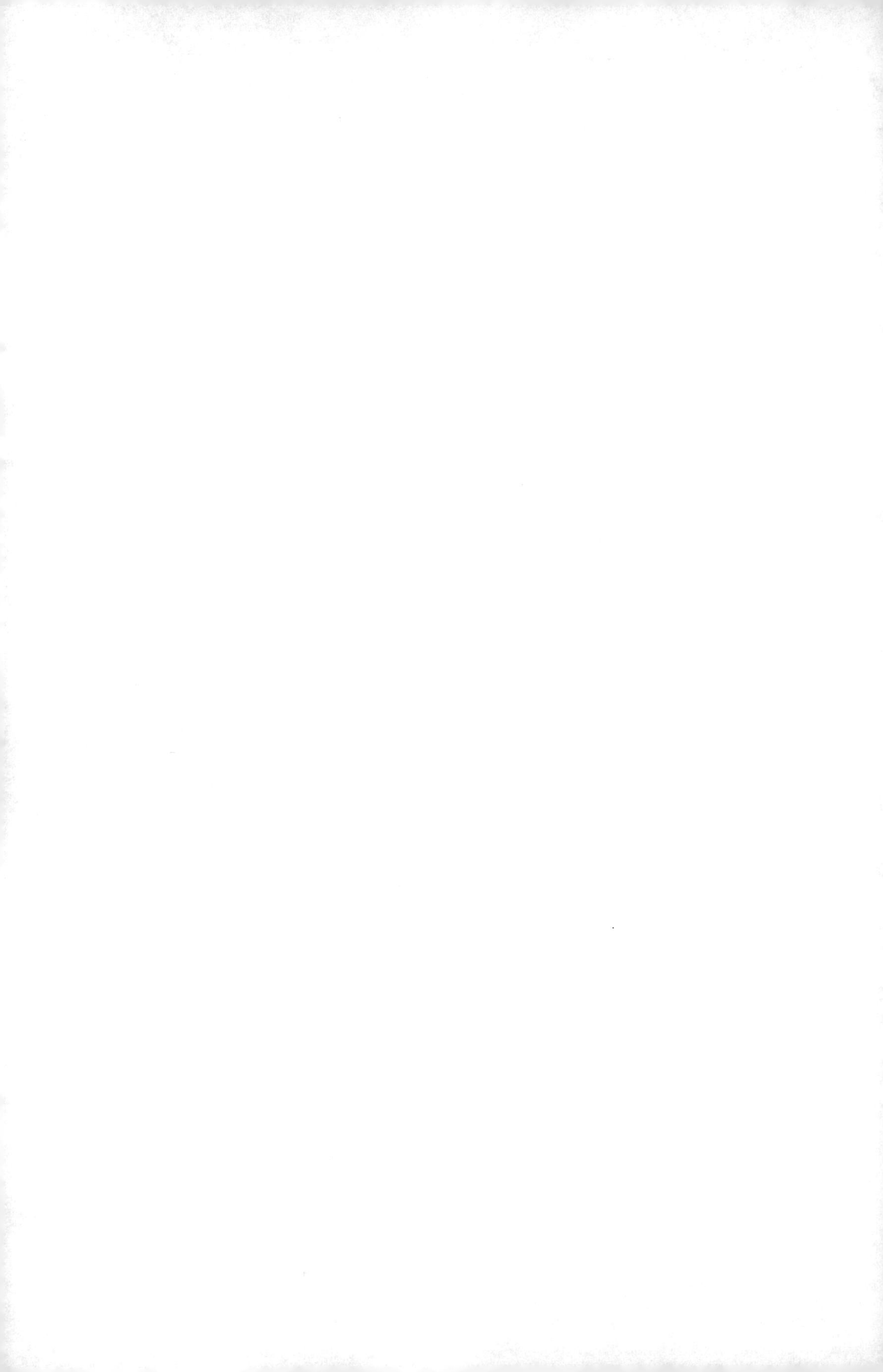

Clinical Epidemiology: A Basic Science for Clinical Medicine

Notice

The indications and dosages of all drugs in this book have been recommended in the medical literature and conform to the practices of the general medical community. The medications described do not necessarily have specific approval by the Food and Drug Administration for use in the diseases and dosages for which they are recommended. The package insert for each drug should be consulted for use and dosage as approved by the FDA. Because standards for usage change, it is advisable to keep abreast of revised recommendations, particularly those concerning new drugs.

I

Diagnosis

1

Clinical Diagnostic Strategies

This first part of the book is about diagnosis, the crucial process that labels patients and classifies their illnesses, that identifies (and sometimes seals!) their likely fates or prognoses, and that propels us toward specific treatments in the confidence (often unfounded) that they will do more good than harm.

This first chapter will provide some definitions and descriptions of the four strategies that we use in clinical diagnosis. The second considers the tactics we use to identify symptoms and signs and how this typically fallible human activity can be made more accurate. The third chapter presents some strategies for deciding whether to seek a given sign or symptom and whether to order a given paraclinical diagnostic test, and the fourth presents a range of simple to complex tactics for interpreting, with power and finesse, these signs, symptoms, and paraclinical diagnostic tests. The final chapter in this section grapples with the rationale and results of our attempts to achieve early diagnosis.

Some Definitions

Discussions about definitions can become so heavy and pedantic that they destroy rather than pique the reader's interest (the first draft of this chapter was no exception!). Nonetheless, and because we identified ourselves as "nominalists" back in the Preface to this 2nd Edition, we need to tell you what we mean when we use certain words.

Most of us, most of the time, see patients because they are sick. We help them most when we recognize that their sickness has three elements [14].

THE DISEASE OR TARGET DISORDER

By this we mean the anatomic, biochemical, physiologic, or psychologic derangement whose etiology (if known), maladaptive mechanisms, presentation, prognosis, and management we read about in medical texts. Although this element is usually called the *disease,* the usefulness of this ambiguous term is hampered by the inability of both patients and health scientists to agree whether even common problems such as hypertension, hay fever, and hemorrhoids are diseases [3]. Accordingly, we shall call this element of a patient's sickness the *target disorder* when it becomes the objective of the diagnostic process.

THE ILLNESS

As a result of having, and responding to, the target disorder, patients exhibit clusters of *symptoms* (manifestations of the target disorder that they themselves perceive, either spontaneously or upon questioning) and *signs* (manifestations perceived by their clinicians during an examination). We shall call this cluster the *illness*.

THE PREDICAMENT

The third element of a sickness is the social, psychological, and economic fashion in which the patient is situated in the environment. David Taylor [14] calls this the *predicament* and we will, too.

The act of clinical diagnosis focuses on the second element of a sickness (the illness), in order to identify the first (the target disorder), while keeping an eye on the third (the predicament). Put more formally, the act of clinical diagnosis is classification for a purpose: *an effort to recognize the class or group to which a patient's illness belongs so that, based on our prior experience with that class, the subsequent clinical acts we can afford to carry out, and the patient is willing to follow, will maximize that patient's health.*

Two logical consequences follow. First, because your diagnosis and "subsequent clinical acts" have their rational basis in our prior, collective experience with *groups* of patients, it follows that the strategies and tactics of understanding the *distribution and determinants of health and disease in groups* (i.e., *epidemiology*) can be useful to you as a clinician. Second, from the point of view of clinical diagnosis, most medical texts* and courses are backward: they start with target disorders and go backward to illnesses, the exact reverse of the diagnostic process.

In proceeding from the illness to the target disorder, the diagnostic process can focus on different elements of the latter. Usually we think of diagnosis proceeding from symptoms and signs to focus on the documentation of maladaptive alterations in structure, function, and/or response to stimuli. Alternatively, especially in primary care, diagnosis can proceed from symptoms and signs to focus on prognosis, and the operative term becomes "watch and wait." Finally, diagnosis may focus on a "therapeutic trial" of identifying the target disorder on the basis of its response to specific therapy.

The foregoing discussion concerns diagnosis in its most common mode. Of course, the same process can be carried out in other modes and for other objectives. We can seek to protect patients, or those around them, by detecting their disorders before they become ill. This presymptomatic diagnosis can be achieved by asking free-living citizens to volunteer for testing (as in shopping plaza screening for hypertension) or by testing for one presymptomatic disorder in a patient who has come to us for help with another, unrelated but symptomatic one (case finding for hypertension in a patient who comes to our office with subdeltoid bursitis). We will discuss these strategies for early diagnosis in Chapter 5.

Moreover, as we'll discuss in greater detail at the beginning of Chapter 4, diagnostic testing sometimes is applied to determine not whether a disorder is present but *how severe* it is (as in testing for target organ damage to the heart, eyes, and kidneys in a patient with diabetes), what its *prognosis* might be (as in

*Exceptions to this rule have grown since the first edition, where we cited portions of only Harrison [9], Harvey [10], and Goroll, May, and Mulley [8]. Books like these pioneered the approach that starts with illnesses (backache, lump in the neck, black stools, convulsions) and only then proceeds to discuss the target disorders (such as herniated disk, thyroid adenoma, duodenal ulcer, meningioma) that could cause them. Recent additions to this list of exceptions are cited on page 356.

bedside tests of left ventricular function after a myocardial infarction), and whether it is responding to therapy (as in the periodic determination of signs, symptoms, and hormone levels in patients previously treated with therapeutic radioiodine).

This chapter is mainly about the clinical diagnosis of symptomatic illness, and we shall now get on with it by considering four strategies for doing so [12].

The Four Strategies of Clinical Diagnosis

STRATEGY #1

Jot down your diagnoses for the patients in Plates 1 to 6.*

Did a single diagnosis leap to mind as you looked at each picture?† If we asked you to tell us why you are sure that Plate 2 is psoriasis, would you launch into a differential diagnosis based on the distribution, configuration, and desquamation characteristics of the dermatitides, or would you simply state: "Because that's what psoriasis looks like!" or "What else could it be?"

If the latter shoe fits, you have been executing the strategy called *pattern recognition.* It is also sometimes called the *gestalt method* or, informally, *Aunt Minnie* (the latter because, if you saw your Aunt Minnie walking down the street, even dozens of meters away and with her back to you, you would instantly know it was she from the length of her stride, the way she swings her arms, that distinctive hat she always wears, and her Wellington boots).

By pattern recognition is meant *the instantaneous realization that the patient's presentation conforms to a previously learned picture (or pattern) of disease.* It is usually visual, and if this book included moving, as well as still pictures, we could have included parkinsonism, myasthenia gravis, catatonia, and rabies.

Pattern recognition can also be auditory, as from the speech of the patient with a cleft or paralyzed palate. Moreover, it has been claimed that the voice of myxedema may permit its diagnosis by telephone. Pattern recognition by odor is less common (humans are not very good at sensing them, and society dictates that we should not give them off) but examples include diabetic acidosis, liver failure, and the "sweaty foot" smell of isovaleric acidemia. Perhaps we now regard sniffing at patients as impolite (at least if they are adults; some neonatologists claim that babies with impending sepsis can be sniffed out). Or, maybe the opportunities to sniff with diagnostic profit are simply diminishing; one of our "attendings" back in medical school diagnosed typhoid fever by sniffing the air as he came onto the big charity wards of that era.

Pattern recognition also can occur through touch, as with the ganglion on the back of the hand, the stony hard cancer of the breast or prostate, or the subcutaneous lipoma. Finally, pattern recognition by taste diagnosed diabetic glycos-

*We hope you are the sort of reader who is willing to study figures and tables, because we will use them throughout this book to present key pieces of evidence. The text, on the other hand, is mostly concerned with inferences about this evidence, and you will not learn how to apply these strategies and tactics if you ignore the figures and tables.

†You can compare your diagnoses with ours by checking the footnote on page 6.

uria in the days before modern chemistry labs and squeamishness took over the testing of urine.*

Pattern recognition is reflexive, not reflective. We do it, but usually cannot explain to others why or how we do it.† Because it is thus "nonverbal" it usually is "learned" on patients, not "taught" in lecture halls, and its use understandably increases with clinical experience.

It can be (and has been!) argued that pattern recognition is only the start, and not the end, of the diagnostic process, and that it results in several, *possible* diagnoses, rather than a single, *certain* one. We maintain that it manifestly does both, and would call as our first witness the country doctor who reaches for the lindane when he sees nits and for the heaviest book in the house when he feels a ganglion. Nonetheless, we shall come back later to pattern recognition as a means for starting a different diagnostic strategy.‡

STRATEGY #2

A patient with chest pain is being worked up by a physician's assistant, who refers to a series of figures, including the one shown in Figure 1-1.

Note that each decision point (or "box") in Figure 1-1 poses one or more unambiguous questions, the responses to which determine the subsequent direction of the diagnostic inquiry. Also note that the individual pathways can terminate in confirmatory tests for the etiology of the pain, in specific management, or in referral to another clinician.

Figure 1-1 is an example of what we call the *multiple-branching* or *arborization* strategy of diagnosis: *the progression of the diagnostic process down but one of a large number of potential, preset paths by a method in which the response to each diagnostic inquiry automatically determines the next inquiry to be carried out and, ultimately, the correct diagnosis.*

The arborization strategy is supremely logical; indeed, it had better be, for its "algorithm" must be spelled out in its entirety before the patient appears. Accordingly, the multiple-branching method must include all relevant causes for or managements of the presenting problem, linking them by pathways that rival the idealized diagnostic process of an expert clinician.

As inferred from the example in Figure 1-1, the multiple-branching method often focuses on symptoms and is used mainly when diagnosis is delegated from those who traditionally have carried it out (e.g., physicians) to those who tra-

*Thomas Willis, the 17th-century physician who described the arterial circle at the base of the brain, wrote that diabetic urine "was wonderfully sweet as if it were imbued with Honey or Sugar" in his chapter, Of the Too Much Evacuation by Urine, and Its Remedy; and Especially of the Diabetes or Pissing Evil, Whose Theory and Method of Curing, Is Inquired Into [15].

†We will show you in Chapter 4 that pattern recognition results when a sign or symptom has a very high specificity for a single disorder and simply does not occur in other disorders. One of our clinical clerks coined a mnemonic, *SpPin*, to remind us that a sign with high *Sp*ecificity, when *P*resent, rules—*in* the disorder.

‡The patients appearing in Plates 1 to 6 have Down syndrome, psoriasis, hyperthyroidism, neurofibromatosis (did you pick up the café au lait spots?), primary syphilis, and herpes zoster of the ophthalmic portion of the fifth cranial nerve, respectively.

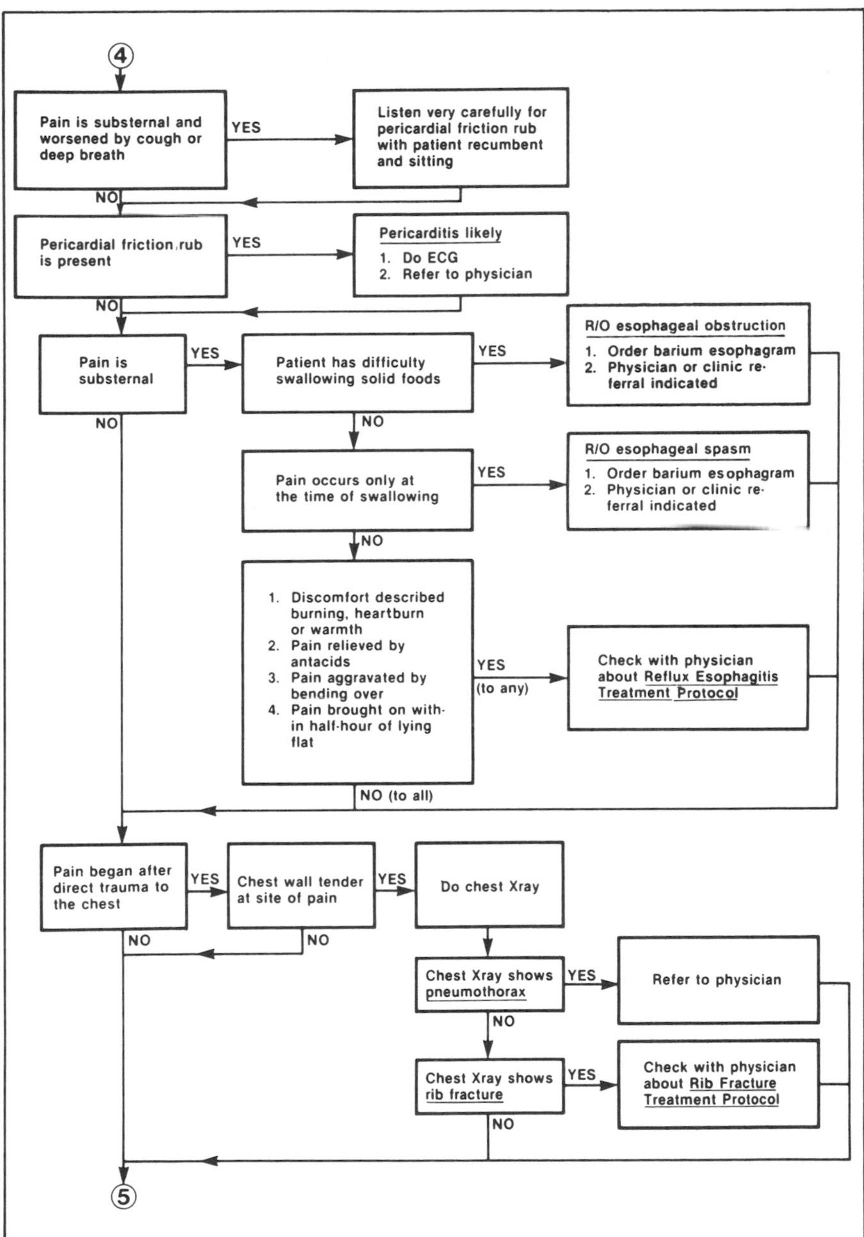

Figure 1-1. Part of a chest pain algorithm. (Courtesy of Harold C. Sox, Jr., M.D.)

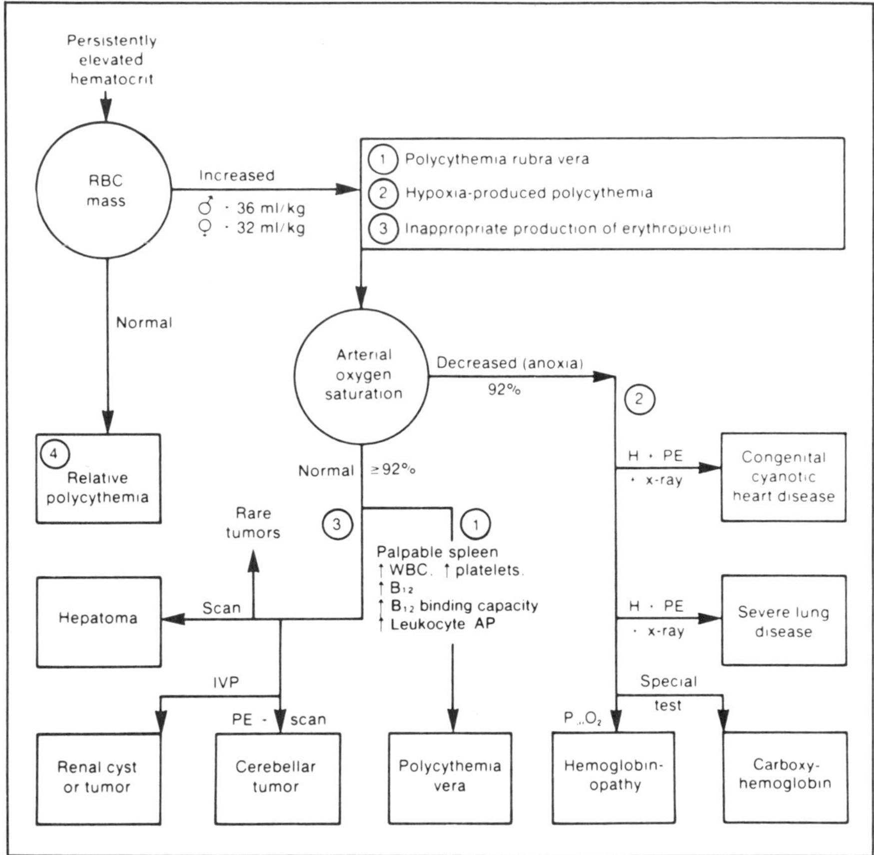

Figure 1-2. Algorithm for a persistently elevated hematocrit. (From P. Cutler, *Problem Solving in Clinical Medicine*. Baltimore: Williams & Wilkins, 1979.)

ditionally have not (e.g., nurses) [13]. Its usefulness, however, extends beyond delegation of responsibility for evaluating presenting symptoms, as shown in Figure 1-2. In this figure, the algorithm deals with a laboratory test result (a persistently elevated hematocrit) rather than a sign or symptom and was prepared to help physicians deal with a relatively uncommon problem, not to help nurse practitioners deal with a relatively common one.

Finally, the multiple-branching method can deal with a very broad array of disorders in which triage, not treatment, is the objective. This would apply in regions where patients and physicians are kept apart by space, time, or money and what is required is a sorting out, at the periphery, of illnesses into those that need (and can benefit from) referral and those that can be cared for locally. An impressive example of this is seen in Figure 1-3. As shown, a very few signs and symptoms distinguish among life-threatening and innocuous nutritional dis-

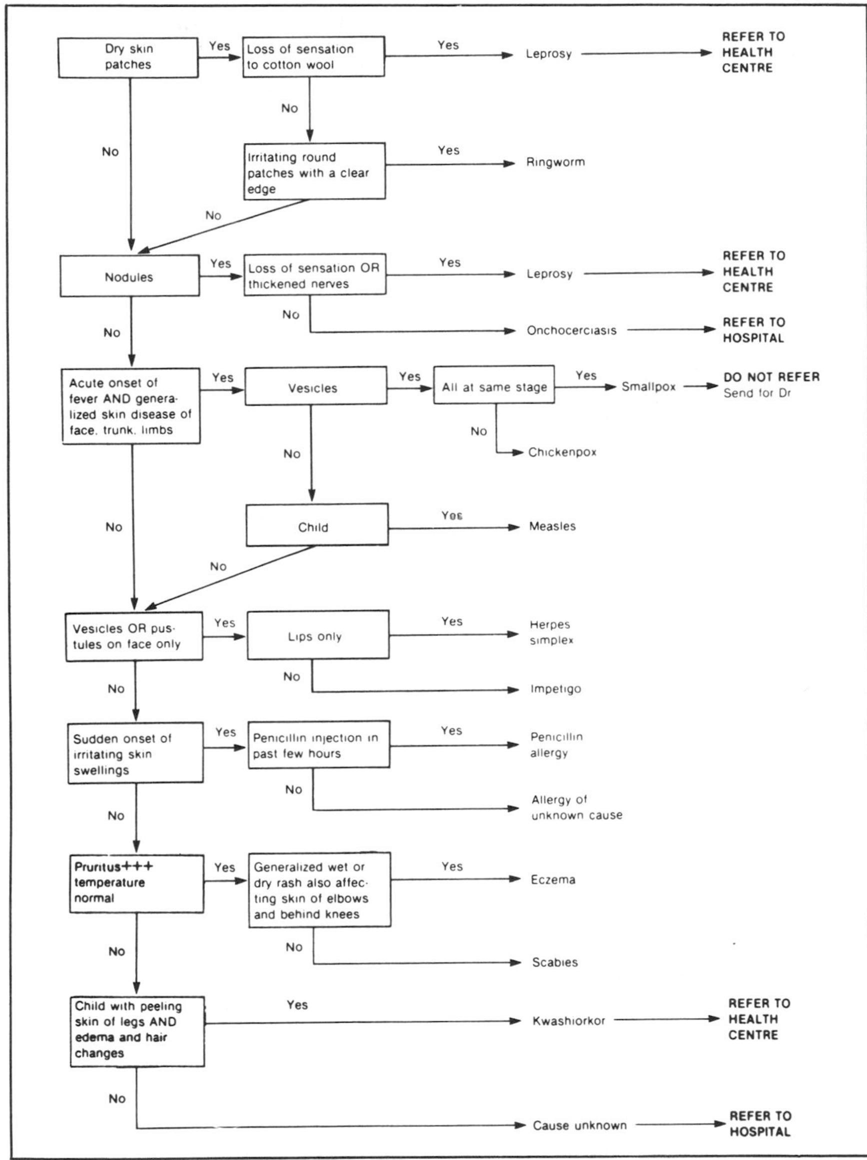

Figure 1-3. An algorithm for skin rash in Tanzania. (From B. J. Essex, *Diagnostic Pathways in Clinical Medicine*. Edinburgh: Churchill Livingstone, 1976. P. 134.)

orders, allergies, and infections (the latter from viruses,* bacteria, fungi, arthropods, and worms). More important, the algorithm distinguishes those patients requiring urgent or early referral from those that can be cared for locally. This last example stresses the *efficiency* of the multiple-branching approach. If you were a high school student faced with two hundred rashes, no laboratory, and the nearest dermatologist four days away, would you pass up an algorithm like this one?

STRATEGY #3

"Go do a complete history and physical."

All of you have received such a command, haven't you? Indeed, most of you could hardly wait until you could turn around and issue the same command to somebody else, couldn't you?†

One of us faithfully followed this command as a shiny new clinical clerk, and the 35-page workups that resulted provoked two contrasting pronouncements from the Chief Resident. The first acclaimed: "These are the best workups ever performed on this service." The second lamented: "But who the hell would ever want to wade through them?" When their author protested, "Didn't you want a complete history and physical?," the Chief Resident (revealing a latent talent for shaggy-dog stories) countered, "Yes, but not *that* complete!"

Anecdotes notwithstanding, complete histories and physicals can be awfully complete, as confirmed by the guides promulgated by different medical schools or published in texts on physical diagnosis. For example, one of the latter points out that "The parts of the medical history follow a standardized sequence, differing only in small details from one institution to another," [5] and goes on to list the components of the past history of infectious disease:

> Dates and complications of measles, German measles, mumps, whooping cough, chickenpox, smallpox, diphtheria, typhoid fever, malaria, hepatitis, scarlet fever, rheumatic fever, chorea, influenza, pneumonia, pleurisy, tuberculosis, bronchitis, tonsillitis, venereal diseases, and others. Give dates of chemotherapy and antibiotic treatment with any reaction to drugs.

Curiously, these same texts express ambivalence about the whole undertaking. For example, the introduction to the foregoing excerpt points out: "Ordinarily, the items in the past history have no great diagnostic value." What is going on here?

What is going on here is called the clinical diagnostic strategy of *exhaustion: the painstaking, invariant search for (but paying no immediate attention to) all*

*The eradication of smallpox renders this task easier, but not by much.

†For those of you who are just starting medical school, this chicken is now being hatched; we are confident that it will come home to roost!

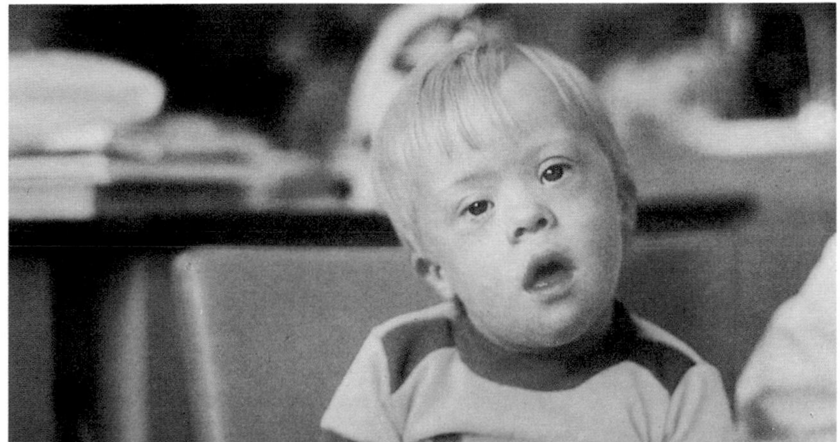

Plate 1

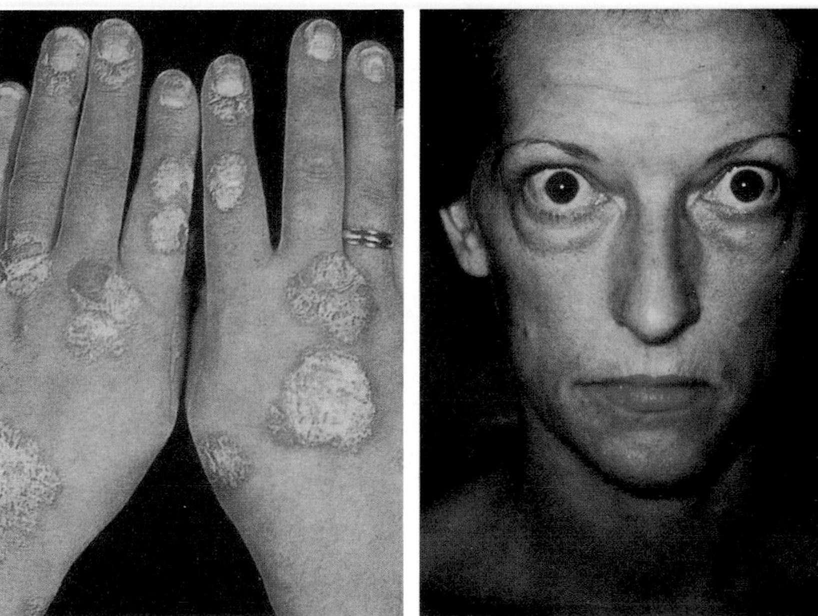

Plate 2

Plate 3

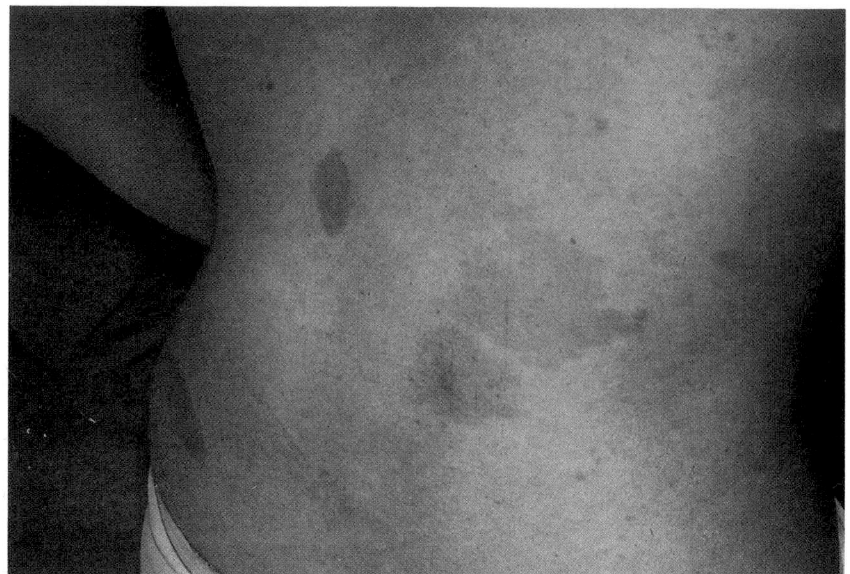

Plate 4

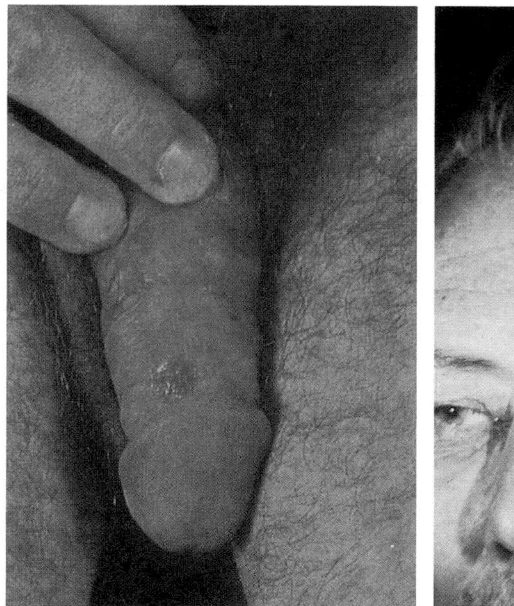

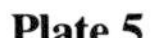

Plate 5

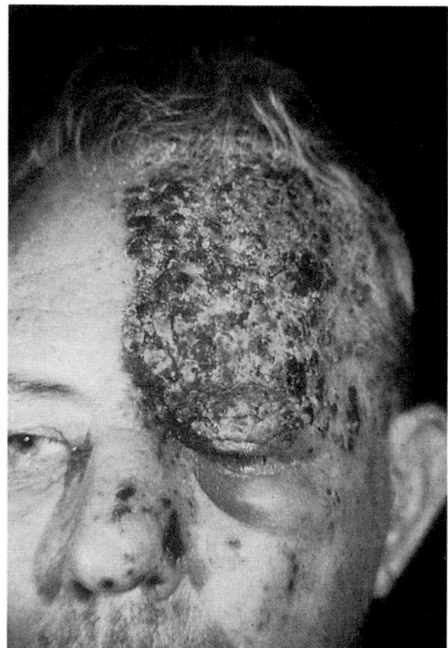

Plate 6

medical facts about the patient, followed by sifting through the data for the diagnosis.

The strategy of exhaustion depicts diagnosis as a two-stage process. First, collect all the data that might possibly be pertinent and, only when this is complete, proceed to the second stage of searching through it for the diagnosis; create the data bank first, and only then pose the diagnostic question.

This explains the confusion of the author of the 35-page workups. If the exhaustion strategy is in use, the more extensive the writeup, the better. This also explains why the method of exhaustion is sometimes referred to as "looking for the pony."*

Most medical students probably think that the strategy of exhaustion is the "right way" to diagnose. So too, unfortunately, do some of their teachers and the authors of some books on clinical diagnosis. It is also tragically true that many clinical laboratories behave as if the method of exhaustion is the "right way," and bury us in unsolicited laboratory test results when we ask for just one or a few tests.†

Not so. The strategy of exhaustion is the method of the novice, and it is abandoned with experience. For example, some of our colleagues have videotaped a random sample of family physicians and internists as they worked up a series of programmed patients [1]. When the tapes were played back and these clinicians were asked why they inquired after specific symptoms and signs, and what they were thinking at each stage of the workup, two curious things happened. First, despite their accurate and efficient diagnoses, many of them started by apologizing for not using the method of exhaustion ("I know I'm not doing this the right way, but my practice is so busy that I've slipped into some shortcuts")!

Second, although the method of exhaustion was never used as the underlying diagnostic strategy, these clinicians often and quite abruptly switched it on, and then off, during their workups. When asked why they executed these snippets of the exhaustion strategy, they reported using it to rule out remote diagnostic possibilities, to establish rapport with the patient, and *to keep the patient occupied while they were thinking about something else*! For the seasoned clinician

*"Looking for the pony" comes from a Christmas tale of two brothers, one of whom was an incurable pessimist and the other, an incurable optimist. On Christmas Day, the pessimist was given a roomful of shiny new toys and the optimist, a roomful of horse shit. The pessimist opened the door to his roomful of toys, sighed, and lamented, "A lot of these are motor driven and their batteries will run down; and I suppose I'll have to show them to my cousins, who'll break some and steal others; and their paint will chip; and they'll wear out. All in all, I really wish you hadn't given me this roomful of toys!" The optimist opened the door to his roomful of horse shit and, with a whoop of glee, threw himself into the muck and began burrowing about in it. When his horrified parents extricated him from the excrement and asked him why on earth he was thrashing about in it, he joyfully cried, "With all this horse shit, there's *got* to be a pony in here somewhere!"

†If this deluge is decreasing at your institution, see if you can determine whether the pressure for change was scientific or financial!

the method of exhaustion is like the vermiform appendix: an unnecessary and occasionally painful vestige.

Incidentally, its laboratory counterpart, the hospital admission screen, has been discredited as well. Timothy Durbridge and his colleagues in Adelaide, Australia [6] randomized 1500 admissions to undergo or not undergo a routine battery of about 50 tests as soon as they arrived, providing the clinicians of experimental patients with all of the results. This exhaustive testing produced no improvement in mortality, morbidity, duration of monitoring, disability, medical opinions of patients' progress, or length of stay. Admission screening did, however, increase the total cost of caring for these patients by about 5% and was followed by lowered patient satisfaction.

Should the complete history and physical be banished from the medical curriculum? For reasons that will become clear shortly, we hold the paradoxical position that all medical students should both be taught *how* to do a complete history and physical and, once they have mastered its components, be taught *never to do one*.

STRATEGY #4

Imagine that your reading of this book is interrupted by the telephone. Your local emergency room is on the line, and, depending on your specialty, the nurse says:

1. "We have a 56-year-old man here with chest pain and shortness of breath." Jot down in this box what is going through your head:

2. "We have an 8-week pregnant, 23-year-old primipara with spotting and severe right-lower-quadrant pain." Jot down what is going through your head in this box:

3. "We have a 2-year-old girl with a fever of 40° C and a red ear, who has just had a grand mal seizure." Jot down what is going through your head in this box:

4. "We have a 12-year-old boy with right-lower-quadrant pain, rebound tenderness, and a white count of twelve thousand." Jot down what is going through your head in this box:

5. "We have just sutured the slashed wrists of a 19-year-old university student." Jot down in this box what is going through your head:

We have read the message about the 56-year-old man with chest pain and shortness of breath to groups totalling several hundred students and clinicians, and their reactions are quite uniform. As soon as they hear this fragmentary information, these students and clinicians respond in one (often both) of two ways. First, they may call out diagnoses, for example, beginning with "myocardial infarction" and "pulmonary embolus," then pause, and then continue with "pneumothorax" and a mix of other intrathoracic catastrophes. Alternatively, they call out management options: "Get him to the coronary unit," "Put him on a monitor," "Admit him to the ward," and so forth.

This is called the *hypothetico-deductive* strategy, the one used by virtually all clinicians, virtually all of the time. It is *the formulation, from the earliest clues about the patient, of a "short list" of potential diagnoses or actions, followed by the performance of those clinical (history and physical) and paraclinical (e.g., laboratory, x ray) maneuvers that will best reduce the length of the list.*

Where do the hypotheses come from? Our colleague and teacher, Moran Campbell [2], suggests that many, if not most, spring from our view of diagnostic labels as "explanatory ideas" that tie our understanding of human biology to the illnesses of our patients. Also, and especially with experience, many hypotheses spring forth by pattern recognition of a sort that generates multiple *possibilities* rather than a single, very high *probability.*

When Howard Barrows, Geoffrey Norman, Victor Neufeld, and John Feightner [1] videotaped random samples of family physicians and internists working up programmed patients with pericarditis, duodenal ulcer, peripheral neuropathy, or multiple sclerosis, they documented that the first hypothesis was generated, on average, 28 seconds after hearing the chief complaint (varying from 11 seconds for the multiple sclerosis patient to 55 seconds for the peripheral neuropathy patient). The correct hypotheses (these clinicians were right about 75% of the time) were generated an average of 6 minutes into these half-hour workups (in less than a minute for the multiple sclerosis patient and less than 90 seconds for the duodenal ulcer patient), and an average of 5.5 hypotheses were generated for each case.

At the same time that they were generating this list of hypotheses, these clinicians were simultaneously performing those bits of history-taking and physical examination that would best help them shorten their list, keeping their working hypotheses at any one time to about three and directing their history and physical to these three working hypotheses. Significantly, a limit of three working hypotheses, plus a fourth for "or something else" had been proposed independently by Moran Campbell [2].

Once clinicians generate a working hypothesis, however, their hypothetico-deductive diagnostic strategy usually departs from its experimental cousin. Whereas experimental science often advances by seeking information (through the "crucial experiment") that will *disprove* a hypothesis, observations on clinicians have documented that most of the symptoms and signs they seek are selected because they *support* rather than refute a working hypothesis. As we shall discover in the next chapter, this focus on weakly confirmatory (rather than refutational or "rule-out") evidence can lead to diagnostic inefficiency and error.

So, seasoned clinicians use the hypothetico-deductive approach. At what stage do medical trainees start to adopt this strategy? When the Barrows group [11] taped and analyzed medical students working up the same programmed patients we described earlier, the results were dramatic. Medical students employ the hypothetico-deductive strategy *on arrival* at medical school! Regardless of their duration in the M.D. program, they generate their first hypothesis 20 to 50 seconds after hearing the chief complaint, generate about six hypotheses in all, and selectively gather historical and physical information to support working hypotheses. The differences between beginning and graduating students (and between students and seasoned clinicians) are quantitative, not qualitative; with additional education and experience, clinicians become more likely to generate the correct hypothesis, to generate it earlier, and to gather more pertinent historical and physical data about their working hypotheses.

On the basis of these and similar studies, we conclude that the hypothetico-deductive model is the most appropriate current description of the diagnostic process as it *is* executed, both by seasoned clinicians and by the earliest trainees. How can we do a better job of it ourselves, and how can we help others learn to improve at it? We think that the solution has two elements. One of these, outside the scope of this book, is a mastery of the dynamic models (but not the inert facts) of structure, function, and response to stimuli that comprise the important teachings of the other basic sciences, for these provide the hypotheses to be tested in the diagnostic process. Thus, a recognition of where models for pain and for cardiopulmonary function intersect leads to the hypotheses of myocardial infarction, pulmonary embolus, pneumothorax, dissecting thoracic aortic aneurysm, and so on in the first patient with chest pain and shortness of breath.

The second element, the focus of the next three chapters, is a mastery of the highly directed but unbiased selection, acquisition, and interpretation of the clinical and paraclinical data that will best shorten the list of hypotheses. Chapters 2 and 3 are mostly about capturing these data from the history, the physical examination, and the various diagnostic laboratories, and Chapter 4 is mostly about their interpretation.

In summary, then, diagnostic approaches can usefully be described as one or a combination of four types: the pattern recognition approach of the seasoned clinician, the multiple-branching method of the delegate, the exhaustion method of the novice, and the most widely used strategy, the hypothetico-deductive approach. All of this provides an opportunity to tie up a loose end. What did we mean when we said that all medical students should be taught *how* to do a complete history and physical but must also be taught *never to do one*? We meant that the complete history and physical is the sum of an all-encompassing set of *subroutines,* each of which can (if performed and interpreted correctly) provide a key test of one or more working hypotheses. We need to know all these subroutines and to keep them at our fingertips so that we can, selectively and efficiently, plug different ones in when and where we need them.

To those of you who are just starting your clinical training, we hope that the foregoing both convinces you of the need to master but not habitually use all the subroutines and also provides you with some additional time during your work-ups to actually get to know your patients. To those of you who are already in clinical practice, we hope that the foregoing both clarifies our earlier statement and also quenches any residual guilt you may still harbor over your abandonment of the "complete history and physical."

References

1. Barrows, H. S., Norman, G. R., Neufeld, V. R., and Feightner, J. W. The clinical reasoning of randomly selected physicians in general medical practice. *Clin. Invest. Med.* 5: 49, 1982.
2. Campbell, E. J. M. Personal communication, 1976.

3. Campbell, E. J. M., Scadding, J. G., and Roberts, R. S. The concept of disease. *Br. Med. J.* 2: 757, 1979.
4. Cutler, P. *Problem Solving in Clinical Medicine.* Baltimore: Williams & Wilkins, 1979. P. 104.
5. DeGowin, E. L., and DeGowin, R. L. *Bedside Diagnostic Examination.* New York: Macmillan, 1969. P. 13, 21.
6. Durbridge, T. C., Edwards, F., Edwards, R. G., and Atkinson, M. An evaluation of multiphasic screening on admission to hospital. Précis of a report to the National Health and Medical Research Council. *Med. J. Aust.* 1: 703, 1976.
7. Essex, B. J. *Diagnostic Pathways in Clinical Medicine.* Edinburgh: Churchill Livingstone, 1976. P. 134.
8. Goroll, A. H., May, L. A., and Mulley, A. G. *Primary Care Medicine.* Philadelphia: Lippincott, 1981.
9. Isselbacher, K. J., Amams, R. D., Braunwalt E., Petersdorf, R. G., and Wilson, J. D. (eds.). *Harrison's Principles of Internal Medicine* (9th ed.). Toronto: McGraw-Hill, 1980.
10. Harvey, A. M., Johns, R. J., McKusick, V. A., Owens, A. H., Jr., and Ross, R. S. (eds.). *The Principles and Practice of Medicine* (20th ed.). New York: Appleton-Century-Crofts, 1980.
11. Neufeld, V. R., Norman, G. R., Feightner, J. W., and Barrows, H. S. Clinical problem-solving by medical students: A cross-sectional and longitudinal analysis. *Med. Ed.* 15: 315, 1981.
12. Sackett, D. L. Clinical diagnosis and the clinical laboratory. *Clin. Invest. Med.* 1: 37, 1978.
13. Sox, H. C., Jr., Margulies, I., and Sox, C. H. Psychologically mediated effects of diagnostic tests. *Ann. Intern. Med.* 95: 680, 1981.
14. Taylor, D. C. The components of sickness: Diseases, illnesses and predicaments. *Lancet* 2: 1008, 1971.
15. Willis, T. In R. H. Major (ed.), *Classic Description of Disease* (3rd ed.). Springfield, Il.: Thomas, 1945. P. 240.

2

The Clinical Examination

Regardless of which of the foregoing diagnostic strategies we employ, we are going to carry out a clinical examination (i.e., a history and physical), however brief, every time we encounter a patient. The accuracy of this clinical examination is crucial, for it serves as the basis for most of our judgments about diagnosis, prognosis, and therapy.

As essential clinical acts, history taking and physical examination receive a lot of attention, mostly in the form of majuscular "how to" texts in physical diagnosis. We have no intention of adding another one here.* Rather, we shall develop three key themes that are usually omitted from such texts: (1) the potential power of clinical observations in determining the diagnosis, prognosis, and therapeutic responsiveness of patients; (2) the magnitude of, and causes for, the errors and inconsistencies of the clinical examination that undermine its power; and (3) ways to minimize these errors and inconsistencies and, thus, realize the full potential of the clinical examination.

The Power of Clinical Observations

Clinical examination is far more powerful than laboratory evaluation in establishing diagnoses, prognoses, and therapeutic plans for most patients in most places. In a general practice, for example, Crombie [11] documented that 88% of diagnoses were established by the end of a brief history and physical exam subroutine. In a general medical clinic, Sandler [50] showed that 56% of cases had been assigned correct diagnoses by the end of the history, and that this figure rose to 73% by the end of the physical examination. Even when patients are referred to specialty centers after exhaustive workups elsewhere, attention is appropriately refocused on the patient's "story" and the physical examination. Indeed, when a colleague in gastroenterology was asked to consult on a patient who already had undergone an extensive battery of endoscopic, radiographic, and biochemical studies elsewhere, he proclaimed: "All that there is left for us to do is a history and physical!"

Advances such as MRI scanning and gene probes have certainly increased our diagnostic power, and the provision of diagnostic tests with "hard numbers" has led to an understandable reliance on the clinical laboratory. However, we must never forget that the clinical data we gather in the examining room and at the bedside are usually much more useful than any which we can obtain by filling

*Indeed, a group of us are developing a "whether and why to" series of articles and book that will describe only those symptoms and signs that have been shown to be precise and accurate; most colleagues, when hearing of our proposed book, predict that it will be a very slender volume!

out laboratory slips and requisitions. To underscore this point we offer the following examples.

Our first illustration of the power of the clinical examination in establishing a diagnosis is derived from ischemic heart disease: the likelihood of clinically important coronary artery stenosis can be determined with a high degree of accuracy on the simple clinical observations of age, sex, and symptoms alone. Careful clinicopathologic studies [15] have now established, for example, that a 60-year-old man referred to a specialist* for exertional retrosternal chest pain that is relieved by 5 to 15 minutes of rest (typical angina) has a 94% probability of exhibiting at least 75% stenosis of at least one artery at angiography. Conversely, a 30-year-old woman with nonanginal chest pain has less than a 1% chance of such coronary stenosis. Whether the man needs angiography depends upon therapeutic possibilities (coronary artery bypass surgery), not diagnostic ones. The diagnosis already has been established, about as certainly as it is reasonable to desire, from the history alone, particularly considering the risk (albeit small) and expense (large) of angiography. In the woman's situation, it would be difficult to justify angiography, as its risk of inducing complications rivals the likelihood that she has significant coronary artery disease. If she is worried about a heart attack she should be exuberantly reassured, and angiography undertaken only if she requires "delabeling." Moreover, although we have a plethora of noninvasive tests that could be applied in such situations, they are similarly unnecessary for diagnostic purposes in these two patients. As we will show you in Chapter 4, these patients' "pretest likelihoods" of coronary artery disease are already so extreme that further tests might, in fact, be misleading. We gain much more information from our clinical observations in the two cases outlined above than we can possibly get from currently available noninvasive tests. Although such tests are helpful when we are uncertain of the patient's diagnosis (for example, when the odds favoring clinically significant coronary artery disease are 50:50 or 60:40), we must learn to trust our clinical examination when it is worthy of this trust.

Our second example has to do with the power of clinical observations in determining prognosis. When Norman Boyd and Alvan Feinstein [6] assessed the relative prognostic value of simple clinical observations versus the more complicated staging by surgery and biopsy in Hodgkin's disease, the surprising results of Table 2-1 emerged.

The four prognostic levels that result from Ann Arbor anatomic staging, shown on the left, present a 5-year survival range of 53% (70% − 17%). By contrast, the right-hand panel of Table 2-1 displays the greater prognostic value of some simple clinical observations such as localized pain or tumor, generalized fatigue, and weight loss. Thus, the small number of patients who had neither systemic nor local symptoms of their disease when first diagnosed had an excellent 5-year prognosis. Patients with local symptoms of long duration (suggesting slow growth of the tumor without distant spread), local symptoms of short du-

*The clinical site is important, as we shall see in Chapter 4.

Table 2-1. Relative prognostic values of anatomic and clinical data in Hodgkin's disease

Prognosis from anatomy only			Prognosis from symptoms only		
Stages*	N	5-Year survival	Stages	N	5-Year survival
I	47	70%	Asymptomatic	5	100%
II	50	60%	Local symptoms, long duration	21	90%
III	63	48%	Local symptoms, short duration	95	59%
IV	24	17%	Systemic symptoms first, then local	34	38%
			Local symptoms first, then systemic	29	14%
		Survival gradient = (70% − 17%) = 53%			Survival gradient = (100% − 14%) = 86%

*Ann Arbor Anatomic Stages. Data modified from N.F. Boyd and A. R. Feinstein. Symptoms as an index of growth rates and prognosis in Hodgkin's disease. *Clin. Invest. Med.* 2:25, 1978.

ration, and systemic symptoms were progressively less likely to survive for 5 years; only 14% of Hodgkin's patients with local, followed by systemic, symptoms prior to diagnosis were alive 5 years later. Thus, the range of survival delineated by a careful clinical history, 86% (100% − 14%), was greater than that generated by the much more laborious anatomic approach, and if these results are confirmed in other, independent series of Hodgkin's patients, their clinical importance will be underscored. Table 2-2 shows the prognosis of these same patients when assessed by a combined Ann Arbor and clinical staging.

Although this combined system outperforms anatomical staging, the best prognostic group generated in this way (patients with no systemic symptoms and only isolated, local disease) did not have as good a prognosis (77%) as the best group (100%) defined on clinical history alone. Thus, a clinical staging system was found superior for the assessment of prognosis in these patients. Of course, no conclusion can be drawn from this study about the value of symptoms in selecting therapeutic interventions, as these were based solely on the Ann Arbor staging. Nonetheless, when we confront the fact that the Ann Arbor staging process is complicated, difficult to apply, invasive, and expensive while clinical staging is immediate, simple, easy to apply, noninvasive, and cheap, standard reliance on the former is indeed paradoxical. Ironically, such is the allure of the scalpel and microscope that we think of the Ann Arbor data as "hard" and the clinical history as "soft." Surely clinical data should be judged by their power, not their appearance!

So, some clinical observations (often very simple ones) are powerful determinants of diagnosis, prognosis, and therapeutic responsiveness. We will bet that this is so for most illnesses and diseases, although you could not tell it from reading most current medical texts, for there the laboratory focus predominates. Clearly, we need to ferret out these key clinical observations, for their identification will sharply increase our effectiveness and efficiency as clinicians. This ferreting-out process will, at the same time, identify the other clinical observa-

Table 2-2. Proportion (and %) of Hodgkin's patients surviving five years, based on a combination of Ann Arbor and symptomatic staging

	Systemic symptoms	
Anatomic stage	Absent	Present
I	33/43 (77%)	0/ 4 (0%)
II	25/37 (68%)	5/13 (38%)
III	21/36 (58%)	9/27 (33%)
IV	1/ 5 (20%)	3/19 (16%)

Survival gradient = (77% − 16%) = 61%

Data modified from N. F. Boyd and A. R. Feinstein. Symptoms as an index of growth rates and prognosis in Hodgkin's disease. *Clin. Invest. Med.* 2:25, 1978.

tions (often laborious ones) that, because they are meaningless or hopelessly imprecise, are simply a waste of time.

For example, a group of orthopedic surgeons have carried out a series of studies of the reproducibility and validity of the clinical assessment of patients referred to an orthopedic clinic with backaches [57]. When two or more clinicians examined each patient, they found that they agreed closely on certain physical findings. We have listed these in Table 2-3.

The degree of agreement on these signs is impressive and was attained through the progressive refinement of clinical criteria, substituting actual measurements for "clinical impressions." Furthermore, some of these physical signs (such as limited flexion and straight-leg raising) are important prognostic findings and therefore are not of mere metric interest.

This same series of studies showed that "eyeballing" detected only the most severe examples of loss of lordosis, list (leaning to one side), and limited flexion; high levels of reliability among observers were achieved only when a measuring tape and explicit criteria were applied. Of equal importance was the documentation that several commonly used clinical signs were so unreliable and unamenable to useful measurement that they had to be completely discarded; these included muscle spasm, guarded movements, and the anatomical localization of tenderness. Thus, this systematic study identified some techniques of clinical assessment that we should adopt and some other techniques that we might as well abandon.

The need for reproducible, reliable clinical measurement goes beyond the requirement for powerful diagnostic, prognostic, and treatment data. We must also avoid being misled by poorly collected or biased clinical observations into making incorrect diagnoses. The consequences of such misdiagnoses can be devastating. For example, two pediatricians [4] tracked down 93 Seattle, Washington, junior-high-school students who had been labeled as having organic heart disease. One of the pediatricians, a cardiologist, examined these students and determined their exercise capacity. The second pediatrician, an epidemiologist who

Table 2-3. Reproducibility of certain physical findings in patients with backache

Observation	Agreement (%)	Probability that agreement was due to chance
Operative scars	100	<0.001
Loss of lordosis (<2 cm)	88	<0.001
List (>1 cm)	78	<0.05
Limited flexion (<5 cm)	91	<0.001
Limited lateral flexion (<3 cm)	70	<0.05
Tenderness		
Lumbar	100	<0.001
Buttock	81	<0.001
Straight-leg raising (<75 degrees)	77	<0.001
Root irritation signs	86	<0.01
Root compression signs	93	<0.001

Data modified from G. Waddell, C. J. Main, E. W. Morris, et al. Normality reliability in the clinical assessment of backache. *Br. Med. J.* 284:1519, 1982.

Table 2-4. The extent of disability in cardiac nondisease

	Heart disease present	Heart disease absent
Restricted physical or social activity	8 (44%)	30 (40%)
Disabling restriction	2	6
Partial restriction	3	9
"Treated differently"	3	15
No activity restriction	10 (56%)	45 (60%)
	18 (100%)	75 (100%)

Data modified from A. B. Bergman and S. J. Stamm. The morbidity of cardiac nondisease in school children. *N. Engl. J. Med.* 276:1008, 1967.

was "blind" to his cardiology colleague's findings, interviewed (but did not examine) each student and his or her family and determined the degree to which their physical or social activity had been restricted. The results of their evaluations are shown in Table 2-4.

Two striking findings emerged from this study. First, physical and social activities were as frequently and as severely restricted among misdiagnosed children with normal hearts as among correctly diagnosed children with congenital or acquired heart disease. Second, because 75 (81%) of the 93 children labeled as having heart disease actually had normal hearts, the amount of disability from cardiac nondisease greatly exceeded that from actual heart disease.

What should we make of all this? Two conclusions strike us as inevitable. First, we need to know what data to seek in our clinical examinations, and what to ignore. Second, when clinical data are relevant, we need to know how to obtain them in a reliable and accurate way. It is this second conclusion that provides the focus for the rest of this chapter.

We will begin this second section with some examples of inconsistencies between the observations of two clinicians who examine the same patient once or when one clinician examines the same patient twice; that is, we shall begin with several examples of *clinical disagreement.* We shall then describe some of the known causes for clinical disagreement, and finally we shall consider methods of reducing disagreement, keeping in mind Feinstein's [22] admonition: "To advance art and science in clinical examination, the equipment a clinician most needs to improve is himself."

How Often Does Clinical Disagreement Occur?

CLINICAL DISAGREEMENTS OVER PATIENTS' HISTORIES

Suppose you see a 46-year-old traveling salesman who has undergone proximal gastric vagotomy and pyloroplasty for duodenal ulcer and are assessing his response to surgery. He is free of pain, has a fair appetite and has not been troubled by nausea, reflux, vomiting, epigastric fullness, or dysphagia. However, you elicit a history of "dumping" severe enough to cause him to cancel occasional business appointments and lose some sales. A recent consultation note from his surgeon, on the other hand, indicates that the dumping is "mild."

A crucial element in our decision whether to recommend surgery for one patient with peptic ulcer is an assessment of the results of similar operations performed on other patients with peptic ulcer. Were their symptoms relieved? Did the procedure result in new, equally disabling symptoms? Were the patients able to return to full function at home and on the job? Accurate estimates of the surgical outcomes of such patients must be based on carefully taken, thorough histories; thus, our conclusions about the value of the operation depend on the skill, objectivity, and consistency with which these histories are obtained.

How consistent are such histories? If two clinicians interviewed the same patient would they agree or disagree about the results of that patient's operation for peptic ulcer? Unfortunately, even seasoned clinicians often disagree. When two senior British surgeons [28], using the same set of clinical criteria, independently interviewed the same group of patients who had undergone operations for peptic ulcer, they agreed on whether the operation had been successful in less than two-thirds of the cases. Thus, at least one of these seasoned clinicians was wrong about the success of a patient's operation at least one-third of the time. Does this mean that we cannot be sure about the claims of superiority for one form of peptic ulcer surgery over another? Well, the clinicians who conducted the British study questioned whether the results of ulcer operations performed at different centers could ever be compared as long as this degree of clinical disagreement persisted. We will come back to this example when we discuss strategies for reducing clinical disagreement.

Other examples of clinical disagreement over patients' histories abound. For example, when three cardiologists [48] interviewed the same 57 men with chest pain, 54% were judged by at least one clinician to have angina pectoris. However, all three cardiologists agreed about the history in only 75% of cases, and when one cardiologist concluded that a given patient had angina pectoris, the other two agreed with him only 55% of the time. In view of the importance of the history in predicting clinically significant coronary stenosis, as illustrated at the start of this chapter, such clinical disagreement is a major concern.

CLINICAL DISAGREEMENTS ABOUT PHYSICAL FINDINGS

Suppose your patient, a 38-year-old executive with primary hypertension, had a pretreatment fifth-phase diastolic blood pressure of 115 mm Hg. After six weeks of step-two therapy (a thiazide and a beta blocker), the diastolic pressure has fallen to 95 mm Hg. Although your examinations of her optic fundi have consistently revealed only early arteriovenous crossing changes, an ophthalmologist who examined her a few days after you last saw her reported a small flame-shaped hemorrhage near the left disc.

Is clinical disagreement less of a problem in the physical examination? The quick answer is "no." Clinicians who examine the same patient often disagree. Indeed, the clinician who examines the same patient twice often disagrees with his or her own earlier findings.

For example, examination of the optic fundus is a universally accepted component of the physical examination of a patient suspected of having cardiovascular disease or diabetes, and in hypertensive patients it may provide a better index of prognosis than measurement of the blood pressure. However, when two clinicians [2] carefully examined the same set of 100 fundus photographs the disagreements documented in Table 2-5 were generated.

Using the Keith-Wagener system of classification they agreed that 46 of these 100 patients had little or no retinopathy (Grade 0 or I) and that a further 32 had moderate or severe retinopathy (Grade II or III). Thus, they agreed with each other about three-quarters of the time, and disagreed about whether patients had retinopathy about one-quarter of the time.

If two clinicians examining the same patient often disagree, what happens when one clinician examines the same patient twice? Clinicians are somewhat

Table 2-5. Agreement between two clinicians examining the same set of 100 fundus photographs

		Second clinician	
		Little or no retinopathy	Moderate or severe retinopathy
First clinician	Little or no retinopathy	46	10
	Moderate or severe retinopathy	12	32

Data modified from N. Aoki, H. Horibe, Y. Ohno, et al. Epidemiological evaluation of funduscopic findings in cerebrovascular diseases: III. Observer variability and reproducibility for funduscopic findings. *Jpn. Circ. J.* 41:11, 1977.

Table 2-6. Agreement between two examinations of the same 100 fundus photographs by one clinician

		Second examination	
		Little or no retinopathy	Moderate or severe retinopathy
First examination	Little or no retinopathy	69	11
	Moderate or severe retinopathy	1	19

Data modified from N. Aoki, H. Horibe, Y. Ohno, et al. Epidemiological evaluation of funduscopic findings in cerebrovascular diseases: III. Observer variability and reproducibility for funduscopic findings. *Jpn. Circ. J.* 41:11, 1977.

more likely to agree with themselves (intraobserver agreement) than with other clinicians (interobserver agreement), but not by much. Table 2-6 summarizes the results of two independent clinical assessments by a single clinician, three months apart, of the same set of 100 fundus photographs.

Overall agreement was high, with 88 (69 + 19) of 100 patients receiving identical assessments on both occasions. Note, however, that even when the clinician knew that a study was in progress, 11 patients judged to have little or no retinopathy when their photographs were first reviewed were judged to have moderate or severe retinopathy when these photographs were reexamined later. Furthermore, it is likely that intraobserver and interobserver agreement would fall even lower under the more natural conditions of routine examinations by less expert observers.

Koran [39] has reviewed many other examples of disagreements among and within clinicians about their clinical observations and conclusions, and the general finding is of highly variable but suboptimal performance. However, although virtually all clinical assessments are inconsistent to some degree, most are demonstrably more consistent than would be expected on the basis of chance. To understand this, and to determine whether strategies for improving clinical agreement are effective, we will have to learn a bit about the measurement of this agreement.*

There are several methods of doing this, and the simplest is to calculate the proportion of cases in which the clinician agreed with himself or with another clinician. Table 2-7 shows this calculation for the situation in which two clinicians reviewed the same 100 fundus photographs.

*To understand this and several other principles that form a basic science for clinical medicine, you will need to overcome any numerophobia and grapple with the numbers that clinicians apply to various clinical measurements. We will help you accomplish this by keeping the mathematics simple and the clinical examples unambiguous, and will carry you through them in small, orderly steps. We will also provide you with plenty of opportunities to test your growing prowess, and will confine the methodological fine points to footnotes.

Table 2-7. Calculation of observed agreement in a 2 × 2 table*

		Second clinician: Little or no retinopathy	Second clinician: Moderate or severe retinopathy	
First clinician	Little or no retinopathy	46	10	56
	Moderate or severe retinopathy	12	32	44
		58	42	100

$$\text{Observed agreement} = \frac{46 + 32}{100} = 78\%$$

*The data in this table are arranged in two horizontal rows and two vertical columns (the totals lie outside the table and are not counted) and such tables are often called "2 × 2" or "two-by-two" tables.

Data modified from N. Aoki, H. Horibe, Y. Ohno, et al. Epidemiological evaluation of funduscopic findings in cerebrovascular diseases: III. Observer variability and reproducibility for funduscopic findings. *Jpn. Circ. J.* 41:11, 1977.

As already discussed, these two clinicians agreed that 46 of these 100 patients had little or no retinopathy, and also agreed that 32 of them had moderate or severe retinopathy; thus, they agreed on (46 + 32)/100 or 78% of these patients. But this description of their agreement is rather superficial, for if the second clinician simply tossed a coin (rather than studied each fundus photograph) and called it "little or no retinopathy" if the coin landed "heads" and "moderate or severe retinopathy" if the coin landed "tails," he would agree with the first clinician part of the time by chance alone. How great would this chance agreement be? The answer is shown in Table 2-8.

The coin-tossing second clinician would call half of the photographs "little or no retinopathy" and the other half "moderate or severe retinopathy." Thus, half (28) of the 56 photographs judged by the first clinician to exhibit little or no retinopathy would also be called "little or no retinopathy" by the coin-tossing second clinician (and thus appear in cell *a* of the table), and half (22) of the 44 photographs judged by the first clinician to exhibit moderate or severe retinopathy would also be called "moderate or severe retinopathy" by the second, coin-tossing clinician (and thus appear in cell *d*). Thus, the agreement between these two clinicians on the basis of chance alone (the sum of cells *a* and *d* divided by the total number of photographs) is (28 + 22)/100 or 50%.

Can we extrapolate this artificial example to a general approach to determining the extent of agreement that we would expect on the basis of chance alone in real clinical situations? Yes, we can.

If we return to Table 2-7, we could determine chance agreement by pretending that the second clinician was once again tossing a coin, but that this time he obtained 58 heads and 42 tails. Thus, he would call a photograph "little or no

Table 2-8. Calculation of chance agreement when a second clinician tosses a coin

		Second clinician (who tosses a coin)		
		Heads (little or no retinopathy)	Tails (moderate or severe retinopathy)	
First clinician (who examines the fundus)	Little or no retinopathy	50% of 56 = 28 (a)	50% of 56 = 28 (b)	56
	Moderate or severe retinopathy	(c) 50% of 44 = 22	(d) 50% of 44 = 22	44
		50/100 = 50%	50/100 = 50%	100

Table 2-9. Calculation of chance agreement in a 2 × 2 table

		Second clinician		
		Little or no retinopathy	Moderate or severe retinopathy	
First clinician	Little or no retinopathy	58% of 56 = 32.5 (a)	42% of 56 = 23.5 (b)	56
	Moderate or severe retinopathy	(c) 58% of 44 = 25.5	(d) 42% of 44 = 18.5	44
		58/100 = 58%	42/100 = 42%	100

Agreement expected on the basis of chance

$$= \frac{a + d}{\text{total}} = \frac{32.5 + 18.5}{100} = 51\%$$

retinopathy" 58% (58/100) of the time and would call it "moderate or severe retinopathy" 42% (42/100) of the time. The result is shown in Table 2-9.

If chance alone were operating, we would expect 58% (32.5) of the 56 photographs judged by the first clinician to exhibit little or no retinopathy would also be called "little or no retinopathy" by the second clinician (and thus appear in cell *a*), and 42% (18.5) of the 44 photographs judged by the first clinician to exhibit moderate or severe retinopathy would also be called "moderate or severe retinopathy" by the second clinician (and thus appear in cell *d*).* Thus, the agreement between these two clinicians that we would expect on the basis of

*The second clinician would have called 58% of the patients in *every* cell (including cell *d*) "little or no retinopathy." However, since cells *c* and *d* correspond to patients with "moderate or severe retinopathy," it is the other 42% of patients who wind up there by chance. We can generate the same table by assuming that the second clinician calls 42% of the patients in every cell "moderate or severe retinopathy," couldn't we? Sure we could.

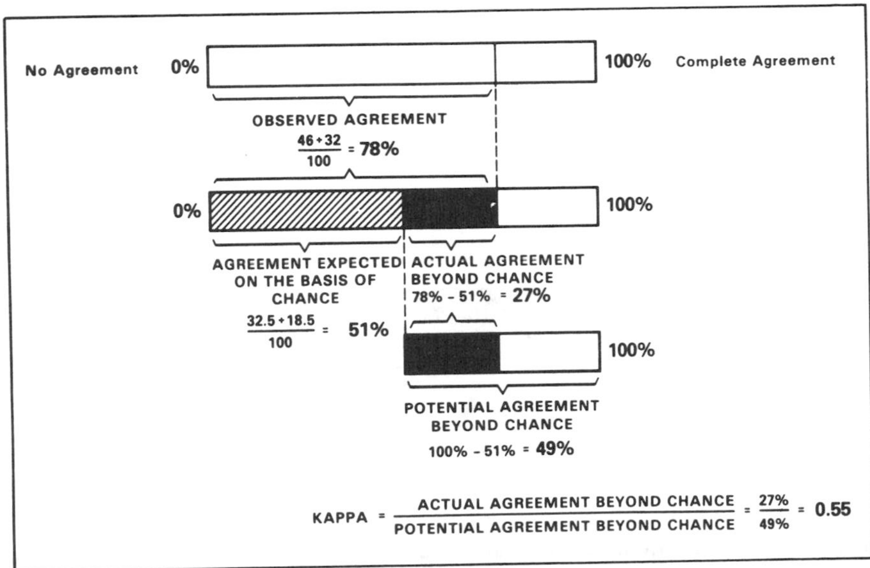

Figure 2-1. Developing a useful index of clinical agreement.

chance alone (the sum of cells *a* and *d* divided by the total number of photographs) is (32.5 + 18.5)/100 or 51%.*

Surprise! The expected agreement is 51%, not 50%, because both clinicians judged that more than half of these photographs showed little or no retinopathy (56% so judged by the first clinician and 58% by the second). Only when one (or both) judged a clinical finding to be present 50% of the time will the expected agreement on the basis of chance equal 50%.

Here is a chance to test your understanding of what we have just done. What percent agreement would you expect on the basis of chance alone if both clinicians judged a clinical finding to be present in 60%, 70%, 80%, and 90% of patients? The answers are in the footnote at the bottom of this page.†

Returning to our example in Table 2-7, the observed agreement was 78% and the expected agreement on the basis of chance alone was 51%. Is there a way of combining these into a clinically useful index? One way to do so is shown in Figure 2-1.

The top bar in Figure 2-1 depicts the observed agreement of 78% between the two clinicians described in Table 2-7. In the middle bar, this 78% is broken down

*If you plan to carry out such calculations yourself, here are two ways to check your work. First, the "expected" values in cells *a, b, c,* and *d* should add up to the same totals as the numbers actually observed. Second, you should get the same "expected" values regardless of whether you use the first or second clinician as the coin-tosser (if the first clinician is the coin-tosser, the expected value in cell *a* is [56/100] × 58 = 32.5).

†The percent agreement expected on the basis of chance alone in these examples is 52%, 58%, 68%, and 82%, respectively.

Table 2-10. Agreement about the level of central venous pressure*

		Resident's reading			
		≤5 cm	6–9 cm	≥10 cm	Total
Clinical clerk's reading	≤5 cm	12	3	0	15
	6–9 cm	5	7	1	13
	≥10 cm	0	6	6	12
	Total	17	16	7	40

*In centimeters of water above the sternal angle.

into its two components, the 51% agreement expected on the basis of chance alone and the remainder (78% − 51% = 27%), the actual agreement beyond chance. In the bottom bar of Figure 2-1, this *actual* agreement beyond chance (27%) is compared with the *potential* agreement beyond chance (100% − 51% = 49%). Finally, the ratio of the actual to potential agreement beyond chance is calculated (27%/49% = .55). The result, .55, represents the proportion of potential agreement beyond chance that was actually achieved, and this proportion goes by the name of "kappa" [25].

Here is another chance to test your understanding of what is being measured here (and to learn something about looking at neck veins at the same time). When one of our colleagues, Deborah Cook, was a chief medical resident she arranged for a series of critically ill patients to undergo three estimates of their jugular venous pressure within the space of an hour (one by a clinical clerk, one by a medical resident, and one by the attending physician), all performed "blind" to the simultaneous, gold standard measurement of central venous pressure obtained from an indwelling central venous catheter [9]. The agreement between the clerks and the residents is shown in Table 2-10. See whether you can calculate a kappa for this table.

The correct answers (and the key calculations) are in the footnote below.*

Are these kappa levels low or high* [40]?† Although most clinicians would consider them disappointingly low, they are at about the usual level for most components of the clinical examination [13]. For example, the proportion of potential agreement beyond chance that is actually achieved is .51 for the pres-

*In Table 2-10, the observed agreement is (12 + 7 + 6)/40 = 62%. The agreement expected on the basis of chance for individual cells is as follows: ≤5 cm = (15 × 17)/40 = 6.4; 6–9 cm = (13 × 16)/40 = 5.2; ≥10 cm = (12 × 7)/40 = 2.1. Therefore, the total agreement expected on the basis of chance is (6.4 + 5.2 + 2.1)/40 = 34%. Thus, the actual agreement beyond chance is 62% − 34% = 28%, and the potential agreement beyond chance is 100% − 34% = 66%. As a result, kappa is 28%/66% = .42.

†Some experts have attached the following qualitative terms to kappas: .0–.2 = "slight;" .2–.4 = "fair;" .4–.6 = "moderate;" .6–.8 = "substantial;" and .8–1.0 = "almost perfect."

ence or absence of a dorsalis pedis pulse [43] and .50 to .62 for the presence or absence of various signs of chronic airflow obstruction [56].*

Table 2-10 allows us to make three other points. First, we can use kappa to look at multiple levels of agreement (low, normal, high) rather than just two (normal, abnormal). Second, if one clinician thought the central venous pressure was low, we would be more concerned if a second clinician thought it was high than if that second clinician thought it was normal (and we note with relief that this never happened in reading neck veins!). Thus, the extent of disagreement is important, and another nice property of kappa is that we can weight the kappa for the degree of this disagreement. As a result, even though the observed agreement for reading neck veins as low, normal, or high might be the same for two pairs of clinicians, the pair who disagree by two levels (one calls the neck veins low and the other calls them high) will generate a lower weighted kappa than the pair who disagree by only one level. Finally, although kappa has provided a helpful way to look at clinical agreement and disagreement, there are other measures that you may come upon in your clinical reading.†

CLINICAL DISAGREEMENTS IN THE INTERPRETATION OF DIAGNOSTIC TESTS

Observations at the bedside are not the only ones that are subject to clinical disagreement. Suppose another patient of yours, a 55-year-old school principal, has undergone annual routine mammography. The report comes back stating "Suspicious for malignancy." You show her mammogram, without disclosing the contents of the report, to another radiologist, who tells you it is "within normal limits."

The problem of clinical disagreement extends to the interpretations of diagnostic tests whenever these interpretations involve humans, as is the case for x rays, ECGs, pathology specimens, and the like. Three examples are summarized in Table 2-11.

As shown in Table 2-11, the interpretation of mammograms, a crucial step in the early detection of curable breast cancer, is subject to the same disagreement as other clinical judgments. Because most mammograms are normal, the agreement expected on the basis of chance alone is very high (in this case, 91%). Thus, the potential agreement beyond chance was only 9%, and the actual agreement beyond chance was 6%. Thus the kappa of 6%/9% = .67. In this example, not only did the radiologists frequently disagree with one another, but one of them failed to recommend referral for women subsequently shown to have breast cancer (8 cases) almost as often as he correctly recommended their referral (11 cases) [8].

*Actually, kappa is affected somewhat by the average frequency (prevalence) of the abnormal sign as well, which is one of the reasons that clinical epidemiologists are still looking for better ways to describe agreement.

†If you want to look into them, you can begin with the book by Joseph Fleiss [25] and then use one of the strategies in Chapter 11 to track this topic forward in time.

Table 2-11. Clinical disagreement in interpreting diagnostic materials

Diagnostic material	Clinical question	Clinicians	Observed	Agreement expected by chance	Kappa
Mammogram[a]	Should this woman be referred for surgical assessment?	Two radiologists examined the same 1214 mammograms	97%	91%	.67
Exercise electrocardiogram (ECG)[b]	Is the ST-T response normal, borderline, or abnormal?	Two cardiologists examined the same ECGs from 38 patients	57%	39%	.30
		One cardiologist twice examined the same ECGs from 38 patients	74%	33%	.61
Peripheral blood film[c]	Does this patient have iron deficiency?	Two pathologists examined the same films from 29 women with iron-deficiency anemia[d]	69%	49%	.39
		One pathologist twice examined the same films from 29 women with iron-deficiency anemia[d]	83%	51%	.65

[a]Data modified from J. Chamberlin, S. Ginks, P. Rogers, et al. Validity of clinical examination and mammography as screening tests for breast cancer. *Lancet* 2:1026, 1975.

[b]Data modified from H. Blackburn, G. Blomgvist, A. Freiman, et al. The exercise electrocardiogram: Differences in interpolation. Report of a technical group on exercise electrocardiography. *Am. J. Cardiol.* 21:871, 1968.

[c]Data modified from V. F. Fairbanks. Is the peripheral blood film reliable for the diagnosis of iron-deficiency anaemia? *Am. J. Clin. Pathol.* 55:447, 1971.

[d]Hemoglobin level 11.6 g/dl or less and serum iron level less than 12.5 μmol/L (70 mg/dl).

Similar disagreements are common in the interpretation of coronary angiograms [14, 59]. When the decision for a coronary bypass operation is in the balance, any degree of diagnostic inconsistency is cause for concern. Equally disturbing is the degree of inconsistency documented in the interpretation of exercise electrocardiograms [5], the second example in Table 2-11, especially when one contemplates the frequency with which they are obtained and the potential impact of their interpretation on the employability, insurability, and social and emotional function of those who undergo them.

The third example in Table 2-11 reveals inconsistencies even among those who have the last word (at least at clinicopathologic conferences). In interpreting blood films, three clinical pathologists exhibited substantial disagreement with each other and with their own prior interpretations of the same blood film [17]. Moreover, in this 1971 study all three failed to report changes suggestive of iron deficiency in 60% of women whose hemoglobin levels varied from 6.8 to 11.6 g/dl and whose serum iron levels were less than 12.5 μmol/L (70 mg/dl). Have we improved since 1971? A study reported 12 years later documented agreement greater than chance for less than half of the features that are commonly sought on a blood smear [34].

The mammography example adds a new dimension to our discussion of clinical disagreement. Whereas the previous examples measured just the agreement between and within clinicians about gastrointestinal symptoms or funduscopic signs, the mammography example adds the dimension of the ultimate diagnosis, confirmed by an accepted "gold standard" of histologic confirmation and subsequent clinical course. As a result, we can now talk about *accuracy* and *bias* as well as *consistency,* and can proceed to a higher level of understanding about the problem of clinical disagreement.

The examples we have described to this point have dwelt mainly upon the amount of agreement between two or more clinicians and between two or more exams by the same clinician on different occasions. These two elements might usefully be termed *interobserver* and *intraobserver consistency.* A general definition of consistency would then be *the extent to which* multiple examinations *of the same patient or specimen agree with one another.* As we have seen, there is not very much consistency for most clinical observations, and we should be searching for ways to increase whatever consistency does exist.

However, you probably already have recognized that a very high degree of consistency among clinicians might not only be difficult to achieve, but, in some instances, might even be achieved at the loss of accuracy. For example, it is often possible to convince neophytes that they hear a fourth heart sound, even in patients with atrial fibrillation (in which case no S_4 is possible). The level of consistency could then be high in such circumstances, but all the observations would be incorrect. This example permits us to introduce two additional concepts: accuracy and bias. The *closeness of a clinical observation to the true clinical state* is termed *accuracy,* and *bias* is *any systematic deviation of an observation from the true clinical state.* Because these additional terms, accuracy and bias, will help us when we discuss strategies to improve the quality of our clinical examinations, we will provide an example to tie them together.

A patient's true level of compliance with medications can be determined by applying a gold standard, such as repeated measurements of serum drug levels. However, when their physicians are asked to rate them as compliant or noncompliant, these ratings are hopelessly inaccurate. In fact, the clinicians studied by Raymond Gilbert and his team [27] were no more accurate than they would be if they simply flipped a coin. However, these same investigations have found that although clinicians' estimates of patient compliance are inaccurate, they are not biased. That is, clinicians overestimate the compliance of some patients and underestimate the compliance of a roughly similar number of other patients. Because their clinical estimates of compliance were not biased, it was not possible to improve the accuracy of these clinicians by having them adjust their estimates (say, by having them adjust their estimates up or down to bring them closer to the truth).

On the other hand, patients' estimates of their own compliance, although reasonably accurate, are generally biased upwards. That is, patients generally overestimate their compliance by about 20% [29]. Accordingly, clinicians who want to know whether patients are taking less than 80% of their medications correct for this bias in patients' estimates by asking them, "Since I saw you last, have you ever missed *any* of your pills?"

As we can see from the foregoing, consistency between and within clinicians is a desirable but insufficient state of affairs; we need accuracy as well, and when inaccuracy is the result of bias we can correct for it if we know its magnitude and direction.

For many clinical assessments there is, alas, no gold standard of accuracy. Thus, neither the accuracy nor the bias of these assessments can be measured directly, and we are left with consistency as the only measure of how well we are performing. Although this state of affairs is not very satisfactory, we can at least strive for consistency in such assessments, realizing that assessments that are not consistent cannot be accurate.

CLINICAL DISAGREEMENTS OVER MAKING DIAGNOSES AND THERAPEUTIC RECOMMENDATIONS

Suppose you are asked to see a 52-year-old accountant with painful joints who has "made the rounds" of three specialists. You find bilateral joint tenderness (but no effusions) affecting his proximal interphalangeal joints, metacarpal joints, wrists, and knees. Except for a marginal rise in his erythrocyte sedimentation rate, his blood tests and radiographs fail to show any diagnostic features of rheumatoid arthritis. Neither high dose aspirin nor three other nonsteroidal agents have provided much relief and his work, mobility, and sleep continue to be hampered. One specialist suggested that a trial of gold or methotrexate would be warranted for what appeared to be seronegative rheumatoid arthritis, whereas the other two judged that he had osteoarthritis and that these two drugs were contraindicated.

Clinical disagreements are most striking when they apply to diagnostic or management decisions. Our arthritic accountant is clamoring for relief and we cannot agree on what he has or how it should be treated. A classic example of this problem was reported several decades ago and had to do with recommending tonsillectomy [3]. Among 389 eleven-year-old school children with intact tonsils who were examined by a group of physicians, tonsillectomy was recommended for 174 (45%). The remaining 215 children, in whom tonsillectomy had not been recommended, were recycled for a second opinion (without revealing the first opinion) and tonsillectomy was recommended for 99 (46%). The remaining 116 children, who by now had been given a clean bill of tonsillar health on two separate occasions, were then examined a third time; tonsillectomy was recommended for 51 (44%) of them! For us, the most remarkable finding in this study was not the inconsistency in the diagnoses and therapeutic recommendations made by these clinicians when they repeatedly examined the same children, but the consistency in the proportion of children for whom tonsillectomy was recommended in each of the three cycles of examinations: 45%, 46%, and 44%.

Although we are quick to laugh off the follies of medical yesteryears, contemporary examples reveal that the situation is unchanged. When three clinical pharmacologists more recently evaluated 60 patients admitted to hospital because their clinicians had diagnosed adverse reactions to medications, alcohol or "recreational" drugs, the pharmacologists agreed on the diagnoses for only half the patients [36]. Furthermore, in one-third of these cases the pharmacologists disagreed with each other about whether any medication- or alcohol-related adverse reaction had occurred at all.

CLINICAL DISAGREEMENTS ABOUT THE QUALITY OF MEDICAL CARE

Finally, the increasing emphasis on medical audits and quality assurance prompts a final example of clinical disagreement from this burgeoning field. In a study by Robert Brook's team [7], seasoned internists were asked to review the records of patients with urinary tract infection, hypertension, or gastric or duodenal ulcer, and to provide a peer judgment about the quality of care they had received. The extent of their agreement beyond chance varied from only .15 to .56 (median .27).

The Etiology of Clinical Disagreement

Having described the magnitude and types of clinical disagreement, plus some general properties of clinical measurements, we are ready to consider the causes for clinical disagreement in the hope that they will point to strategies for improving the accuracy as well as the consistency of our clinical measurements and conclusions. These causes may usefully be categorized according to their source: the examiner, the examined, and the examination (summarized in Table 2-12).

THE EXAMINER

Biologic Variation in the Senses

Clinical examination invariably begins with the senses—sight, hearing, touch, smell, and (rarely) taste. Variations in the acuity and appreciation of the senses

Table 2-12. The etiology of clinical disagreement

The Examiner
1. Biologic variation in the senses
2. The tendency to record inference rather than evidence
3. Ensnarement by diagnostic classification schemes
4. Entrapment by prior expectation
5. Simple incompetency
The Examined
1. Biologic variation in the system being examined
2. Effects of illness and medications
3. Memory and rumination
4. Toss-ups
The Examination
1. Disruptive environments for the examination
2. Disruptive interactions between examiners and examined
3. Incorrect function or use of diagnostic tools

(e.g., colorblindness, presbyopia, and presbycusis) will lead to disagreements between clinicians. Less widely acknowledged, however, is a factor responsible for inconsistencies in the results of examinations performed by the same clinician: biologic variation in the examiner's senses. This has been documented in a study [26] contrasting how the same physicians perform when rested and when tired (summarized in Table 2-13).

In this study the ability of interns to detect simple cardiac arrhythmias, such as atrial and ventricular premature beats and supraventricular tachycardia, on the same electrocardiogram rhythm strip, deteriorated markedly following a busy night on call (mean sleep duration 1.8 hours), and was accompanied by substantial declines in perception, cognition, and mood.

The Tendency to Record Inference Rather Than Evidence

This cause of clinical disagreement has been discussed in detail by Feinstein [22, 23]. Patients' descriptions of their symptoms and the appearance, sound, and feel of their physical findings enter the clinician's consciousness as sensory evidence. Because the diagnostic process translates and synthesizes this evidence into one or more inferences, it is understandable that the latter tend to serve as the medium of exchange between clinicians and in medical records. Thus, we tend to speak of "pleuritic" rather than "inspiratory" chest pain and of "hematuria" rather than "reddish" urine. In replacing evidence by inference, however, we run the risk of increasing diagnostic error; for although clinicians often agree about sensory evidence, they often disagree about the inference to be drawn from it.

Confining the clinical record to inferences has another important drawback: it may both misdirect the diagnostic process and obscure the original starting point. For example, one of us was once asked to see a man with polycystic kidneys, drug-resistant hypertension, multiple prior drug reactions, and a newly devel-

Table 2-13. Effect of lack of sleep on clinical acumen

	Rested	Fatigued
Mean hours of sleep prior to testing	7.0	1.8
Mean number of symptoms		
Physiologic (weakness, nausea, etc.)	1.1	5.4
Perceptual (trouble focusing eyes, etc.)	0.1	1.4
Cognitive (difficulty concentrating, etc.)	1.4	4.6
Mean number of errors on ECG interpretation	5.2	9.6

Data modified from R. C. Friedman, J. T. Bigger, and D. S. Koranfield. The intern and sleep loss. *N. Engl. J. Med.* 285:201, 1971.

oped skin rash. The rash quickly was judged to be due to drugs and it was this inference, rather than a detailed description of the skin lesions, that appeared in the clinical notes. The next 6 weeks were spent painstakingly altering, one at a time, the patient's antihypertensive medications, and the failure of his skin rash to clear was taken only to represent that the offending drug had not yet been removed from his complex antihypertensive regimen.

It was only when a total, but totally unsuccessful, revision of all his drugs was completed that the original inference was reexamined and the inadequacy of the original inference realized. The diagnostic process was started all over again, the compatability of the original evidence with tinea corporis was recognized, appropriate fungal studies were carried out (with confirmatory results), and proper therapy was initiated. A hasty inference had closed this clinician's mind to other possibilities, wasting several weeks in a fruitless treatment of the wrong diagnosis. This risk needs to be kept in mind any time we use the diagnostic strategy of pattern recognition, or if we accept a single hypothesis too quickly when using the hypothetico-deductive approach.

Ensnarement by Diagnostic Classification Schemes

Current diagnostic classification schemes can increase the risk of clinical disagreement in two ways. First, they often provide arbitrary, hazy, and frequently inconsistent "break points" in a smooth and continuous distribution of an attribute such as blood pressure, body mass, or glucose tolerance. As a result, we engage in fruitless arguments over whether a patient is "really" hypertensive, obese, or diabetic. The related issues in, and perversions of, the definition of "normalcy" are discussed in the next chapter.

Second, clinical disagreement arises when different diagnostic criteria are applied to the same clinical entity by different groups of clinicians. Consider "heart attack." Depending on which group of physicians you talk to, it can be any of five different entities! To the anatomic pathologist, "heart attack" is an *anatomic* diagnosis, requiring specific gross and microscopic changes in the myocardium. To the clinical chemist, on the other hand, "heart attack" is often a *biochemical* diagnosis, requiring an appropriately timed elevation of one or more cardiac enzymes in blood specimens drawn from the patient. To the electrocardiographer, however, "heart attack" is an *electrophysiologic* diagnosis, requiring (in the case of a transmural infarction, for example) injury currents, Q waves, and ST-T changes in serial electrocardiograms. Not to be outdone, to some self-styled preventive cardiologists, "heart attack" is an *etiologic* diagnosis, consisting of hyperlipidemia, tobacco addiction, a Type A personality, a bad family history, physical inactivity, and the like.*

Finally, to the clinician who gets out of bed in the middle of the night to attend the patient with a "heart attack," it is a *clinical* diagnosis consisting of certain symptoms (pain, breathlessness, sweating, etc.) and signs (gallop, rales, premature ventricular contractions, and so forth).

Thus, "heart attack" can be an anatomic, a biochemical, an electrophysiologic, an etiologic, or a clinical diagnosis. Although these different definitions can and often do converge, many heated and unresolved arguments about whether given patients "really" have had heart attacks take place along the way, and often the disagreements arise from ensnarement by different diagnostic classification schemes. The analogy to the argument among the blind men over the essence of an elephant comes to mind, but in our diagnostic situation we are dealing not just with the beast's legs, flanks, trunk, and tail, but with his footprints and effluvia as well.

Entrapment by Prior Expectation

We tend to find what we expect or hope to find. The power and consistency of this cause for clinical disagreement were well demonstrated in the tonsillectomy example described earlier [3]. As you will recall, clinicians consistently recommended tonsillectomy for about 45% of the same children they had judged not to need this operation on one or even two recent prior examinations.

That expectation still influences clinical diagnosis is evident in the electronic age. The introduction of fetal heart monitoring provided a golden opportunity to demonstrate the power of expectation (and hope!) on the clinical examination. In an early study of monitoring by Day, Madden, and Wood [12], the results of the monitoring were kept from the clinicians who were following a group of women in labor. The accuracy of the clinical assessments was later determined in comparison with the monitor's results. Now, everybody knows that the "normal" fetal heart rate is 140 beats per minute and, sure enough, when the fetal heart monitor registered heart rates of 130 to 150 there was close agreement with the clinicians' notations in the charts. However, when the monitor documented fetal heart rates over 150 beats per minute, clinicians tended to record them as lower (more "normal") than they actually were. Similarly, when the monitor

*Those to whom this definition of the diagnosis appears farfetched should simply recall the recurring, widespread advertisement in clinical journals of the 1970s that captioned a picture of a smiling, healthy-looking, middle-aged man with the chilling title "This man is ill and doesn't know it." Page 2 of the ad revealed his diagnosis: "He has seriously elevated lipid levels." Ironically these ads recommended clofibrate, a drug later shown to increase the mortality of such individuals [46].

documented fetal heart rates below 130 per minute, the clinicians tended to record them as higher (again, more "normal") than they actually were. It is reasonable to argue that these clinicians not only *expected* the fetal heart rates to be normal, but *hoped* that they would be normal as well; abnormally high or low fetal heart rates spell trouble for both patients and clinicians.

Hope must play a powerful role in determining the results of all sorts of clinical examinations, especially when the abnormal finding produces anguish for our patients (has the tumor recurred?) or more work for an already overburdened clinician (does this patient need a hypertension workup?). However biased, the desire to deny even the obvious and to "watch and wait" in such cases is certainly understandable, though often clinically dangerous.

Simple Incompetency

Finally, clinical disagreement is inevitable when examiners do not know where and how to look, listen, touch, smell, and taste or how to interpret what they see, hear, feel, smell, and taste.

Sometimes the results are merely hilariously harmless. One of us recalls a fellow intern who proudly showed an annular carcinoma he had just found on one of his first sigmoidoscopies; when it was suggested that the lesion was, in fact, an eroded cervix his mortification was matched by the patient's bemused relief (and a subsequent endoscopy "through proper channels" was normal).

Other times, the results can have tragic consequences. The misinterpretation of physiologic heart murmurs that led to the diagnosis of organic heart disease in the normal children back in Table 2-4 is an example of overinterpretation of normal findings. The underinterpretation of abnormal findings also can lead to unfortunate clinical disagreement, as may well have been the case in the fetal heart-monitoring example.

Since none of us has met practicing clinicians who aspire to incompetence in clinical examination, we conclude that something about the teaching, learning, and especially the maintaining, of clinical skills may ultimately be at fault here. Given the proportion of clinicians we encounter, even at advanced stages of training, who tell us that no one has ever watched them execute a history and physical examination, we have a way to go in helping learners master these skills at the outset. More surprising, we may need to place much more emphasis on clinical skills in CME curricula. One of our Chief Residents recently found that clinical clerks outperformed attending physicians in estimating central venous pressure from neck veins [9], and a 1989 review of the clinical skills literature suggested that basic clinical skills may not improve beyond graduation from medical school [45].

THE EXAMINED

Biologic Variation in the System Being Examined

Most clinicians recognize that clinical attributes such as weight, blood pressure, and pulse will vary from hour to hour and day to day, depending on such factors as position, diet, fluid intake, stress, exercise, and so forth. Furthermore, we acknowledge that if the blood pressure is surprisingly high or low one day, by "regression toward the mean" [49], it will tend to return to a more usual level on a subsequent examination; this is why we require several visits before we are willing to diagnose moderate hypertension. However, we may not realize that this same biologic variation is also the rule for many "exact" measurements, including electrocardiograms, left ventricular end-diastolic pressures, and ejection fractions [42, 53]. It follows that such variation will lead to inconsistencies in the clinical descriptions of patients and, when the variation crosses a critical boundary, in diagnoses.

Effects of Illness and Medications

This cause of disagreement operates when the target disorder or its treatment affect the patient's ability to provide a cogent and accurate history, or alter the clinical manifestations of disease. In some situations the effect is permanent; thus, strokes often impair memory or communication, and, in many hypertensive patients, the blood pressure returns to normal following a myocardial infarction. In other circumstances, the changes are temporary, as in the effects of heart failure on cardiac auscultation or the effects of alcohol (and its withdrawal) on the clinical history. Similarly, because analgesics may mask the physical signs and cloud the recall of patients with acute abdomens, their use is contraindicated until a diagnosis is established.

Memory and Rumination

Patients, especially those with chronic or serious illnesses, tend to ruminate over past events in search of a cogent cause for their troubles. Repeated history taking reinforces this rumination, may cause the patient to consult records or other family members, and often reorganizes scattered memories into orderly patterns of recalled events. Thus, serial histories may exhibit substantial evolution or other change, resulting in blatant disagreements over the occurrence or timing of important prior health events (and not inconsiderable consternation of students and house officers during professorial rounds).

Toss-ups

When clinicians disagree over which of two management regimens is better for a given patient, it just may be that the regimens under dispute are equally efficacious (or useless!). The mechanisms of disease underlying the patient's disorder may be resistant to all interventions, on the one hand, or equally responsive to both, on the other. This cause for disagreement has been named the *toss-up* [37], and we shall reexamine it again in each of the next two chapters.

THE EXAMINATION

Disruptive Environments for the Examination

The environment in which the examination is carried out can affect both senses and sensibilities. Attempts at cardiac auscultation on jetliners are futile, and the noise levels in some emergency rooms effectively swamp all but the loudest Korotkoff sounds. Artificial or dim lighting can render the detection of jaundice or cyanosis impossible. A shivering patient in a cold examining room will welcome neither a prolonged clinical interview nor the cold steel of diagnostic instruments. Finally, privacy may be a prerequisite for the disclosure of information about the family (e.g., epilepsy, consanguinity, or insanity), the operative history (e.g., an illegal abortion), or exposure to sexually transmitted disease.

Disruptive Interactions Between Examiners and Examined

Although effective communication between clinicians and patients is widely acknowledged as a prerequisite for appropriate management in both behaviorally [32] and biologically oriented [38] clinical journals, the effect of faulty communication on clinical disagreement has not often been quantified. A study of a random sample of 155 patient interviews conducted in a private family doctor's practice revealed that one-fifth of the interviews failed to unearth important features, such as melena or urinary frequency, in the history of the patient's present illness or in the past history [52]. Surprisingly, the investigators found that such lapses were greatest not when patients were at odds with their physicians, but when they lavished their physicians with excessive praise. Furthermore, patients from different ethnic backgrounds are known to focus their symptoms onto different body sites; the failure of clinicians to recognize this and the social distance between them and their patients has been offered as one explanation for the wide variations in the incidence of nonorganic diagnoses reported among different ethnic groups living in identical physical, social, and economic environments [60].

Moreover, the effects of patient apprehension on the acquisition of clinical information in an unfamiliar setting can be substantial, as any clinician knows who has attempted to reassure a frightened patient labeled hypertensive in a shopping plaza screening program. Similarly, painful examinations, such as palpation of a tender abdominal mass, may alter or obscure important clinical findings.

Incorrect Function or Use of Diagnostic Tools

A mercury manometer with a low reservoir or a defective anaeroid manometer with a hidden pinstop can give falsely low blood pressure readings. Indeed, Perlman and his colleagues [47] found 40 (13%) of 310 anaeroid manometers examined in seven hospitals in Michigan to produce errors of 7 mm Hg in comparison with mercury manometers. Use of an inappropriate sphygmomanometer cuff width or the too-rapid deflation of a cuff can also lead to systematic errors, and some individuals have been shown to choose certain terminal numbers (digits 8, 0, or 2) over others (digits 4 or 6) when reporting blood pressure measurements [35]. Similar faults have been identified in the manufacture, maintenance, and use of other diagnostic tools, classic examples being switched leads, wrong calibration, and/or wrong speed on ECG tracings.

How to Avoid Clinical Disagreement and Learn from One's Mistakes

In the previous sections of this chapter, we considered the potency of some clinical observations and the impotence of others, presented methods for refining the measurement properties of these observations, and documented sources of disagreement and error in clinical assessments. In this final section we will consider six strategies to prevent or minimize the occurrence of clinical disagreement.

WHEN DOES CLINICAL DISAGREEMENT REALLY MATTER?

Improving the consistency and accuracy of our clinical observations requires at least an initial investment of time and effort while we perfect our approach. Assuming that none of us has a reserve of time to dip into for this sort of activity, it is obvious that we must be efficient about this process. To begin, we might well review the clinical observations we commonly make and eliminate from our repertoire those assessments that are not of value, such as our own judgment of the patient's compliance with the regimen we prescribed [27]. As a more general tactic, we have already suggested that the "method of exhaustion" be abandoned as a diagnostic approach. In a similar vein, we should reserve strategies for reducing clinical disagreement for those crucial items in the patient's history, physical examination, and diagnostic evaluation that are important to that patient's diagnosis, management, or prognosis, as illustrated in the following cases.

A 50-year-old patient of yours is to undergo elective cholecystectomy and on hospital admission he states that he thinks he "may have had a heart attack a few months ago." In this case, both the fact and timing of this cardiac event are crucial. If he did have a myocardial infarction and it occurred within the previous 3 months, his risk of having another one postoperatively approaches 30% [54], whereas postponing his elective operation until 6 months after his infarct reduces this risk to about 4%.

Our second case involves a child with scarlatina, fever, and arthralgia, who has a questionable new heart murmur. The cardiac examination is crucial in this case. If this child does have carditis, the Jones criteria [55] for acute rheumatic fever are met, with all their implications for recurrence, prognosis, and antistreptococcal prophylaxis.

In our final case, a young athlete develops calf-swelling following immobilization for torn knee ligaments and a venogram reveals "equivocal" evidence of deep vein thrombosis in the ipsilateral thigh. In this case, the interpretation of the venogram is crucial. If this patient has proximal deep vein thrombosis, the season is over and a course of full-dose, intravenous heparin, plus three months of oral anticoagulants, is required [33].

In these cases a specific item in the history, in the physical examination, or in the interpretation of a diagnostic test has a crucial effect on the patient's prognosis and treatment. When such crucial elements arise in the clinical evaluation of a patient, steps must be taken to prevent or at least minimize both inaccuracy and inconsistency in determining their presence and significance.

Strategies for preventing or minimizing clinical disagreement are summarized in Table 2-14; they have been taken from several sources [13], including an important series by Feinstein [19–22].

Table 2-14. Six strategies for preventing or minimizing clinical disagreement

1. Match the diagnostic environment to the diagnostic task
2. Seek corroboration of key findings
   a. Repeat key elements of your examination
   b. Corroborate important findings with documents and witnesses
   c. Confirm key clinical findings with appropriate tests
   d. Ask "blinded" colleagues to examine your patient
3. Report evidence as well as inference, making a clear distinction between the two
4. Use appropriate technical aids
5. "Blind" your assessments of raw diagnostic test data
6. Apply the social sciences, as well as the biologic sciences, of medicine

Match the Diagnostic Environment to the Diagnostic Task

Select a site with the appropriate light, heat, silence, and privacy for the diagnostic tasks to be carried out. This may mean moving the patient to a more suitable place; if such transport becomes a routine prerequisite for a proper clinical examination, modification of the examining room is in order.

Seek Corroboration of Key Findings

This can be accomplished in four ways:

REPEAT KEY ELEMENTS OF YOUR EXAMINATION. The justification for repeating your history and physical goes well beyond the hope that "something may turn up." First, your patient, jogged by the earlier interview, may now have recalled and reorganized important historical events or key cardinal symptoms. Indeed, this phenomenon may partially explain why the "attending" physician's history is often more informative than the initial history elicited by the clinical clerk.

Second, biologic variation and, especially, regression toward the mean (the tendency for extreme laboratory results or physical findings to revert toward less extreme values on repeated examination [49] may have occurred in the body systems under scrutiny, permitting a more clear-cut decision on whether prior findings (such as blood pressure) were or were not normal. Third, if you carried out the previous examination when you were fatigued, a second examination when you are rested may uncover key findings previously missed. Finally, a repeat examination may disclose key items that simply were overlooked on an earlier exam, a phenomenon that is well documented in reading chest x rays [58].

CORROBORATE IMPORTANT FINDINGS WITH DOCUMENTS AND WITNESSES. Key items in the history and physical are often documented in prior clinical or health records. Did your patient have neonatal asphyxia? Was she diabetic during her first pregnancy? Did he receive anticoagulants when taken sick on his holiday? Often these key items can be confirmed at once with a well-placed telephone call or a perusal of old records. In one study, in which current histories were compared with old hospital records, it was found that even dramatic events such as hematemesis and melena were often forgotten or fabricated [10].

Other important information, such as the features of transient neurologic deficits or prior medication use, can often be confirmed by talking with family members or other witnesses. Indeed, patients can improve on their histories by keeping symptom diaries. Such an approach has been shown to substantially decrease the underreporting of bowel symptoms revealed during routine histories [41].

Finally, the comparison of present with past diagnostic test results (especially roentgenograms) can do much to eliminate clinical disagreements over the presence, duration, and progression of important disease processes.

CONFIRM KEY CLINICAL FINDINGS WITH APPROPRIATE DIAGNOSTIC TESTS. As noninvasive diagnostic tests such as ultrasound and body scanning become more widely available (and, we hope, more reproducible!), and as the safety and acceptability of invasive tests such as fiberoptic endoscopy, mediastinoscopy, peritoneoscopy, and culdoscopy improve, clinicians can increasingly look to procedures other than autopsy for confirmation of their findings and diagnoses. As we shall see in the final section of this book, this strategy of confirmation can be of considerable value in one's continuing education in clinical diagnostic skills as well as in patient care. However, when applying this strategy you have to decide whether and how much to tell those who will carry out these confirmatory tests, as we shall now discuss.

ASK "BLINDED" COLLEAGUES TO EXAMINE YOUR PATIENT. It is often useful to ask a colleague to repeat a key portion of a history or physical to determine whether your observations are confirmed. Such a strategy has been shown to be quite valuable, for example, in the evaluation of patients with suspected valvular heart disease [18]. For this strategy to be useful, however, it is vital that the second examiner be told only of the area to be interrogated or examined, and not of your tentative conclusion. Thus, your request should be "Listen to his heart and tell me what you think," rather than "I think this man has aortic stenosis. Please listen and tell me whether you agree." To preface a request for a repeat examination with a statement of your own conclusions downgrades the second examination from a test of clinical agreement to a test of friendship.

Report Evidence as Well as Inference

When clinical notes convey the sensory events ("right parasternal heave, loud S_1 and P_2, faint opening snap, grade 2/6 decrescendo early diastolic murmur with presystolic accentuation best heard at the apex") as well as the corresponding inference ("mitral stenosis"), several benefits accrue. First, agreement between examinations and examiners increases. For example, Feinstein [23] has documented substantially greater agreement among clinicians for the acoustic elements of cardiac diagnoses than for the diagnoses themselves. Similarly, the British surgeons [28] cited at the beginning of this chapter showed that a thorough discussion and agreement about the piece of evidence required for a conclusion that ulcer surgery had been successful tended to improve agreement on this inference.

Second, the recording of evidence as well as inference often provides crucial information for comparison with later findings, and so provides a far sounder basis for judging the course and progression of the patient's disease. Third, communication among the multiple clinicians who may be practicing team care on the same patient is obviously enhanced. Finally, the recording of evidence permits clinicians to retrace their steps back to the initial clinical data when subsequent diagnostic tests or events prove that the original diagnostic inference was wrong.

Use Appropriate Technical Aids

Although the stethoscope is universally accepted as a technical aid to auscultation, the same cannot be said for aids to other important clinical measurements. Measurements of distance and size still rely on fingerbreadths, imaginary landmarks (such as the midclavicular line), eggs, fruits, and vegetables, despite a consensus that the use of a tape measure or ruler leads to more precise and useful clinical data. Similarly, although the ECG is a routine technical aid for the confirmation and quantitation of cardiac arrhythmias, we often ignore opportunities for the useful application of other technical aids. For example, the "blood pressure" cuff does not measure blood pressure at all; it measures air pressure. Thus, it can be used to quantify abdominal tenderness (quite helpful when following an acute abdomen [51], especially when sharing clinical responsibilities with other team members), to measure grip or other muscle strength in arthritis [30], or as a crude oscillometer in the bedside evaluation of peripheral vascular disease.

Care must be taken to avoid the ersatz accuracy that may result when we replace human judgment with numbers or "hard copy." For example, although it seems sensible that the use of calipers should improve clinical agreement about the degree of arterial stenosis on coronary cineangiograms, a group of our colleagues showed that the "eyeball" method of interpretation generated statistically significantly higher kappas! [31]. However, when we can document an important clinical sign by the quick application of an inexpensive technical device that improves the accuracy or consistency of clinical measurement, we ought to do so.

Arrange for Independent Interpretation of Observational Diagnostic Test Data

Many of the diagnostic tests we order, such as ECGs, radiographs, biopsy specimens, and the like, require observational assessment and interpretation. These assessments can be easily biased by prior expectation (remember the fetal heart rate example?). This risk is particularly high when these data are interpreted by the same clinician who previously examined the patient, without the aid of an independent "blind" observer. Clinicians who interpret their own tests without independent confirmation are likely to find exactly what they expect—whether it is there or not. Common situations in which this occurs are emergency rooms, when speed may be of the essence and the clinician may not want, or be able, to wait for a second opinion, and doctors' offices that have their own ECG, x ray, and other diagnostic machines. Although interpretation by the examining clinician may be a matter of necessity in some circumstances, this should be followed by independent interpretation later.

Of course, "blindness" of the test interpreter can be taken too far. The clinical pathologist will not apply the special stains unless the rare diagnosis that requires them is noted on the request. Clearly, there must be effective communication between the clinician and the test reader if they are to achieve the correct interpretation of the test for the patient in question. Less clear, however, is the amount of information that the independent observer should have on hand when a test is interpreted. Perhaps the best trade-off between blindness and senselessness is the one suggested by David Spodick [53], who has emphasized the benefits of writing two independent interpretations of every ECG, the first one with no information save the patient's age and sex, and the second one with pertinent clinical information at hand. We will return to this point later, and extensively so, when we consider interpretation of diagnostic tests. For now, we simply suggest that the "expectation bias" be reduced by having a second person, preferably a diagnostic test expert, interpret observational test data.

Apply the Social Sciences, as Well as the Biologic Sciences, of Medicine

The clinician who takes pains to listen to the patient and to pay close attention to the physician-patient relationship is doing much more than practicing the art of medicine: the clinician is practicing good scientific medicine. An understanding of the impact of interpersonal and behavioral factors upon both diagnosis and management is central to the practice of scientific medicine. If we fail to recognize such basic elements as the relation between "not liking" given patients, assigning them bad prognoses, and prescribing them multiple drugs [16], we are at risk of reducing the quality of our clinical care.

In 1970, Anderson and his colleagues [1] in the Department of Medicine at King's College Hospital Medical School identified eight skills that are required to obtain an accurate and useful history (Table 2-15).

Most of these skills are overtly behavioral, and it is encouraging to discover that the application of empathetic responses to patients can be learned as well as inherited [24]. This is not to say that the creation of a warm clinician-patient relationship always improves the quality of a medical history. Indeed, as we already pointed out, one study has documented that patients who most admire and respect their clinicians may withhold key information on the occurrence and severity of the side effects of medication [52].

What we do stress, however, is the need for us all to critically appraise the effects of the way that we talk with patients as well as the content of what we talk about. For example, the interviewing strategies of attentiveness (acknowledging patients' concerns and understandings and taking them seriously), facilitation (encouraging patients to tell their stories in their own words), and collaboration (recognizing and supporting patients as partners in care), published by Mishler and his colleagues [44] almost 20 years after the list in Table 2-15, deserve our continued scrutiny as they undergo empiric testing for their benefits to clinicians and patients.

In closing this chapter, we return to some good advice from Alvan Feinstein [22]: "To advance art and science in clinical examination, the equipment a clinician most needs to improve is himself." We ought to be educated as well as humbled when our patient's subsequent clinical course, operation, or autopsy

Table 2-15. Eight skills required to obtain an accurate and useful history

The Ability to:
Establish understanding
Establish information
Interview logically
Listen
Interrupt
Observe nonverbal cues
Establish a good relationship
Interpret the interview

Modified from J. Anderson, D. L. Day, M. A. C. Dowling, et al. The definition and evaluation of the skills required to obtain a patient's history of illness: The use of videotape recordings. *Postgrad. Med.* 46:606, 1970.

shows us that we erred in our original diagnosis. Indeed, if we were to carry out a more systematic documentation of our own successes and failures in diagnosis, we could both identify areas in which we need to improve our clinical skills and find out whether we are making progress in reducing our rate of clinical disagreement.

This documentation is but one element of an approach to reviewing our clinical performance that ought to serve as the starting point for our continuing self-education. We have devoted the final third of this book to this and other aspects of "keeping up to date" and you may want to jump ahead to Chapter 10 on Performance Review. On the other hand, you may choose to concentrate on strategies for deciding which symptoms, signs, and laboratory tests are worth capturing, in which case you will want to proceed to the next chapter on the selection of diagnostic tests.

References

1. Anderson, J., Day, D. L., Dowling, M. A. C., et al. The definition and evaluation of the skills required to obtain a patient's history of illness: The use of videotape recordings. *Postgrad. Med.* 46: 606, 1970.
2. Aoki, N., Horibe, H., Ohno, Y., et al. Epidemiological evaluation of funduscopic findings in cerebrovascular diseases. III. Observer variability and reproducibility for funduscopic findings. *Jpn. Circ. J.* 41: 11, 1977.
3. Bakwin, H. Pseudodoxia pediatrica. *N. Engl. J. Med.* 232: 691, 1945.
4. Bergman, A. B., and Stamm, S. J. The morbidity of cardiac nondisease in school children. *N. Engl. J. Med.* 276: 1008, 1967.
5. Blackburn, H., Blomgvist, G., Freiman, A., et al. The exercise electrocardiogram: Differences in interpretation. Report of a technical group on exercise electrocardiography. *Am. J. Cardiol.* 21: 871, 1968.
6. Boyd, N. F., and Feinstein, A. R. Symptoms as an index of growth rates and prognosis in Hodgkin's disease. *Clin. Invest. Med.* 2: 25, 1978.
7. Brook, R. H. *Quality of Care Assessment: A Comparison of Five Methods of Peer Review.* Washington: Government Printing Office. DHEW HRA-74-3100, 1973.
8. Chamberlain, J., Ginks, S., Rogers, P., et al. Validity of clinical examination and mammography as screening tests for breast cancer. *Lancet* 2: 1026, 1975.

9. Cook, D. J. Clinical assessment of central venous pressure in the critically ill. *Am. J. Med. Sci.* 299: 175, 1990.
10. Corwin, R. G., Krober, M., and Roth, H. P. Patients' accuracy in reporting their past medical history, a study of 90 patients with peptic ulcer. *J. Chronic Dis.* 23: 875, 1971.
11. Crombie, D. L. Diagnostic process. *J. Coll. Gen. Practit.* 6: 579, 1963.
12. Day, E., Madden, L., and Wood, C. Auscultation of foetal heart rate: An assessment of its error and significance. *Br. Med. J.* 4: 422, 1968.
13. Department of Clinical Epidemiology and Biostatistics, McMaster University, Hamilton, Ontario. Clinical Disagreement: II. How to avoid it and how to learn from one's mistakes. *Can. Med. Assoc. J.* 123: 613, 1980.
14. Detre, K. M., Wright, E., Murphy, M. L., et al. Observer agreement in evaluating coronary angiograms. *Circulation* 52: 979, 1975.
15. Diamond, G. A., and Forrester, J. S. Analysis of probability as an aid in the clinical diagnosis of coronary artery disease. *N. Engl. J. Med.* 300: 1350, 1979.
16. Ehrlich, H. J., and Bauer, M. L. Therapists' feelings toward patients and patient treatment outcomes. *Soc. Sci. Med.* 1: 283, 1967.
17. Fairbanks, V. F. Is the peripheral blood film reliable for the diagnosis of iron deficiency anaemia? *Am. J. Clin. Pathol.* 55: 447, 1971.
18. Feinstein, A. R., and DiMassa, R. The unheard diastolic murmur in acute rheumatic fever. *N. Engl. J. Med.* 260: 1331, 1959.
19. Feinstein, A. R. Scientific methodology in clinical medicine: I. Introduction, principles and concepts. *Ann. Intern. Med.* 61: 564, 1964.
20. Feinstein, A. R. Scientific methodology in clinical medicine: II. Classification of human disease by clinical behavior. *Ann. Intern. Med.* 61: 757, 1964.
21. Feinstein, A. R. Scientific methodology in clinical medicine: III. The evaluation of therapeutic response. *Ann. Intern. Med.* 61: 944, 1964.
22. Feinstein, A. R. Scientific methodology in clinical medicine: IV. Acquisition of clinical data. *Ann. Intern. Med.* 61: 1162, 1964.
23. Feinstein, A. R. *Clinical Judgment.* Baltimore: Williams & Wilkins, 1967.
24. Fine, V. K., and Therrien, M. E. Empathy in the doctor-patient relationship: Skill training for medical students. *J. Med. Educ.* 52: 757, 1977.
25. Fleiss, J. L. *Statistical Methods for Rates and Proportions* (2nd ed.) New York: Wiley, 1981. Pp. 217–234.
26. Friedman, R. C., Bigger, J. T., and Koranfield, D. S. The intern and sleep loss. *N. Engl. J. Med.* 285: 201, 1971.
27. Gilbert, J. R., Evans, C. E., Haynes, R. B., and Tugwell, P. Predicting compliance with a regimen of digoxin therapy in family practice. *Can. Med. Assoc. J.* 123: 119, 1980.
28. Hall, R., Horrocks, J. C., Clamp, S. E., et al. Observer variation in assessment of results of surgery for peptic ulcer. *Br. Med. J.* 1: 814, 1976.
29. Haynes, R. B., Taylor, D. W., Sackett, D. L., et al. Can simple clinical measurements detect patient noncompliance? *Hypertension* 2: 757, 1980.
30. Helewa, A., Goldsmith, C. H., and Smythe, H. A. The modified sphygmomanometer—an instrument to measure muscle strength: A validation study. *J. Chron. Dis.* 34: 353, 1981.
31. Holder, D. A., Johnson, A. L., Stolberg, H. O., et al. Inability of caliper measurement to enhance observer agreement in the interpretation of coronary cineangiograms. *Can. J. Cardiol.* 1: 24, 1985.
32. Hoorneart, F., and Pierloot, R. Transference aspects of doctor-patient relationship in psychosomatic patients: I. *Br. J. Med. Psychol.* 49: 261, 1976.
33. Hull, R., Delmore, T., Genton, E., et al. Warfarin sodium versus low-dose heparin in the long-term treatment of venous thrombosis. *N. Engl. J. Med.* 301: 855, 1979.
34. Jen, P., Woo, B., Rosenthal, P. E., Bunn, F., et al. The value of the peripheral blood

smear in anemic patients; the laboratory's reading v. a physician's reading. *Arch. Intern. Med.* 143: 1120, 1983.
35. Kantor, S., Winkelstein, W., Jr., Sackett, D. L., et al. A method for classifying blood pressure: An empirical approach to the reduction of misclassification due to response instability. *Am. J. Epidemiol.* 84: 510, 1966.
36. Karch, F. E., Smith, C. L., Kerzner, B., et al. Adverse drug reactions—a matter of opinion. *Clin. Pharmacol. Ther.* 19: 489, 1976.
37. Kassirer, J. P., and Pauker, S. G. The toss-up. *N. Engl. J. Med.* 305: 1467, 1981.
38. Kirscht, J. P. Communication between patients and physicians. *Ann. Intern. Med.* 86: 499, 1977.
39. Koran, L. M. The reliability of clinical methods, data and judgments. *N. Engl. J. Med.* 293: 695, 1975.
40. Landis, R. J., and Koch, G. G. The measurement of observer agreement for categorical data. *Biometrics* 33: 159, 1977.
41. Manning, A. P. How trustworthy are bowel histories? Comparison of recalled and recorded information. *Br. Med. J.* 2: 213, 1976.
42. McAnulty, J. H., Kremkau, E. L., and Rosch, J. Spontaneous changes in left ventricular function between sequential studies. *Am. J. Cardiol.* 34: 23, 1974.
43. Meade, T. W., Gardner, M. J., Cannon, P., et al. Observer variability in recording the peripheral pulses. *Br. Heart J.* 30: 661, 1968.
44. Mishler, E. G., Clark, J. A., Ingelfinger, J., Simon, M. P. The language of attentive patient care. *J. Gen. Int. Med.* 4: 325, 1989.
45. Nishikawa, J., and Sackett, D. L. Do fundamental clinical skills improve beyond graduation from medical school? *Clin. Res.* 37: 525A, 1989.
46. Oliver, M. J., Heady, J. A., Morris, J. N., and Cooper, J. W.H.O. cooperative trial on primary prevention of ischaemic heart disease using clofibrate to lower serum cholesterol: mortality followup. *Lancet* 2: 379, 1980.
47. Perlman, L. V., Chiang, B. N., Kellor, J., et al. Accuracy of sphygmomanometers in hospital patients. *Arch. Intern. Med.* 125: 1000, 1970.
48. Rose, G. A. Ischemic heart disease. Chest pain questionnaire. *Milbank Mem. Fund. Q.* 43: 32, 1965.
49. Sackett, D. L. Clinical diagnosis and the clinical laboratory. *Clin. Invest. Med.* 1: 37, 1978.
50. Sandler, G. The importance of the history in the medical clinic and the cost of unnecessary tests. *Am. Heart J.* 100 (Part 1): 928, 1980.
51. Shafer, N. Technique for quantitating abdominal pain. *J.A.M.A.* 201: 558, 1967.
52. Snyder, D., Lynch, J. J., and Gruss, L. Doctor-patient communication in a family practice. *J. Fam. Pract.* 3: 271, 1976.
53. Spodick, D. H. On experts and expertise: The effect of variability in observer performance. *Am. J. Cardiol.* 36: 592, 1975.
54. Steen, P. A., Tinker, J. H., and Tarhan, S. Myocardial reinfarction after anesthesia and surgery. *J.A.M.A.* 239: 2566, 1978.
55. Stollerman, G. H., Markovitz, M., Taranta, A., et al. Jones criteria (revised) for guidance in the diagnosis of rheumatic fever. *Circulation* 32: 664, 1965.
56. Stubbing, D. C., Matthew, R. N., Roberts, R. S., and Campbell, E. J. M. Some physical signs in patients with chronic airflow obstruction. *Am. Rev. Resp. Dis.* 125: 549, 1982.
57. Waddell, G., Main, C. J., Morris, E. W., et al. Normality reliability in the clinical assessment of backache. *Br. Med. J.* 284: 1519, 1982.
58. Yerushalmy, J., Harkness, J. T., Cope, J. H., et al. The role of dual reading in mass radiography. *Am. Rev. Tuberc.* 4: 443, 1950.
59. Zir, L. M., Miller, S. W., Dinsmore, R. E., et al. Interobserver variability in coronary angiography. *Circulation* 53: 627, 1976.
60. Zola, I. K. Pathways to the doctor—from person to patient. *Soc. Sci. Med.* 7: 677, 1973.

3

The Selection of Diagnostic Tests

The two previous chapters focused on generating diagnostic hypotheses and capturing clinical data about them. But which clinical data are worth capturing? The answer to this question is what this chapter is all about.

Before presenting the criteria that will help you decide whether a given bit of diagnostic data is worth capturing, we want to reemphasize two points raised in earlier chapters. First, diagnostic data go far beyond those that are generated in the clinical chemistry laboratory, the radiology department, or the pathology service. In fact, as we showed you at the start of the previous chapter, the clinical data obtained by taking a thoughtful history and performing a purposeful physical examination are far more powerful than anything obtained in the diagnostic laboratory and are usually quite sufficient to establish a definitive diagnosis.

Second, although we usually think of gathering diagnostic data in an effort to make a diagnosis, the same data may also be sought for four different (but interrelated) purposes:

1. To judge the *severity* of the illness rather than, or in addition to, its cause. Thus, we search for heart failure in a patient suspected of having a myocardial infarction, both to strengthen our diagnostic hypothesis and to estimate the severity of the cardiac damage. We'll return to this purpose at the end of this chapter.
2. To predict the *subsequent clinical course and prognosis* of the illness and the patient. This purpose is closely linked to the preceding one, and is served when we search for local extensions and distant metastases from a newly diagnosed primary cancer.
3. To estimate the *likely responsiveness to therapy* in the future. This is why we search for surgically curable lesions in newly detected hypertension, or for estrogen receptors in newly diagnosed breast cancer.
4. To determine the *actual response to therapy* in the present. So, we now repeat some of the same thyroid function studies we previously used to establish the diagnosis of thyroid disease, but now in order to determine the adequacy of, compliance with, and responsiveness to the therapy we instituted as a result of our initial diagnosis.

Regardless of the reason for seeking "diagnostic" data, the overriding criterion to use when deciding which data to seek should be the *usefulness* of a given piece of diagnostic data to the clinician who seeks it and the patient who generates it. Moreover, it is the front line clinician who, in deciding that a given clinical sign, symptom, or other diagnostic test will be pursued, bears the responsibility for insuring this usefulness. The conscientious clinician, therefore, must somehow find and appraise evidence on the usefulness of commonly employed diagnostic data. This admonition both challenges contemporaneous clin-

Table 3-1. Eight guides for deciding the clinical usefulness of a diagnostic test

1. Has there been an independent, "blind" comparison with a "gold standard" of diagnosis?
2. Has the diagnostic test been evaluated in a patient sample that included an appropriate spectrum of mild and severe, treated and untreated, disease, plus individuals with different but commonly confused disorders?
3. Was the setting for this evaluation, as well as the filter through which study patients passed, adequately described?
4. Have the reproducibility of the test result (precision) and its interpretation (observer variation) been determined?
5. Has the term *normal* been defined sensibly as it applies to this test?
6. If the test is advocated as part of a cluster or sequence of tests, has its individual contribution to the overall validity of the cluster or sequence been determined?
7. Have the tactics for carrying out the test been described in sufficient detail to permit their exact replication?
8. Has the utility of the test been determined?

ical training (to the extent that trainees are too often taught *what* to think and do, rather than *how* to think and *why* to do) and presents the conscientious clinician with a huge task: the critical appraisal of the usefulness of each clinical measurement that we make. This task becomes all the greater when we recognize the rate at which new diagnostic tests and whole new diagnostic technologies are presented to us.

What, then, is the busy clinician to do? Two things, and this book will try to help with both of them. First, the final section on keeping up will help the busy clinician become more efficient at finding, sifting, assessing, storing, and learning relevant clinical information. Second, this chapter will help the busy clinician learn how to decide which diagnostic data are worth pursuing.

This latter decision can be made in two ways. First, the busy clinician can leave the critical appraisal to "the experts" and simply seek out or avoid diagnostic data on the basis of the recommendations of others. We all do this when faced with what is (for us) a rare presenting problem, and this certainly makes sense. To track down and critically appraise the diagnostic options for an illness we encounter only twice a decade is a waste of our time, and it is sensible to indiscriminately mime the diagnostic actions of respected colleagues who encounter such illnesses twice a week. But what about the illnesses *we* encounter twice a week? This chapter is written to help busy clinicians critically appraise the diagnostic options in such illnesses (both those options available today and those that will become available in the future).

Such a critical appraisal should be triggered every time we are told that a given piece of clinical data is really useful in diagnosing (or ruling out) a disorder that we commonly encounter (or at least consider) in our clinical practice. The clinical data at issue could be a symptom or other element of the patient's history, a physical sign, or a laboratory test, and we could be told about its importance by a teacher, a colleague, a consultant, a diagnostic laboratory, a textbook, a clinical journal, or a visiting fireman.

Critical appraisal begins with getting our hands on evidence about the usefulness of the clinical sign, symptom, or other diagnostic test. Although such evidence is sometimes presented in a textbook or clinical article, it often is merely summarized or interpreted at a continuing education session or in conversations with colleagues, consultants, and those who operate diagnostic laboratories. Because we must examine the actual evidence in order to decide whether the claims of diagnostic usefulness are justified, we must not hesitate to ask these advocates to give it to us (or at least tell us where to find it).

In deciding whether a given sign, symptom, lab test, image, or other information is useful, clinicians can assess the available evidence by using the eight guides listed in Table 3-1, which are derived from a number of sources [4, 10, 12, 20, 25, 27, 29].

Has There Been an Independent "Blind" Comparison with a "Gold Standard" of Diagnosis?

Patients shown (by application of an accepted reference test or "gold standard" of diagnosis such as a biopsy) to have the target disorder of interest, plus a second group of patients shown (by application of this same gold standard) not to have the target disorder, should have undergone the specific interview, physical examination, or other diagnostic test, and had it interpreted by clinicians who did not know (that is, they were "blind" to) whether a given patient really had the disorder. Afterward, these diagnostic test results should have been compared with the gold standard.

The strategies and tactics for this comparison are covered in detail in the next chapter. In brief, they run as follows: First, the gold standard refers to a definitive diagnosis attained by biopsy, surgery, autopsy, long-term follow-up, or other acknowledged standard. If you cannot accept the gold standard (within reason, that is—nothing is perfect!), then you should question whether the diagnostic data are worth capturing.*

What if there is no gold standard in the traditional sense? For example, we have no definitive (as yet) biopsy or laboratory test for AIDS (as opposed to infection with the HIV virus), and there is no gold standard for disorders such as asthma. What should we look for then? One approach is to select one or more logical consequences of the target disorder and make these the gold standard. Thus, the methacholine challenge test [23] is advocated as a good diagnostic test for asthma because patients who react to inhaled methacholine also manifest the logical consequences of asthma: impaired peak flow measurements, worsening following the inhalation of cold air, and improving following inhaled steroids and beta agonists. These logical consequences often are called *constructs* by researchers who study diagnostic tests, and you may see this approach referred to as construct validity.

*Of course, the gold standard must not include the diagnostic test result as one of its components, for the resulting "incorporation bias" invalidates the comparison [27].

Another way to decide whether a diagnostic test is worthwhile when there is no gold standard is simply to ask whether patients are better off as a result of undergoing it. Indeed, you very well might want to ask this question about any diagnostic test, regardless of whether there was a gold standard or not. We agree, and will be discussing this in this chapter, under the heading "Has the Utility of the Test Been Determined?"

If you do accept the gold standard, then consider the diagnostic test: Does it have something to offer that the gold standard does not? For example, is it less risky, less uncomfortable or embarrassing for the patient, less costly, or applicable earlier in the course of the illness? Diagnostic data obtained from the clinical history or physical examination are especially important in this regard, for they are immediately available. Again, if the proposed diagnostic test offers no theoretical advantage over the gold standard, why read further?

If you have stuck with the diagnostic test through all of the preceding discussion, you should then compare the test results with the gold standard and form a judgment about the overall validity of the diagnostic test, using whichever of the approaches (yellow, green, blue, brown, or black belt) from the next chapter that you prefer. If the rule-in and rule-out levels, predictive values, likelihood ratios, and the like look promising, you can proceed further. If, on the other hand, the new test is no better than existing ones, it would have to be safer, easier, quicker, less painful or embarrassing, or less expensive for you to decide to use it. Using a new diagnostic test just because it is new is flashy but dumb.

Suppose that you already know that your patient has coronary heart disease, but want to determine the extent of his left ventricular dysfunction. When you cannot or do not want to have the patient undergo the gold standard (in this case, at least an echocardiogram and maybe even a ventriculogram), you must look for a quicker, easier measure of disease severity.

When a diagnostic test is used to determine the degree of severity of a disease or illness (rather than just its presence or absence), the comparison with the gold standard can become very complex. In terms of what you will encounter in the next chapter, such comparisons usually invoke at least the brown belt (e.g., multilevel likelihood ratios), and often the black belt (e.g., correlation coefficients or even multiple regression). Although you can learn how to carry out many of these calculations in Chapter 4, in Chapter 3 we are supposed to help you interpret calculations already carried out by others, so we had better introduce some of them here. The example to be used is from the clinical examination, rather than the clinical laboratory, because the same principles apply in both situations.

Consider the clinical examination of neck veins as a diagnostic test for the severity of raised central venous pressure. As you may recall from Chapter 2, Deborah Cook arranged for fifty critically ill patients to undergo three estimates of their jugular venous pressure within the space of an hour (one by a clinical clerk, one by a medical resident, and one by the attending physician), all of whom were blind to the simultaneous, gold standard measurement of central venous pressure obtained from an indwelling central venous catheter [3]. In reading about the ability of this clinical examination to describe the severity of these patients' hemodynamic derangement, what calculations might you encounter?

The simplest would be a description of how well the clinical examination identified low (say, 5 cm or less) or high (say, 10 cm or more) central venous pressure (CVP). The sensitivity* for the former was 82% to 100% (that is, when the CVP was truly low by catheter, the clinical examination would detect that fact 82% to 100% of the time), but for the latter only 30% to 60% (with specificities [the proportions of those without the abnormal pressures who were correctly labeled by the examiners] for both of about 80%), telling us that the exam is better at identifying patients with truly low rather than truly high central venous pressures. But both these clinicians' estimates of central venous pressure and the gold standard itself ranged all the way from 1 cm to 20 cm, and the simple analyses, in which both the clinical exam (diagnostic test) and the gold standard are classified as above or below a single cut-point, do not tell us as much as we want to know about gauging the severity of the derangement. What other measures might we encounter?

We will briefly describe two other measures that readers might encounter, with the suggestion that you consult your favorite statistics book if you want to understand them more thoroughly. First, you might find that the authors had developed several (rather than just two) categories of severity. In our example, Deborah Cook employed not one, but two cut-points for both the examiner's opinion and the central line, creating three levels of central venous pressure for each: low (5 cm or less), medium (6 cm–9 cm), and high (10 cm or more). It then became possible for her to show how well the clinicians' estimates of low, medium, and high pressure agreed with the central line, using the kappa statistic we met in the previous chapter [9]. As you recall, kappa tells us the degree of agreement that has occurred (in this case, between the clinical exam and the central line) over and above that which would have occurred by chance alone. Although usually employed as a measure of precision, when the comparison is between a diagnostic test and a gold standard kappa becomes a measure of accuracy. And as shown in the last chapter, a weighted kappa can take into account the degree of disagreement, generating a higher score when disagreements are close than when they are far apart. In our example, the medical students' readings (of low, normal, or high pressure) showed the best agreement with the central line (.73) and the attending physicians' readings the worst (.54)!

A second measure that you might encounter in your reading displays the correlation between the actual numbers generated by the diagnostic test and the gold standard, treating them as continuous variables rather than as two or more broad categories. A common description of this sort is the correlation coefficient (often called the *Pearson correlation coefficient*). Correlation coefficients express the extent to which, when the diagnostic test result goes up, the gold standard goes

*Don't panic! If you do not understand these brief definitions of *sensitivity* and *specificity*, they will be explained in detail in the "green belt" section of the next chapter.

up as well (and vice versa).* When this relation is strong, the correlation coefficient, like kappa, approaches +1.0; when this relation is weak, the correlation coefficient falls toward .0; and when the diagnostic test and the gold standard results go in opposite directions (that is, the higher the diagnostic test result, the lower the gold standard result), the correlation coefficient becomes negative and approaches −1.0. In our example, the Pearson correlation coefficients between clinicians' reports and the central line are +.74 for the medical students, +.71 for the residents, and +.65 for the attending physicians. Are these correlation coefficients high? Well, at least they are positive! Another way of answering this question is to consider the extent to which the different values obtained from the central line (in statistical terms, the variation in central line readings) have been detected (in statistical terms, explained) by the clinical exam. This is done by squaring the correlation coefficient, and in our example we find that 55% ($.74^2$), 50% ($.71^2$), and 42% ($.65^2$) of the variation in the central line results can, indeed, be explained by the clinical exam. Such r^2 values greater than 50% are respectable, and when artificially ventilated patients (in whom the examination is more difficult) were excluded, they rose as high as 81%.

One of the shortcomings of the Pearson correlation coefficient is that it cannot detect situations in which one set of readings is *systematically* lower or higher than the other. Thus, if my clinical estimates of central venous pressure were always 5 cm lower than the true readings provided by the central line, the Pearson correlation coefficient for my agreement would be as high as that of a less experienced colleague whose clinical estimates were bang on. A way of overcoming this shortcoming that you may encounter in your reading is the "intraclass correlation coefficient." It penalizes *systematic* errors in the diagnostic test result and would, quite appropriately, assign me a lower score than my younger, unbiased colleague.† Moreover, it can be interpreted (as slight to almost perfect) just like a kappa.

Other, fancier methods of comparing severity tests with their corresponding gold standards exist, but since they share the correlation coefficient's intent of expressing the extent to which the test results agree with the gold standard, they will not be discussed here.

Having checked and found an appropriate comparison with a gold standard (for either the target disorder or its severity), what about the element of "blindness"? This simply means that those who are carrying out or interpreting the diagnostic test should not know whether the patient being tested really does or does not have the target disorder of interest; that is, they should be "blind" to each patient's true disease status. Similarly, those who are applying the gold standard should not know the diagnostic test result from any patient. It is only

*A nice additional property of the Pearson correlation coefficient is that the two sets of results need not be in the same units of measure; that is, one could use it to compare changes in length (e.g., liver height in the right midclavicular line) with changes in area or volume (e.g., on a liver scan).

†We hope it is intuitively clear to you that the two sets of results *do* need to be in the same units of measure for the intraclass correlation coefficient to be employed.

when the diagnostic test and gold standard are applied in a blind fashion that we can be assured that conscious or unconscious bias (in this case the "diagnostic suspicion" bias) has been avoided. As you may recall, this bias was discussed in the previous chapter on the clinical examination.

The foregoing discussion applies exactly as presented when a sign, symptom, or other diagnostic test is used to diagnose the cause of a patient's illness, the severity of that illness, and the patient's response to therapy. When used to predict the patient's subsequent clinical course and prognosis or the patient's likely responsiveness to therapy, however, the clinician considering the usefulness of such diagnostic data also should be guided by the rules of evidence that apply to making prognoses, and these are given in Chapter 6.

Has the Diagnostic Test Been Evaluated in a Patient Sample That Included an Appropriate Spectrum of Mild and Severe, Treated and Untreated, Disease, Plus Individuals with Different but Commonly Confused Disorders?

Florid disease (such as long-standing rheumatoid arthritis) usually presents a much smaller diagnostic challenge than the same disease in an early or mild form, and the real value of a clinical sign, symptom, or other diagnostic test often lies in its discriminating value in equivocal cases. Moreover, the apparent diagnostic value of some tests actually resides in their ability to detect the manifestations of therapy (such as radiopaque deposits in the buttocks of ancient syphilitics), rather than those of the target disorder, and the potential user must be satisfied that the two are not being confused.

Finally, just as a duck is not often confused with a yak, even in the absence of chromosomal analyses, the ability of a diagnostic test to distinguish between disorders not commonly confused with one another in the first place is scant endorsement for its widespread application. The key value of a diagnostic test often lies in its ability to distinguish among otherwise commonly confused disorders, especially when their prognoses or therapies differ sharply. It is this discriminating property that makes the TSH family of determinations so helpful in sorting out tense, anxious, tremulous, perspiring patients into those with abnormal thyroid function and those with other disorders.

Was the Setting for This Evaluation, as Well as the Filter Through Which Study Patients Passed, Adequately Described?

The proportion of hypertensives with surgically curable lesions varies almost tenfold, depending on whether the same diagnostic tests are applied to hypertensives in a general practice or in a tertiary care center. Because a test's predictive value changes with the prevalence of the target disorder, the article or other evidence advocating the test ought to tell you enough about the study site and patient selection filter to permit you to calculate the diagnostic test's likely predictive value among patients in your own practice.

The selection of control subjects who do not have the target disorder of interest should be described as well. Although laboratory technicians and janitors may be appropriate control subjects early in the development of a new diagnostic test (especially with the declining use of medical students as laboratory animals), the definitive comparison with a gold standard demands equal care in the selection of patients with and without the target disorder. The clinician who contemplates using the diagnostic test deserves some assurance that differences in the test's results are due to a mechanism of disease and not simply to differences in the general health, diet, mobility, age, sex, and so on of case and control subjects.

Has the Reproducibility of the Test Result (Precision) and Its Interpretation (Observer Variation) Been Determined?

As you learned in Chapter 2 on clinical diagnosis, the validity of a diagnostic test demands both the absence of systematic deviation from the truth (that is, the absence of bias) and the presence of precision (the same test applied to the same, unchanged patient must produce the same result). The description of a diagnostic test ought to tell potential users how well they can expect the test results to be reproducible. This is especially true when expertise is required in performing the test (for example, ultrasound exhibits enormous variation in the quality of its results when performed by different operators) or in interpreting it (as you may recall from Chapter 2, observer variation is a major problem for tests involving x rays, electrocardiography, and the like).

Has the Term *Normal* Been Defined Sensibly as It Applies to This Test?

If the article or other source uses the word "normal," its authors should tell you what they mean by it. Moreover, you should satisfy yourself that their definition is clinically sensible. Several different definitions of normal are used in clinical medicine, and we would contend that several of them produce more harm than good. We have listed six definitions of normal in Table 3-2 and acknowledge our debt to Tony Murphy for pointing out most of them [24, 25].

Perhaps the most common definition of normal assumes that the diagnostic test results (or some arithmetic manipulation of them) for everyone, or for a group of presumably normal people, or for a carefully characterized "reference" population, will fit a specific theoretical distribution known as the *normal* or *Gaussian* distribution. One of the nice properties of this Gaussian distribution is that, by definition, its mean plus- or minus-two standard deviations encloses 95% of its contents, leaving 2.5% at each of its upper and lower ends. For this reason, the "mean plus- or minus-two standard deviations" became a tempting way to define the normal several years ago, and came into general use.

It is too bad that it did, for three logical consequences of its use have led to enormous confusion and the creation of a new field of medicine: the diagnosis of nondisease [21]. First, diagnostic test results simply do not fit the Gaussian

Table 3-2. Six definitions of normal in common clinical use

Property	Term	Consequences of its clinical application
The distribution of diagnostic test results has a certain shape	Gaussian	Ought to occasionally obtain minus values for hemoglobin, etc.
Lies within a preset percentile of previous diagnostic test results	Percentile	All diseases have the same prevalence. Patients are normal only until they are worked up
Carries no additional risk of morbidity or mortality	Risk factor	Assumes that altering a risk factor alters risk
Socially or politically aspired to	Culturally desirable	Confusion over the role of medicine in society
Range of test results beyond which a specific disease is, with known probability, present or absent	Diagnostic	Need to know predictive values that apply in your practice
Range of test results beyond which therapy does more good than harm	Therapeutic	Need to keep up with new knowledge about therapy

distribution (actually, we should be grateful that they do not; the Gaussian distribution extends to infinity in both directions, necessitating occasional patients with impossibly high hemoglobins and others on the minus side of zero!). Second, if the highest and lowest 2.5% of diagnostic test results are called abnormal, then all diseases have the same frequency, a conclusion that is also clinically nonsensical.

The third harmful consequence of the use of the Gaussian definition of normal is shared by its more recent replacement, the *percentile*. Recognizing the failure of diagnostic test results to fit a theoretical distribution such as the Gaussian, some laboratorians have suggested that we ignore the shape of the distribution and simply refer (for example) to the lower (or upper) 95% of test results as normal. Although this percentile definition does avoid the problems of infinite and negative test values, it still leads to the conclusion that all diseases are of equal prevalence and still contributes to the "upper-limit syndrome" of nondisease because its use means that the only "normal" patients are the ones who are not yet sufficiently worked up [25].

This inevitable consequence arises as follows: If the normal range for a given diagnostic test is defined as including the lower 95% of diagnostic test results, then the probability that a given patient will be called "normal" when subjected to this test is 95% or .95. If this same patient undergoes two independent diagnostic tests (independent in the sense that they are probing totally different organs or functions), the likelihood of this patient being called normal is now (.95) × (.95) = .90. So the likelihood of any patient being called normal is .95 raised to the power of the number of independent diagnostic tests performed on him. Thus, a patient who undergoes 20 tests has only .95 to the 20th power, or about one chance in three, of being called normal; a patient undergoing 100 such tests has only about six chances in one thousand of being called normal at the end of the workup.*

Other definitions of normal, in avoiding the foregoing pitfalls, present other problems. The *risk factor* approach is based on studies of precursors or statistical predictors of subsequent clinical events; by this definition, the normal range for serum cholesterol or blood pressure consists of those levels that carry no additional risk of morbidity or mortality. Unfortunately, however, many of these risk factors exhibit steady increases in risk throughout their range of values; indeed, before the current controversy about whether extremely low cholesterol levels constitute risk factors for cancer, it was suggested that the "normal" serum cholesterol (defined by cardiovascular risk) might lie below 3.9 mmol/L (150 mg%) [16]. Another shortcoming of this risk factor definition becomes apparent when we examine the consequences of acting upon a test result that lies beyond the normal range: Will altering a risk factor really change risk? For example, although obesity is a risk factor for hypertension, controversy continues over whether weight reduction improves mild hypertension. One of us led a randomized trial in which we peeled 4.1 kilograms (on average) from obese, mildly hypertensive women with a behaviorally-oriented weight reduction program (control women lost less than one kilogram) [13]. Despite both their and our efforts (the cost of the experimental group's behaviorally-oriented weight reduction program came to $50 per kilo), there was no accompanying decline in blood pressure.

A related approach defines the normal as that which is *culturally desirable,* providing an opportunity for what H. L. Mencken called "the corruption of medicine by morality" through the "confusion of the theory of the healthy with the theory of the virtuous" [22]. One sees such definitions in their benign form at the fringes of the current life-style movement (e.g., "It is better to be slim than fat," and "Exercise and fitness are better than sedentary living and lack of fitness.") [18] and in its malignant form in the health care system of the Third Reich. Such a definition has the potential for considerable harm and also may serve to subvert the role of medicine in society.†

Two final definitions are of high relevance and utility to the clinician because they focus directly on the clinical acts of diagnosis and therapy. The *diagnostic* definition identifies a range of diagnostic test results beyond which a specific

*This consequence of such definitions helps explain the results of the previously noted (Chap. 1, p. 14) randomized trial of hospital admission multitest screening that found no patient benefits, but increased health care costs, when such screening was carried out [7].

†Mencken offered a similarly pungent point of view on the latter: "The true aim of medicine is not to make men virtuous; it is to safeguard and rescue them from the consequences of their vices" [22].

target disorder is (with known probability) present. It is this definition that is used in the first guide to critically appraising a diagnostic test: comparison with a gold standard. The "known probability" with which a target disorder is present is known formally as the positive predictive value (and you will meet it in the next chapter under both this name and its aliases, the posterior probability or posttest likelihood of disease following a positive test). This diagnostic definition is the one we shall emphasize here and in the next chapter, where we will show you that the known probability of a target disorder being present or absent depends on where we set the limits for the normal range of diagnostic test results. This definition has real clinical value and is a distinct improvement over the definitions described above. It does require, however, that clinicians keep track of diagnostic ranges and cutoffs.

The final definition of normal sets its limits at the point beyond which specific treatments have been shown conclusively to do more good than harm. This *therapeutic* definition is attractive because of its link to action. The therapeutic definition of the normal range of blood pressure, for example, avoids the hazards of labeling patients as diseased unless they are going to be treated. Thus, in the early 1960s the only levels of blood pressure conclusively shown to benefit from antihypertensive drugs were those in excess of 130 mm Hg (phase V). Then, in 1967, the first of a series of United States Veterans Administration randomized trials demonstrated the clear advantages of initiating drugs at 115 mm Hg, and the upper limit of normal blood pressure, under the therapeutic definition, fell to that level [33]. In 1970, the upper limit for normal blood pressure was lowered to 105 mm Hg with the publication and acceptance of the second Veterans Administration trial report [34] and the debate on whether the upper limit for this therapeutic definition should be lowered to 90 mm Hg that was underway as the first edition of this book went to press [1, 15, 26, 32] still rages as we publish the second edition. Obviously, the use of this therapeutic definition requires that clinicians keep abreast of advances in therapeutics and helps to integrate all three sections of this book.

When appraising evidence about the usefulness of a (new) diagnostic test, then, you should satisfy yourself that the authors have defined what they mean by normal and that they have done so in a sensible and clinically useful fashion.

If the Test Is Advocated as Part of a Cluster or Sequence of Tests, Has Its Individual Contribution to the Overall Validity of the Cluster or Sequence Been Determined?

In many conditions, an individual diagnostic test examines but one of several manifestations of the underlying disorder. For example, in diagnosing deep vein thrombosis the impedance plethysmograph examines impaired venous emptying whereas the ^{125}I-fibrinogen leg scan examines the turnover of coagulation factors at the site of thrombosis [14]. Furthermore, plethysmography is much more sensitive for proximal than for distal venous thrombosis, whereas the reverse is true for leg scanning. As a result, these tests are best applied in sequence: If impedance plethysmography is positive, the diagnosis is made and treatment begins at once; if the plethysmography is negative, leg scanning begins and the diagnostic and treatment decision awaits its results.*

This being so, it is clinically nonsensical to base a judgment of the value of leg scanning on a simple comparison of its results, all alone, against the gold standard of venography. Rather its agreement with venography among suitably symptomatic patients with negative impedance plethysmography is one appropriate assessment of its validity and clinical usefulness. Another valid assessment would compare the combination of leg scanning and impedance plethysmography with the gold standard of venography.

In summary, any single component of a cluster of diagnostic tests should be evaluated in the context of its clinical use.

Have the Tactics for Carrying Out the Test Been Described in Sufficient Detail to Permit Their Exact Replication?

If the proponents of a diagnostic test have concluded that you should use their test, they have to tell you how to do it, and this description should cover patient issues as well as the mechanics of performing and interpreting the test. Are there special requirements for fluids, diet, or physical activity? What concomitant drugs should be avoided? How painful is the procedure and what is done to relieve this? What precautions should be taken during and after the test? How should the specimen be transported and stored for later analysis? These tactics and precautions must be described if you and your patients are to benefit from (and not be needlessly harmed by) this diagnostic test.

Has the Utility of the Test Been Determined?

The ultimate criterion for a diagnostic test or any other clinical maneuver is whether the patient is better off for it. Is a treatable disorder identified? Is the need for still further investigation reduced? Do patient and clinician benefit from the reduction of uncertainty?

In this regard, a diagnostic test can be thought of as a technology that ideally involves a sequence of development and testing, beginning with establishing its technical capability (that is, its ability to perform to specification in a highly controlled laboratory setting). If the test succeeds there, it proceeds to considerations of the range of its possible uses, followed by the determination of its diagnostic accuracy for each. This major phase of test development deserves the attention it receives in this chapter for it serves as the basis for the test's clinical application, described in Chapter 4.

But there are other issues to consider. As our growing concerns for costs and benefits are matched by our growing abilities to study them, we are now begin-

*The sensibility of this sequence is independent of the fact that plethysmography can be interpreted at once, whereas ^{125}I-fibrinogen leg scanning requires an initial wait for incorporation of the isotope into the active clot.

ning to see reports of the effect of introducing a new diagnostic test on clinicians, on management decisions, and even on patient outcomes. These reports sometimes confirm and extend our individual observations that the accuracy of a diagnostic test is no guarantee of its clinical usefulness.* Even if accurate, a test result may fail to change the probabilities for competing diagnoses sufficiently to alter our treatment plan or, if it does, induce a reluctant patient to accept the change. And if there is no effective treatment available, the harmful effects of knowing the diagnosis may exceed those of the ignorance (of diagnosis or prognosis) that preceded the test, especially, as shown in Chapter 5, if the test achieves the early diagnosis of symptomless, untreatable disease. Even when false-negative and false-positive test results are rare, they can devastate; consider the consequences of a false-negative mammogram for a treatable breast cancer, or a false-positive serology for HIV. Finally, the test procedure itself, especially if provocative or invasive, will occasionally go awry and harm individual patients more than it helps them. These adverse consequences may more than outweigh any positive contribution to health status resulting from what is otherwise an accurate test.

On the other hand, there may be good reasons to perform accurate diagnostic tests that influence neither therapy nor even mortality. For example, we often order tests that can only marginally reduce uncertainty in the hope that they will reduce the anxiety of our patients (and ourselves!). Harold Sox [30] and his colleagues randomized half of a group of patients presenting with apparently noncardiac chest pain to undergo creatine phosphokinase determinations and electrocardiograms, and found that they showed less short-term disability than control patients who did not have these studies. That this reassurance can extend to patients' families was shown by Taylor [31] and his colleagues when they randomized the wives of men undergoing exercise tests following myocardial infarctions either to sit in the waiting room, to watch the test, or to climb on the treadmill and work at their husbands' peak exercise level for three minutes. As their involvement increased, experimental wives not only wound up progressively more confident in their husband's physical and cardiac capabilities than the control wives who sat in the waiting room, but also were better at predicting how their spouses would perform in repeat exercise tests up to six months later.

Of course, anxiety reduction may be no greater following the performance of negative diagnostic tests than it would be following other, easier interventions. For example, Richard Deyo randomized patients with innocent-appearing back pain to receive immediate x rays or an informative chat with a nonclinician about low back pain and the benefits versus risks of back x rays (with roentgenograms only if they failed to improve) [5]. Those undergoing immediate x rays wound up no less symptomatic or more satisfied than those in the "education" group. A final, less benign reason for ordering diagnostic tests that make patients no better off is when their performance makes the clinician better off (in money or

*In this regard, we think it is a shame that the term *diagnostic efficacy* has crept into the literature, especially since it is used as a synonym for accuracy rather than utility.

prestige), a practice Relman [28] has labelled an "entrepreneurial fever" among physicians. This fever may explain why, for example, nonradiologists with their own x-ray machines use diagnostic x rays on almost twice as many patients as nonradiologists who must send their patients elsewhere to have these studies done [2].

From the foregoing, you can see why you need to know whether a diagnostic test improves the lot of patients who undergo it. But what sort of evidence should you seek on this issue? A useful diagnostic test does three things: It provides an accurate diagnosis, supports the application of a specific efficacious treatment, and ultimately leads to a better clinical outcome for the patient. Although evidence on the latter is the most powerful, it is also the most difficult to find, and you will usually find only information on how accurate the test is and how it influences management.

Are these substitutes of accuracy and management ever sufficient as surrogates for clinical outcomes? We would suggest that they are, but only under special circumstances. If, for example, a new diagnostic test is shown to be more accurate (or equally accurate, but safer or cheaper) than an established test for a diagnosis well known to trigger treatment with a regimen known (through evidence from the randomized therapeutic trials you will learn how to assess in Chapter 7) to improve clinical outcomes for patients, then it is safe to play the "substitution game" and accept accuracy information as a valid substitute for outcomes. When looking at this evidence, one would be wise to consider the possibility that the diagnostic test identified a different spectrum of disease with different responsiveness to treatment. For instance, leg scanning is an adequate alternative to venography for deep vein thrombosis below the knee, but clots restricted to this area do not require anticoagulation.

Even better than information on accuracy alone would be evidence on the next step, showing that the new test led to the initiation of appropriate therapy. How might this evidence be presented to you? In its simplest form, it might be a report simply reviewing patient records and judging whether the diagnostic test altered patient management. This sort of evidence is deservedly unconvincing, for it can only guess at what would have been done if the test had not been available.

More convincing would be a report that asked physicians about their management plans both before and after the new test was performed, documenting any changes in these plans that could be attributed to the new test. For example, Eisenberg and colleagues [8] investigated residents who were looking after critically ill patients about to undergo right heart catheterizations in an intensive care unit. The residents were asked both to predict the result of this diagnostic study and to state how they would manage the patient if it were not performed. When these predictions and statements were compared with subsequent clinical notes, it was discovered that the former were seldom accurate and that subsequent therapy differed from that planned before the catheterization in 58% of patients.

However, even these "before-after" studies are necessarily artificial ("What would you do before I give you the information I'm going to give you?"), and you may want to continue your search for better evidence on the utility of a diagnostic test. The best evidence you could find would be a randomized trial in which patients were randomly allocated to alternative diagnostic plans, only one of which included the diagnostic test of interest. Thus, routine practice might be compared to the routine plus the new, as in two randomized trials of fetal heart monitoring in which low-risk women in labor were randomized to receive, or not receive, the addition of continuous fetal heart-rate monitoring to detect fetal distress [17, 35]. Neither trial demonstrated benefit either to mother or fetus, and both suggested that mothers of monitored babies underwent more interventions.

Alternatively, you may find a randomized trial in which a new test is evaluated as a possible replacement for an existing test, as when a fetal biophysical profile derived from dynamic ultrasound was compared with that resulting from conventional nonstress tests in another group of pregnant women [19]. Expectant mothers were randomized to receive just one of these two procedures, and the results were reported to their physicians in a fashion that blinded them to which test had been performed. This trial found no differences in neonatal outcomes, although the additional ability of ultrasound to detect fetal anomalies was seen as a potential advantage. Our own group is currently conducting a randomized trial which compares mediastinoscopy with computed tomography as diagnostic tests for mediastinal spread in patients with potentially operable carcinoma of the lung in order to determine which approach reduces needless thoracotomy. As discussed in Chapter 5, this rigorous sort of evidence is increasingly demanded when the decision is being made whether to seek the early diagnosis of asymptomatic diseases like cancer. In their full form, these reports include information on the clinical outcomes of patients.

Is it necessary to be this demanding about evidence on a diagnostic test's utility? We think that it is, based on what has been found in such studies. For example, when patients with acute upper gastrointestinal bleeding were randomized to receive upper gastrointestinal endoscopy or barium radiography, the diagnostic yield of the endoscopy was clearly higher, confirming "conventional wisdom" about its superiority [6]. There were, however, identical rates of operation following these alternate diagnostic tests (18.1% in the endoscopy group and 18.2% in the radiography group) and deaths were actually higher (though not statistically significantly so) following endoscopy (8.4% vs. 7.6%, respectively), provoking continuing debate on the utility (as opposed to mere accuracy) of endoscopy in upper g-i bleeding. And another report showed that although determining radionuclide ejection fractions after myocardial infarction clearly provided additional information about cardiac function, it did not change management or reduce the subsequent incidence of heart failure [11]. Given the discomfort and risk of diagnostic procedures, to say nothing of the way that they compete for scarce resources, we think that you are justified in demanding evidence that they improve patient outcomes before they become widely disseminated.

The following guides may help you interpret reports of trials of the utility of diagnostic tests. First, you should be satisfied that the appropriate role of the new diagnostic test was what was studied. If its potential usefulness is as an addition to conventional testing, experimental patients should have received both the conventional and new tests (and control patients only the conventional). If, on the other hand, the new test is proposed to replace an existing method, experimental patients should have received only the new test (and control patients only the conventional).

Second, all clinically relevant outcomes of undergoing the diagnostic test should be reported. For example, when the execution of a test requires a delay in the initiation of definitive therapy (while the procedure is being rescheduled, the test is incubating, or the slides are waiting to be read) the consequences of this delay should be described. Outcomes of particular relevance in trials of diagnostic tests include complications from more invasive procedures and especially their psychologic impacts (e.g., the reassurance value of negative test results) on both patients and clinicians. These psychologic impacts are often subtle and complex, as well as very important, and can be profoundly influenced by the manner in which test results are presented to patients (often as a consequence of their reassurance value for the clinician).

Third, the patients included in such studies of diagnostic technology must be appropriate. For example, their probability of having the target disorder should neither be so likely that the test is unnecessary, nor so unlikely that even an excellent test could never show its usefulness. Fourth, you should satisfy yourself that statistically significant results are also clinically important, and that statistically nonsignificant results are not simply the inevitable consequences of either enrolling patients in whom the test could not influence therapy or outcome, or of enrolling too few patients to detect an important difference if it did occur. Fifth, you should consider whether the diagnostic test, if useful, is feasible in your practice. Finally, as with any other report, you should be satisfied that all patients who entered the study were accounted for at its conclusion.

By applying the preceding guides you should be able to decide whether or not a sign, symptom, or other diagnostic test will be useful in your practice, or whether it still has not been evaluated properly. Depending on the context in which you are considering the test, one or another of the eight general guides will be the most important one and you can go right to it. If it has been met in a credible way, you can go on to apply the others; if the most important guide has not been met, you can discard that evidence and go on to other more pertinent evidence. In this way, you can improve the efficiency with which you use your scarce study time.

When trying to pick the most useful of an array of competing signs, symptoms, and other diagnostic tests for the same target disorder, these guides provide you with a basis for comparing them with each other. On the basis of this comparison, you can pick the one or the few that will best meet your clinical requirements, and can spare yourself, your patient, and those who ultimately foot the bill from the execution of needless procedures.

The eight guides we have presented here also constitute fair questions to ask anybody who is advocating the pursuit of specific signs, symptoms, or other data in an effort to diagnose a given illness. The application of these guides will permit you to generate a "short list" of useful diagnostic data to seek for the illnesses you encounter. These guides should also help you decide when and whether to replace or supplement your current diagnostic pursuits with new ones.

Having decided which signs, symptoms, and other diagnostic data to pursue, how should you interpret the results of this pursuit? That is what the next chapter is all about.

References

1. Australian National Blood Pressure Study Management Committee. The Australian therapeutic trial in mild hypertension. *Lancet* 1: 1261, 1980.
2. Childs, A, and Hunter, E. Non-medical factors influencing use of diagnostic x-ray by physicians. *Med. Care* 10: 323, 1972.
3. Cook, D. J. Clinical assessment of central venous pressure in the critically ill. *Amer. J. Med. Sci.* 299: 175, 1990.
4. Department of Clinical Epidemiology and Biostatistics, McMaster University, Hamilton, Ontario. How to read clinical journals: II. To learn about a diagnostic test. *Can. Med. Assoc. J.* 124: 703, 1981.
5. Deyo, R. A., Diehl, A. K., and Rosenthal, M. Reducing roentgenography use. Can patient expectations be altered? *Arch. Intern. Med.* 147: 141, 1987.
6. Dronfield, M. W., Langman, M. J. S., Atkinson, M., et al. Outcome of endoscopy and barium radiography for acute upper gastrointestinal bleeding: Controlled trial in 1037 patients. *Br. Med. J.* 284: 545, 1982.
7. Durbridge, T. C., Edwards, F., Edwards, R. G., and Atkinson, M. An evaluation of multiphasic screening on admission to hospital. Précis of a report to the National Health and Medical Research Council. *Med. J. Aust.* 1: 703, 1976.
8. Eisenberg, P. R., Jaffe, A. S., and Schuster, D. P. Clinical evaluation compared to pulmonary artery catheterization in the hemodynamic assessment of critically ill patients. *Crit. Care Med.* 12: 549, 1984.
9. Fleiss, J. L. *Statistical Methods for Rates and Proportions* (2nd ed). New York: Wiley, 1981. P. 217.
10. Galen, R. S., and Gambino, S. R. *Beyond Normality: The Predictive Value and Efficiency of Medical Diagnoses.* New York: Wiley, 1975.
11. Gjorup, T., Kelbaek, H., Vestergaard, B., et al. Prospective, randomised, double-blind study of radionuclide determination of left-ventricular ejection fraction in acute myocardial infarction. *Lancet* 1: 583, 1986.
12. Griner, P. F., Mayewski, R. J., Mushlin, A. I., and Greenland, P. Selection and interpretation of diagnostic tests and procedures: Principles and application. *Ann. Intern. Med.* 94 (Part 2): 553, 1981.
13. Haynes, R. B., Harper, A. C., Costley, S. R., et al. Failure of weight reduction to reduce mildly elevated blood pressure: A randomized trial. *J Hypertension* 2: 535, 1984.
14. Hull, R., Hirsh, J., Sackett, D. L., et al. Combined use of leg scanning and impedance plethysmography in suspected venous thrombosis. An alternative to venography. *N. Engl. J. Med.* 296: 1497, 1977.
15. Hypertension Detection and Followup Cooperative Group. Five-year findings of the Hypertension Detection and Followup Program: I. Reduction in mortality of persons with high blood pressure including mild hypertension. *J.A.M.A.* 242: 2562, 1979.
16. Kannel, W. B., Dawber, T. R., Glennon, W. E., and Thorne, M. C. Preliminary report: The determinants of clinical significance of serum cholesterol. *Mass. J. Med. Technol.* 4: 11, 1962.
17. Kelso, I. M., Parsons, R. J., Lawrence, G. F., et al. An assessment of continuous fetal heart rate monitoring in labor. *Amer. J. Obstetrics Gynecol.* 131: 526, 1978.

18. Lalonde, M. *A New Perspective on the Health of Canadians. A Working Document.* Ottawa: Government of Canada, 1974.
19. Manning, F. A., Lange, I. R., Morrison, I., and Harman, C. R. Fetal biophysical profile score and the nonstress test: a comparative trial. *Obstetrics Gynecol.* 64: 326, 1983.
20. McNeil, B. J., Varady, P. D., Burrows, B. A., and Adelstein, S. J. Measures of clinical efficacy: Cost-effectiveness calculations in the diagnosis and treatment of hypertensive renovascular disease. *N. Engl. J. Med.* 293: 211, 1975.
21. Meador, C. K. The art and science of nondisease. *N. Engl. J. Med.* 272: 92, 1965.
22. Mencken, H. L. *A Mencken Chrestomathy.* Westminster: Knopf, 1949.
23. Method for Diagnosis of Asthma. *Med. Lett. Drugs Ther.* 19: 60, 1987.
24. Murphy, E. A. The normal, and the perils of the sylleptic argument. *Perspect. Biol. Med.* 15: 566, 1972.
25. Murphy, E. A. *The Logic of Medicine.* Baltimore: Johns Hopkins, 1976.
26. Peart, W. S., and Miall, W. E. MRC working party on mild to moderate hypertension. MRC mild hypertension trial. *Lancet* (Letter) 1: 104, 1980.
27. Ransohoff, D. F., and Feinstein, A. R. Problems of spectrum and bias in evaluating the efficacy of diagnostic tests. *N. Engl. J. Med.* 299: 926, 1978.
28. Relman, A. R. Dealing with conflicts of interest. *N. Engl. J. Med.* 313: 749, 1985.
29. Sackett, D. L. Clinical diagnosis and the clinical laboratory. *Clin. Invest. Med.* 1: 37, 1978.
30. Sox, H. C. Jr., Margulies, I., and Sox, C.H. Psychologically mediated effects of diagnostic tests. *Ann. Intern. Med.* 95: 680, 1981.
31. Taylor, C. B., Bandura, A., Ewart, C. K, et al. Exercise testing to enhance wives' confidence in their husbands' cardiac capability soon after clinically uncomplicated acute myocardial infarction. *Am. J. Cardiol.* 55: 635, 1985.
32. United States Public Health Service Hospitals Cooperative Study Group. Smith, W. M. Treatment of mild hypertension: Results of a ten-year intervention trial. *Circ. Res.* 40 (Suppl.): 98, 1977.
33. Veterans Administration Cooperative Study Group. Effects of treatment on morbidity in hypertension: I. Results in patients with diastolic blood pressures averaging 115 through 129 mm Hg. *J.A.M.A.* 202: 1028, 1967.
34. Veterans Administration in Cooperative Study Group. Effects of treatment on morbidity in hypertension: II. Results in patients with diastolic blood pressures averaging 90 through 114 mm Hg. *J.A.M.A.* 213: 1143, 1970.
35. Wood, C., Renou, P., Oats, J., et al. A controlled trial of fetal heart rate monitoring in a low-risk obstetric population. *Amer. J. Obstetrics Gynecol.* 141: 527, 1981.

4

The Interpretation of Diagnostic Data

The two previous chapters focused on generating diagnostic hypotheses and capturing clinical data about them. This chapter will focus on strategies and tactics for interpreting diagnostic data, both the clinical data that come from the history and physical exam (where, as you should recall, the vast majority of diagnoses are confirmed) and the paraclinical data that come from the clinical chemistry lab, the x-ray department, the pathology service, and the other diagnostic laboratories.

The importance of clinical data deserves emphasis. Although most explanations of how to interpret diagnostic data confine themselves to laboratory reports, the same principles, strategies, and tactics apply equally to items of the clinical history and findings on the physical examination. Moreover, *symptoms and signs usually generate far more powerful tests of diagnostic hypotheses than we can ever derive from the clinical laboratory*. So, although we shall use a lab test, the determination of creatine kinase, as the recurring example for illustrating the different ways of interpreting diagnostic data that follow, we shall help you remember their wider applicability by including several examples from the history and physical examination as well. Furthermore, although we shall employ a "diagnostic" definition of normal throughout this chapter, these same strategies and tactics apply to the "therapeutic" definition as well. We may interpret the signs, symptoms, and test results of patients with clinically suspected deep vein thrombosis in terms of either the likelihood that they truly have deep vein thrombosis or the likelihood that they truly will benefit from anticoagulant therapy.

There has been a great deal written about the interpretation of diagnostic tests, and it is easy to drown in the associated graphs, tables, curves, formulas, and technical jargon. We have tried to remove the unessential, pedantic bits and have synthesized the rest into five bite-sized chunks, each of which is self-contained, digestible at a single sitting, and contains some features that can be put to good clinical use. The first chunk, for example, is a simple but powerful one that is done entirely with pictures and uses no math or new technical jargon. The later chunks become progessively complex and require you to learn some new terminology and use some math, finally needing a hand calculator. To help you keep track, we have also labeled these chunks with the hierarchy of belts that are awarded students of the martial arts:*

Chunk #1 Yellow Belt: Doing it with pictures
Chunk #2 Green Belt: Doing it with a simple table

*In view of the onslaught of new diagnostic tests and the barrages of unsolicited laboratory results that assault the front-line clinician, the analogy to the art of self-defense is particularly appropriate!

Chunk #3	Blue Belt:	Doing it with a complex table
Chunk #4	Brown Belt:	Doing it with simple math in your head
Chunk #5	Black Belt:	Doing it with more complex math on a hand calculator.

You can stop with whatever chunk you want, and you can even skip from the yellow belt to the brown belt. Black belts (and their patients!) will get the most out of diagnostic data, but even yellow belts can benefit.

Chunk #1 Yellow Belt: Doing It with Pictures

At the Royal Infirmary in Edinburgh, all patients under age 70 who are suspected of having had a myocardial infarction within the previous 48 hours are admitted to the coronary care unit. Like most coronary units, this one became crowded shortly after it opened in 1966,* and those in charge recognized the need to differentiate, as quickly as possible, between those patients who actually had myocardial infarction (and ought to stay in the unit) and those who did not (and could be transferred elsewhere) [40].

The staff thought that rises in the level of creatine kinase (CPK in those days, CK now) might help them diagnose myocardial infarction sooner than measurements of enzymes that rose later, like aspartate aminotransferase (SGOT in those days, AST now). Accordingly, they measured CK on admission and the next two mornings on 360 consecutive patients who were admitted to their coronary unit and lived long enough to have blood samples taken. A clinician who was "blind" to the CK results reviewed the electrocardiograms, clinical records, and autopsy reports of all three hundred and sixty admissions.†

Patients with pathologic Q waves, ST elevation, and subsequent T-wave inversions or positive autopsies were called "very probable" infarcts and those with less diagnostic ECG changes (usually just ST- and T-wave abnormalities) were labeled "possible." These two groups totaled 230; the remaining 130 patients were judged not to have myocardial infarcts.‡

When they examined the highest CK levels attained by each of the 230 patients who did have infarcts and the 130 patients who did not, the results looked like Figure 4-1.

At the upper end of the CK scale, 35 patients in whom an infarct was present,

*Why use such an old example? Because this study meets the guides described in the previous chapter, because it illustrates so many key principles in the interpretation of diagnostic tests, and because the colleagues who reviewed the first edition of this book urged us not to fix things that ain't broke.

†If you are not sure why it is crucial that this clinician was "blind" to the CK results, we would suggest that you go back to the previous chapter and review the first guide for deciding whether to use a particular diagnostic test.

‡Note that the "gold standard" may not always generate two clear-cut groups with, and without, the target disorder. There may be one or even several middle groups who "probably" or "possibly" have the target disorder. In this case, it made sense to handle the middle group as if they had infarcts, and we'll come back to this general issue when we discuss the other belts.

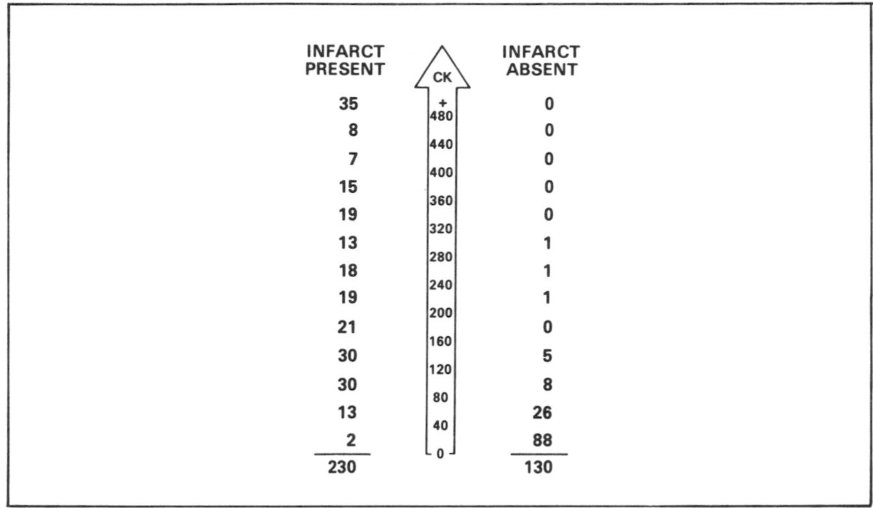

Figure 4-1. Maximum CK levels when myocardial infarction is present and absent: raw data.

but none in whom an infarct was absent, had maximum levels of 480 international units (IU) or higher. At the lower end of the scale, only two patients in whom infarcts were present, but 88 in whom infarcts were absent, had maximum CK levels less than 40 IU.*

Although we could proceed directly from here to a discussion of "diagnostic levels of CK," let us convert these sets of numbers to pictures that will be easier to follow. First, we will convert these numbers to percentages that will make them easier to compare (and will come in handy later on). This is done for you in Figure 4-2.

In Figure 4-2, the 35 infarct patients with maximum CK levels 480 or higher constituted 15% of all infarct patients, whereas the 88 patients without infarcts whose maximum CK levels were below 40 comprised 67% of the patient group in whom infarcts were absent.†

Because most clinicians find graphs and other pictures easier to deal with than tables of numbers, we have carried on one step farther and converted the percentages of Figure 4-2 to the bar chart shown in Figure 4-3.

*Alas, creatine kinase is measured in different ways in different clinical laboratories (the determinations used in this study were carried out in the mid-1960s, using a commercial preparation at 30° C). As a result, it's very unlikely that you can directly apply the CK levels and interpretations that appear here to your own practice and hospital. You can talk to your local clinical chemist to see whether there's a way to translate these numbers to fit your local situation, but most of you have access to CK-MB results as well. Perhaps this example will cause you to reconsider how often you really need this latter information!

†Yes, we know that $^{88}/_{130}$ is closer to 68% than 67%, but we want those three patients who have rather high CK levels but no infarcts to be represented as 1% each, so we have to round things off to keep the total percentage at 100%.

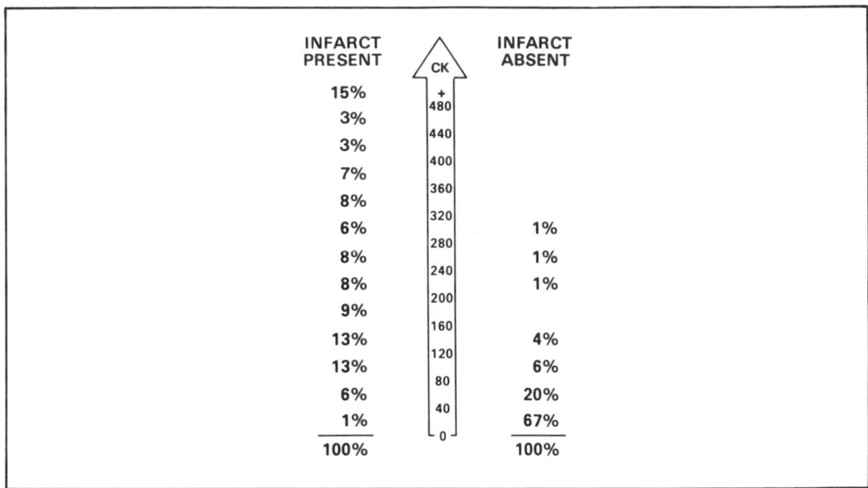

Figure 4-2. Maximum CK levels when myocardial infarction is present and absent: raw data converted to percentages.

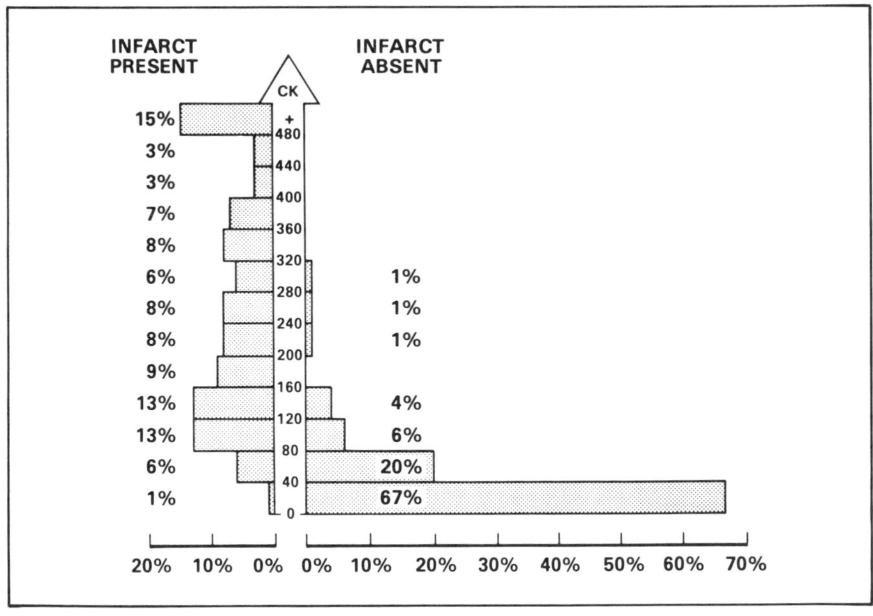

Figure 4-3. A bar chart of maximum CK levels when myocardial infarction is present and absent.

Now the percents are easier to comprehend. The CK levels among patients with infarcts peak once between 80 and 160 IU (the "possible" infarct group, by the way) and again beyond 480 (a group of "very probable" infarcts). On the right-hand side, patients in whom infarcts are absent are clustered down below 40 IU.

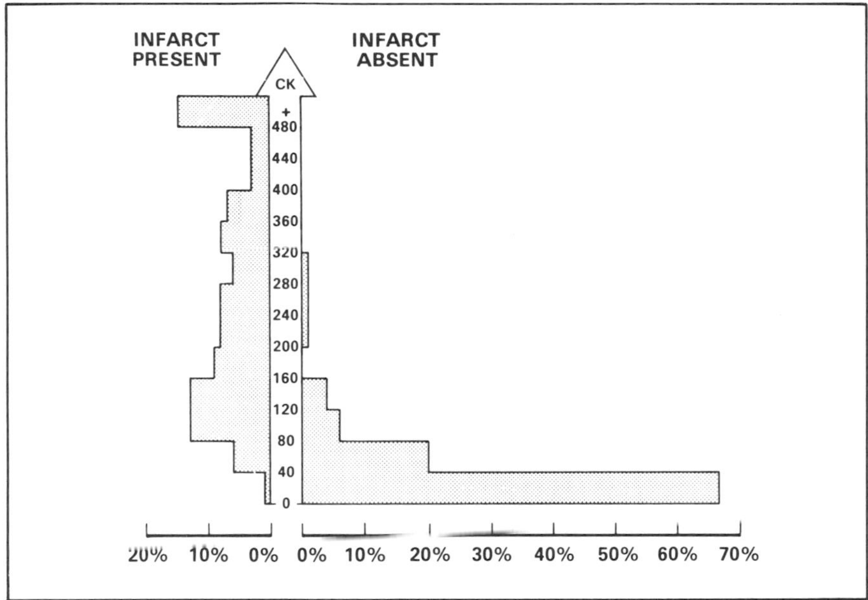

Figure 4-4. A histogram of maximum CK levels when myocardial infarction is present and absent.

Finally, the numbers and lines between the bars can be removed; the uncluttered final result appears in Figure 4-4. Unfortunately, like most clinical data, there is a fair degree of overlap; maximum CKs from less than 40 all the way up to 320 were found both when infarcts were present and when they were absent. Nonetheless, can we take advantage of the fact that *only* infarct patients exhibited maximum CK levels of 320 or more? Sure, we can. We could set a dividing line (or cutoff) between normal and abnormal CK levels at 320 IU and produce the situation shown in Figure 4-5.

By setting the cutoff (which we have labeled *y*) at 320 IU, we can be confident that *every* suspected infarct patient (in the absence of skeletal muscle damage from resuscitation, I-M injection, etc.) with a CK level of 320 or higher has a myocardial infarction. So, when the level is 320 or more, we can "rule in" an infarct.

Have we gained much by selecting a cutoff, above which only infarct patients will reside? Yes and no. On the one hand, we can confidently diagnose at least some infarct patients and manage them accordingly. On the other hand, this rule-in cutoff captures only about one-third ([35 + 8 + 7 + 15 + 19]/230 = 37%) of the 230 infarct patients, and cannot distinguish the remaining 63% of them from all those without infarcts. Thus, of the total 360 coronary care unit admissions (230 with and 130 without infarcts), we have achieved a firm diagnosis (referring back to Figure 4-1) in (35 + 8 + 7 + 15 + 19)/360, or 23% of all admissions.

A second problem with this "absolute" cutoff, beyond which only infarct

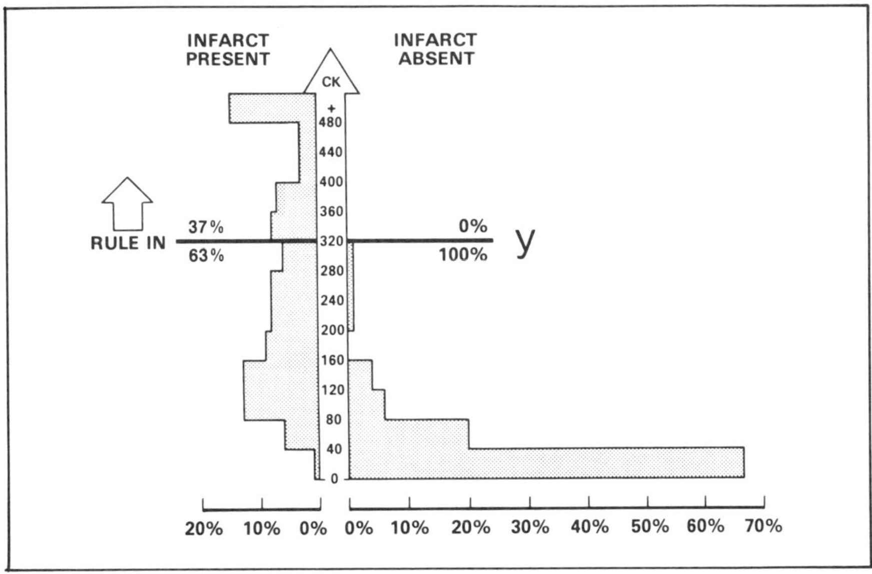

Figure 4-5. An absolute cutoff for maximum CK levels in myocardial infarction.

patients lie, becomes apparent when we think about the *next* 360 admissions to the unit, and the next 360 after them. Will they generate an identical range of CK results?

Almost, but not quite. Subsequent groups of patients will, on average, behave like this first group. Mild infarcts will cluster between 80 and 160 IU and severe ones at or beyond 480 IU, and patients without infarcts will bunch up below 40 IU. However, the *range* of CK results can only become *larger*, never smaller, as more patients are examined. The more patients we encounter, the more likely we are to find patients who, although they have neither myocardial infarctions nor skeletal muscle damage, exhibit higher and higher CK results. Such patients will be quite rare, comprising no more than 1% or at most 2% of the total, but they will occur and the more patients we see, the greater our chances of encountering these "outliers." As a result, if we stick with an "absolute" definition of our rule-in cutoff *y*, beyond which *only* infarct patients reside, we shall be forced to move the cutoff to ever more extreme levels; inevitably, this *y* cutoff will help us diagnose an ever-shrinking portion of the patients we encounter.

Is there a way out of this dilemma? Yes, if we relax our cutoff just a little bit. Bearing in mind that extreme values will be quite rare (comprising only 1% to 2% of all observations), what would happen if we revised our cutoffs so that they exclude 99% of patients with and without infarcts, rather than all 100% them? The very useful result is shown in Figure 4-6.

Now, the rule-in cutoff *y,* by shifting to allow the highest 1% of patients who do not have infarcts to slip above the cutoff, has lowered the cutoff to 280 IU and now encompasses 42% rather than just 37% of all the infarcts. Moreover, a second cutoff has appeared by allowing in the lowest 1% of infarct patients. This

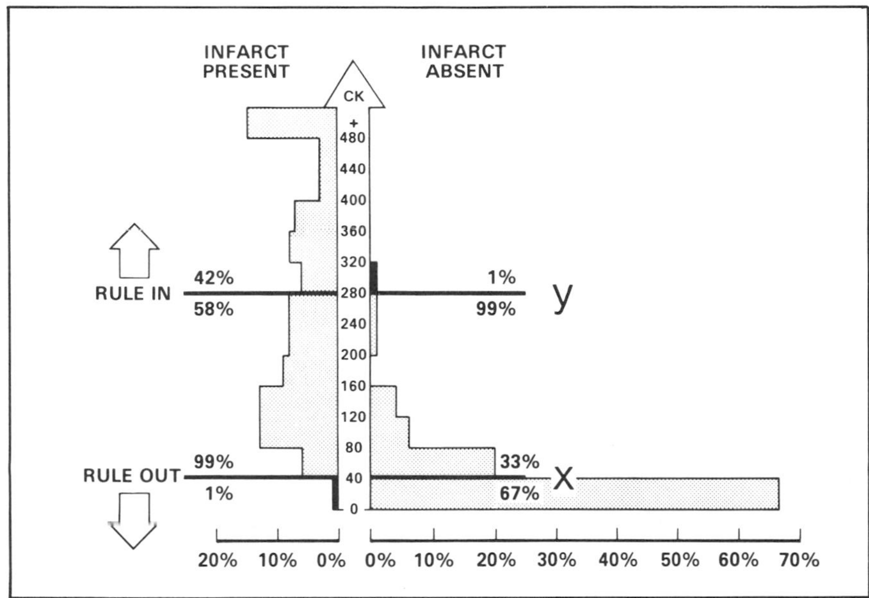

Figure 4-6. A 99% cutoff for maximum CK levels in myocardial infarction.

second cutoff, which we have labeled *x*, can be used to rule out myocardial infarction when the maximum CK remains below 40 IU. Below this cutoff lie only 1% of infarcts, but 67% of patients without infarcts, so we have gained a great deal. Referring again to Figure 4-1, of our 360 original patients we can rule in or rule out myocardial infarction in (35 + 8 + 7 + 15 + 19 + 13 + 88/360, or 51% of them, at the cost of missing two infarcts (whose maximum CKs were less than 40 IU) and overdiagnosing one patient who was infarct-free (but had a CK level at or above 280 IU). Thus, these simple rule-in and rule-out levels could handle more than half the patients who presented with clinically-suspected myocardial infarction!*

There is nothing sacred about choosing a 99% cutoff; it could be 98%, 96%, or 99.5% if you wished. The major factor in deciding where to set it should be your clinical judgment about what is best for the patients concerned. For example, if the treatment for a disorder was innocuous and overdiagnosis produced neither shame nor anguish among those patients who were falsely labeled, you might want to relax the rule-in cutoff *y* to exclude only 95% of patients who do not have the target disorder. On the other hand, if patients really suffered from being labeled with the target disorder (e.g., cancer, venereal disease, schizophrenia), the rule-in cutoff *y* should be set very high so that it excludes 99% or 99.5% of the nondiseased. And, if early diagnosis and therapy were essential

*When you get to the green belt, you will learn what these cutoffs mean in terms of sensitivity and specificity and will meet the terms suggested by our clinical clerks for their application at the bedside: "SpPin" and "SnNout!"

for satisfactory clinical outcomes, as in many neonatal screening programs (e.g., phenylketonuria, neonatal hypothyroidism), you would want a sufficiently low rule-out cutoff x so that its use captures virtually or absolutely all patients with the target disorder (this is why so many babies who screen positive for these disorders are found, on further testing, to be normal; we do not want to miss any cases).

Let us briefly consider how these rule-in and rule-out cutoffs fit into the diagnostic strategies we described in Chapter 1. First, the rule-in cutoff y is the one we invoke when we are diagnosing by pattern recognition, is it not? We are seeking confirmation that our "snap" diagnosis was correct.

Second, when we are using the hypothetico-deductive strategy, we should be seeking those symptoms, clinical signs, and lab tests that help us shorten our list of hypotheses. Although rule-in cutoffs (y) may help, we will gain more from using rule-out cutoffs (x) here, for they will more commonly be encountered and, when found, will *eliminate* hypotheses from our lists. This attention to rule-out cutoffs also will help us overcome our current tendency, described in Chapter 1, to pursue the merely compatible, rather than decisive signs and test results.

So there you are. If you understood the foregoing you should award yourself a yellow belt in diagnosis. It can all be done with pictures and does not call for any new terminology or math.

In summary, to do it with pictures:

1. Pick symptoms, signs, or tests where the overlap between patients who do and do not have the target disorder is as small as possible. If you do not know which symptoms, signs, or tests these are, ask your clinical, radiologic, or laboratory colleagues who claim to be expert in the relevant subspecialty (and quickly learn whether they are!).
2. See if you can find pictures like Figures 4-3 to 4-6; if not, you should be able to construct them from raw data such as that in Figure 4-1 (just follow the steps we carried out in generating the later figures in the series). The patient groups from which these pictures are generated should not just be bunches of classic cases, on the one hand, and robust, young medical students, on the other; most of us can tell the difference between these two groups without any diagnostic tests at all! As you should recall from the previous chapter, the patient groups should be those in whom the target disorder is really suspected as a legitimate entry in the list of hypotheses.
3. Decide whether you want to set strict (99%) or loose (95%) cutoffs for your rule-in and rule-out levels, (remembering that you can mix them and, for example, set y at 100% and x at 95%).
4. Add these cutoffs to the pictures and identify the diagnostic test results that correspond to the rule-in y and rule-out x cutoffs.
5. If you carry a pocket notebook of normal values, you can add your rule-in and rule-out cutoffs to the other "pearls" therein. As we will show you in Chapter 10, these cutoffs (especially when they apply to symptoms and signs) can form one starting point for reviewing your own clinical performance.

Straightforward though it may be, you cannot help but have noticed that "doing it with pictures" leaves a big bunch of patients in the middle, with too much of a symptom, sign, or lab result to rule out the target disorder, but not enough of it to rule the target disorder in (comprising the "intermediate" and "indeterminate" test results described by David Simel and his colleagues) [38]. There are two different ways to handle this large group of patients in the middle, so you now must make a decision on where to go from here. If you want to learn (more) about sensitivity (and SnNout), specificity (and SpPin), predictive value, ROC curves,* and all that, you can continue to read this book in sequence and proceed through the green and blue belts on simple and complex tables. If, on the other hand, you already know as much about these things as you care to know and want to leap ahead to a very powerful strategy (whose use has increased rapidly since the first edition of this book), skip the green and blue belts and go directly to the brown belt (page 119), where you will learn more about how to use likelihood ratios to interpret symptoms, signs, and laboratory test results.

Chunk #2 Green Belt: Doing It with a Simple Table

In Figure 4-7, we have swung the patients with myocardial infarctions (the solid line) over to the same side as the patients without myocardial infarctions (the dotted line). Note that the two lines cross at 80 IU. Selecting this value of 80 IU as the cutoff, we can then flip the infarct patients back where they were and generate Figure 4-8.†

By placing the cutoff at 80 IU, above which the CK test result will be decreed positive and below which it is negative, we have created four groups of patients: (*a*) infarct patients with positive test results (the true-positives); (*b*) patients who, although they do *not* have infarcts, have positive test results (the false-positives); (*c*) infarct patients with negative test results (the false-negatives); and (*d*) patients without infarcts whose test results are negative (the true-negatives).

The CK test has correctly classified patients from groups *a* and *d*. Group *a* tests are positive and are telling the truth; such patients (and such test results) are often referred to as "true-positives." Similarly, group *d* negative test results also are telling the truth; they do not have infarcts, and they are called "true-negatives."

The CK test result, however, has provided a false picture of patients from groups *b* and *c*. In group *b* the test result is positive but the patients do not have infarcts, so these patients and their test results are called "false-positives." In

*ROC is an acronym for *R*eceiver (or *R*esponse) *O*perating *C*haracteristic and comes from the early days of radar and other imaging strategies when interpreters had to distinguish "signals" caused by airplanes from the "noise" caused by other sources.

†There are, of course, lots of ways to select cutoffs. A useful property of this particular cutoff is that it minimizes the number of patients who are falsely labeled as having a given target disorder (when they don't) or as not having it (when they do).

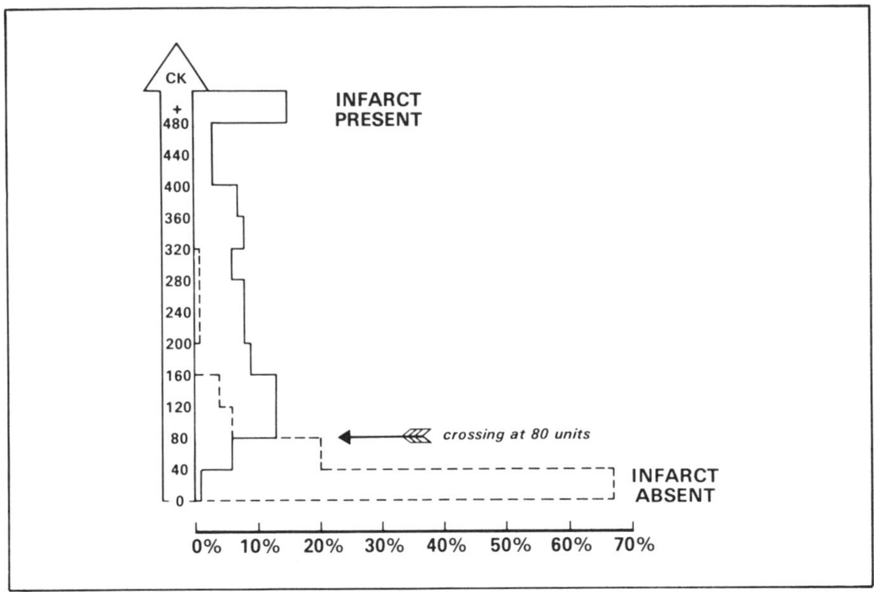

Figure 4-7. The intersection of CK values for patients in whom myocardial infarction is present or absent.

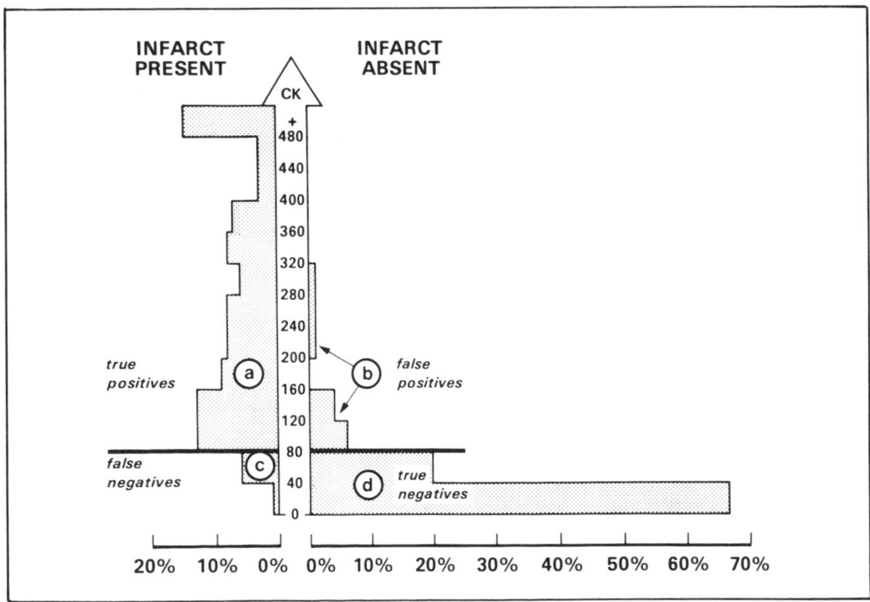

Figure 4-8. Use of an 80 CK IU cutoff in the diagnosis of myocardial infarction.

Table 4-1. Doing it with a simple table

		Myocardial infarction	
		Present	Absent
CK test result	Positive (≥ 80 IU)	True-positive a	b False-positive
	Negative (< 80 IU)	c False-negative	d True-negative

group *c*, the other false picture is created; group *c* patients have infarcts but their test results are negative, so they are called "false-negatives."

These relationships can also be shown by using a simple ("2 × 2" or "four-fold") table and, since that is what this chunk is all about, we have generated Table 4-1.

Table 4-1 corresponds exactly to Figure 4-8: patients with infarcts are on the left, those without infarcts are on the right. The upper half of the table concerns positive CK test results, the lower half negative results. The four inner squares, called cells, are labeled *a, b, c,* and *d* because they correspond exactly to groups *a, b, c,* and *d* of Figure 4-8.*

Once you are comfortable thinking about the table (rather than the pictures of the previous chunk), we can proceed to place patients into it. Go back to Figure 4-1 and add our 80 IU cutoff to it (this simply calls for a horizontal line that cuts right through the number 80 on the CK scale). Among infarct patients, all those who are above this cutoff (true-positives) belong in cell *a* of our new table, and infarct patients below the cutoff (false-negatives) go into cell *c*. On the other side, for patients who do not have infarcts, those above the cutoff are false-positives and belong in cell *b*, and those below the cutoff are true-negatives and belong in cell *d*. When we did this ourselves, the results looked like Table 4-2.

Using this cutoff on these patients, we have 215 true-positive infarct patients with positive test results in cell *a*, 16 false-positive patients with positive test results but no infarcts in cell *b*, 15 false-negative infarct patients with negative test results in cell *c*, and 114 true-negative patients with no infarcts and negative test results in cell *d*. Having filled the table, we can now carry out some simple manipulations on it and generate some clinically useful indexes of the value of doing CK determinations on patients in whom we suspect myocardial infarction. This "doing it with a simple table" is started in Table 4-3.

*We will follow the orientation of rows and columns shown in Table 4-1 throughout this book, but you will come across articles that switch the locations of affected and unaffected patients, rotate the whole table 90 degrees, and so forth. It is important, therefore, to check out how such tables are oriented and arranged before trying to interpret them.

Table 4-2. Filling a simple table

		Myocardial infarction	
		Present	Absent
CK test result	Positive (≥ 80 IU)	35 8 7 15 19 13 18 19 21 30 + 30 215 a	1 1 1 5 + 8 16 b
	Negative (< 80 IU)	c 13 + 2 15	d 26 + 88 114
	Total	230	130

Table 4-3. Getting ready to generate some indexes of clinical usefulness

		Myocardial infarction		
		Present	Absent	
CK test result	Positive (≥ 80 IU)	215 a	16 b	231 a+b
	Negative (< 80 IU)	c 15	d 114	c+d 129
		a+c 230	b+d 130	a+b+c+d 360

Table 4-3 has continued the addition we started in Table 4-2 and now shows:

$(a + c)$: The total number of patients with infarcts, regardless of their test results = 230

$(b + d)$: The total number of patients who do not have infarcts, regardless of their test results = 130

$(a + b)$: The total number of patients with positive test results, this time regardless of whether they have infarcts = 231

$(c + d)$:	The total number of patients with negative test results, regardless of whether they have infarcts = 129
$(a + b + c + d)$:	The grand total of all patients investigated = $(a + c) + (b + d)$ or $(a + b) + (c + d)$ = 360.

So what? What have we gained by converting our attractive pictures into this squat table? As it happens, we have made possible the elucidation of two very important insights about signs, symptoms, and laboratory tests. First, this table approach permits us to describe, in a very concise, snug, and easily remembered way, how "good" these clinical data are at helping us decide whether patients have the target disorder. Second, this table approach permits us to recognize a crucial fickleness of diagnostic data which, unless we understand it, causes us to waste a great deal of time, money, and diagnostic effort.

Let us start with the concise description of how "good" the CK test (or, for that matter, any diagnostic test) really is. To help us remember the various measures of how good a test is and to assist us in communicating these to each other, a set of technical terms has been developed to designate each of them, and we shall introduce these along the way.

In Table 4-3, we find the positive and negative results of the diagnostic test in the upper and lower horizontal rows, respectively, of the table. The vertical columns represent what the patients "really" have, based on all the other information about them, including autopsy findings. Because this other information was judged to be "harder" or more certain than the CK result, the vertical columns of this and similar tables is spoken of as representing the gold standard. In Table 4-3 the gold standard of serial electrocardiograms, clinical course, and autopsy results tells us whether the patients *really* do or do not have infarcts.*

How good is the CK test among patients with infarcts? Well, among 230 who had infarcts—that is $(a + c)$ at the bottom of the left-hand column—the 215 patients in cell a had positive test results, and 215/230 or $(a)/(a + c)$ comes to .93 or 93%. Thus, 93% of infarct patients had positive CK tests, and the shorthand term for this property is *sensitivity*. Although you will usually see the term *sensitivity* used to indicate this "positivity in disease" or *proportion of patients with the target disorder who have a positive test result,* the term sensitivity has other scientific meanings,† and you might want to use some of the synonyms for $a/(a + c)$. They include:

1. *The PiD rate* (with apologies to the gonococcus and other causes of "Pelvic Inflammatory Disease"), for "Positivity in Disease." This synonym has the advantage of being an acronym (its initials remind you of its definition).

*As we've already pointed out, the selection and definition of gold standards is arbitrary and often represents a consensus of contemporaneous experts. Although current gold standards tend to be defined in terms of pathologic anatomy, they are evolving to include major elements of the subsequent clinical course and prognosis of patients with differing diagnostic test results.

†The other meaning for *sensitivity* with which you are probably most familiar is the ability of an analytic method to detect minute amounts of some target substance.

2. *The true positive rate* or *TP rate,* based on cell *a* as the home for the true-positive test results. This term is often used in more advanced discussions of diagnosis (you will meet it if you study for the blue belt), but suffers (along with sensitivity) from not making it clear what the denominator for the rate should be; it is supposed to be $(a + c)$ or (true-positives plus false-negatives).

Recognizing that the measure of a diagnostic test's ability to detect a target disorder when it is present can go by any of three names (sensitivity = PiD rate = TP rate), you can take your pick and relabel the subsequent tables and discussions to suit yourself.

So much for a test's ability to detect the target disorder when it is present. What about the complementary ability to correctly identify the absence of the target disorder? Look again at Table 4-3. Among 130 patients who did not have infarcts (that is $[b + d]$ at the bottom of the second column), the 114 patients in cell *d* had negative test results, and 114/130 or $(d)/(b + d)$ is .88 or 88%.* Thus, 88% of patients who did not have infarcts had negative CK tests, and the shorthand term for this property is *specificity.*

Again, although specificity is the most commonly used term for this property it, too, has another scientific meaning,† and you might want to use synonyms for $(d)/(b + d)$:

1. *The NiH rate* (with apologies to Bethesda, home of the U.S. *N*ational *I*nstitutes of *H*ealth), for "Negativity in Health." Another acronym, the "H" is not always correct, for, although it refers to patients who do not have the target disorder, they are not necessarily healthy.
2. *The true negative rate* or *TN rate*, based on cell *d* as the home for the true negative test results. It is the counterpart of the TP rate and has similar advantages and disadvantages.

As with sensitivity, pick the term you find most sensible for $(d)/(b + d)$ and use it, (remembering that specificity = NiH rate = TN rate = $(d)/(b + d)$. Table 4-4 summarizes where we have come so far.

So, the CK test has a sensitivity (PiD rate, TP rate) of 93% and a specificity (NiH rate, TN rate) of 88%. Is this good or bad? How does it compare with other diagnostic data? To help you find out, we have summarized the sensitivities and specificities of ten symptoms, signs, or laboratory tests, and these appear in Table 4-5.

Table 4-5 contains many lessons for us. The first entry shows how useful a careful, directed history can be in identifying virtually everybody who will have a positive upper gastrointestinal series; indeed, in situations or places with scarce resources, such an approach has been used to decide who does not need to

*The 1% discrepancy between Figures 4-2, 4-3, and 4-6 and this value of 88% is due to rounding to whole percents in the earlier figures.

†The other scientific meaning for *specificity* is the ability of an analytic method to detect a single target substance and no others.

Table 4-4. The sensitivity and specificity of the CK test in myocardial infarction

		Myocardial infarction		
		Present	Absent	
CK test result	Positive (≥ 80 IU)	215 a	b 16	231 a + b
	Negative (< 80 IU)	c 15	d 114	c + d 129
		a + c 230 Sensitivity = PiD rate = TP rate = $\frac{a}{a + c} = \frac{215}{230}$ = 93%	b + d 130 Specificity = NiH rate = TN rate = $\frac{d}{b + d} = \frac{114}{130}$ = 88%	a + b + c + d 360

undergo the barium study, applying the rule of SnNout: if a sign, symptom, or other diagnostic test has a sufficiently high *Sen*sitivity, a *N*egative result rules *out* the target disorder. The second entry reminds us of the power of a simple history, in this case a series of four questions about alcohol use called the CAGE [6].* Not only does the history outperform the clinical laboratory; if you set a high cutoff (three or four positive answers, rather than just one) you can invoke the rule of SpPin: if a sign, symptom, or other diagnostic test has a sufficiently high *Sp*ecificity, a *P*ositive result rules *in* the target disorder. As we noted earlier, we invoke SpPin when we carry out pattern recognition; high specificity is another way of saying that "nothing else looks like this."

Note that here in the green belt we happily sacrifice specificity to invoke SnNout, and sacrifice sensitivity to invoke SpPin (in fact, we moved the cutoff in order to invoke SpPin for the CAGE). Is there any way to have your SnNout and SpPin it, too? There is, but you will have to go for your blue or brown belt to learn how.

The third entry, on the corneal reflex, reminds us that we can use diagnostic data to determine prognosis as well as diagnosis. The fourth, on spontaneous retinal vein pulsation, is special to us because it was the one that prompted one of our clinical clerks to invent the term SnNout (and prompted us to come up with SpPin) as ways to remember the practical and powerful bedside applications of the classroom definitions of sensitivity and specificity. We are constantly on the look-out for SnNouts on our clinical services, for their application permits

*Have you ever felt you should *C*ut down on your drinking?; Have people *A*nnoyed you by criticizing your drinking?; Have you ever felt bad or *G*uilty about your drinking?; Have you ever had a drink first thing in the morning to steady your nerves or to get rid of a hangover (*E*ye-opener)?

Table 4-5. Sensitivities and specificities for some diagnostic tests

Reference	Target disorder (and gold standard)	Type of patient	Diagnostic data	Sensitivity PiD rate TP rate	Specificity NiH rate TN rate
[28]	Ulcer, hiatus hernia, abnormal motility, or other important finding (by radiography)	Patients referred for an upper gastrointestinal series	History of ulcer, over age 50, pain relieved by food or milk, or pain after eating	95% SnNout?	30%
[6]	Alcohol dependency or abuse (by extensive clinical investigation)	Medical and orthopedic inpatients	Gama-glutamyl transpeptidase	54%	76%
			Mean corpuscular volume	63%	64%
			Liver function tests	37%	81%
			"Yes" to 1 or more of the 4 CAGE questions	85%	81%
			"Yes" to 3 or more of the 4 CAGE questions	51%	99.7% SpPin!
[27]	Recovery with moderate to no disability (by follow-up)	Patients with nontraumatic coma	Corneal reflex	92%	35%
[26]	Increased intracranial pressure (by lumbar puncture, surgery, or imaging)	Patients and volunteers	Absence of spontaneous pulsation of the retinal vein	100% SnNout!	85%
[20]	Iron deficiency anemia (by bone marrow aspiration)	Consecutive hospital admissions >65 years old	Red cell protoporphyrin	68%	68%
			Mean red cell volume	72%	68%
			Transferrin saturation	62%	86%
			Serum ferritin	82%	90%
[23]	Deep vein thrombosis (by venography)	Patients with symptoms suggesting deep vein thrombosis	One or both of impedance plethysmography and ^{125}I-fibrinogen leg scanning	92%	92%
[17]	Pancreas cancer (by biopsy, surgery, or autopsy)	Patients with symptoms or signs suggesting cancer of the pancreas	Ultrasound (when successful)	70%	85%
			CT scan	85%	90%
			Endoscopic retrograde cholangio-pancreatography (when successful)	95%	97%

us to shorten hypothesis-lists, avoid expensive and invasive investigations, and speed our patients on to diagnosis, therapy, and home.

The entry in Table 4-5 on the diagnosis of deep vein thrombosis reveals how a combination of two different diagnostic tests can be used, and the entries for pancreatic cancer show how sensitivity and specificity can be used to compare different diagnostic tests for the same condition (there are more powerful ways to make this comparison, and you'll meet them when you go for your blue belt). Finally, the last entry illustrates another use of diagnostic tests: confirmation of a diagnosis among patients with positive screening tests.

But wait a minute! All of this talk about sensitivity and specificity (PiD rates and NiH rates; TP rates and TN rates) solves the wrong problem! When we use diagnostic tests clinically, we *do not know* who actually has and does not have the target disorder; if we did, we would not need the diagnostic test! Our clinical concern is not a vertical one of sensitivity and specificity, but a horizontal one of the meaning of positive and negative test results. Let's go back to Table 4-3 and sort these out.

The top row of Table 4-3 displays 231 positive test results (shown by the $(a + b)$ total. Of these, the 215 in cell a did, indeed, have infarcts. Accordingly, $(a)/(a + b)$ or 215/231 or .93 or 93% of patients with positive CK test results had infarcts. This is the *proportion of patients with positive test results who have the target disorder* and its shorthand name is the *positive predictive value*. Its synonyms are:

1. The *predictive value of a positive test* (a rather longer way of saying the same thing!).
2. The *posttest likelihood* of the target disorder following a positive test*. This mouthful is one that you may not want to use now, but will encounter if you go for your brown belt.
3. The *posterior probability of the target disorder following a positive test*. This is another brown-belt set of terms.
4. The *posttest probability of the target disorder following a positive test* is the term we shall use here.

The second row of Table 4-3 displays 129 negative test results (shown by the $[c + d]$ total). Of these, the 114 in cell d did not have infarcts. Thus, $(d)/(c + d)$ or 114/129 or .88 or 88% of patients with negative CK test results did not have infarcts. This *proportion of patients with negative test results who do not have the target disorder* goes by the shorthand name of *negative predictive value*. Its synonyms are analogous to ones we have just met:

*Unlike sensitivity, specificity, predictive values, or probabilities (which can be expressed as decimals or percentages), likelihoods are expressed as odds. Because odds will be foreign to many readers, we will use them sparingly, and often will describe patients in terms of their pretest and posttest probabilities of a target disorder.

1. The *predictive value of a negative test*
2. The *posttest likelihood* of *not* having the target disorder following a negative test
3. The *posterior probability* of *not* having the target disorder following a negative test*
4. The *posttest probability* of *not* having the target disorder following a negative test

We have updated Table 4-3 to include all of these terms, and it appears as Table 4-6.

Now that looks much more useful clinically!† Over 90% of patients with CK results of 80 IU or more have infarcts, and almost 90% of patients with CK results less than 80 IU do not have infarcts. Right? Not quite! This is where we gain the second very important insight about diagnostic data: their fickleness.

The predictive values of diagnostic signs, symptoms, and laboratory tests are *not* constant, but *must* change with the proportion of patients who actually have the target disorder among those who undergo the diagnostic evaluation. To show you why this is so, let us go back and start with an additional feature of Table 4-6.

Table 4-6 contains 360 patients consecutively admitted to a coronary care unit with suspected myocardial infarction. Of these 360 patients (who, by the way, represent the sum of cells a, b, c, and d), 230 or $(a + c)$ turned out to have myocardial infarctions. That is $(a + c)/(a + b + c + d)$ or 230/360 or .64 or 64%. This proportion of patients with the target disorder among all tested patients, $(a + c)/(a + b + c + d)$, also has a few names: *prevalence*, the *pretest likelihood of the target disorder*, the *prior probability of the target disorder* or the *pretest probability of the target disorder*. We will use the terms prevalence and pretest probability for now; you will meet the others if you go for your brown belt.

Now, suppose that a group of clinicians at another hospital that did not have a coronary care unit were so impressed with the CK test's performance in Edinburgh that they decided to use it routinely in *all* their hospital admissions (save those with skeletal muscle trauma) in whom myocardial infarction was even remotely entertained. Of course, we would expect the prevalence or pretest probability of myocardial infarction to be far lower among these general admissions than in the coronary unit. The proportion $(a + c)/(a + b + c + d)$ might be 10% rather than 64%.

*You might want to use the complement of this term, the posttest probability, posterior probability, or posttest probability *of having the target disorder* following a negative test. This is the rate $c/(c + d)$ or, in this case, $15/129 = .12$ or 12%, and you will note that 12% (calculated here) plus 88% (just calculated in the text) = 100%. You may not want to use this now, but a memory of its origin will come in handy when (and if) you take up the brown belt.

†Incidentally, the fact that sensitivity and positive predictive value (both 93%), and specificity and negative predictive value (both 88%), are identical is happenstance, due to the fact that cells b and c are virtually equal. This is rarely the case, and you should not draw any generalizations from it.

Table 4-6. The sensitivity, specificity, and predictive values of the CK test in myocardial infarction among coronary care unit admissions

		Myocardial infarction			
		Present	Absent		
CK test result	Positive (≥ 80 IU)	215 (a)	16 (b)	231 (a + b)	Positive predictive value = Predictive value of a positive test = Posttest likelihood or posterior probability of disease = $\frac{a}{a+b} = \frac{215}{231} = 93\%$
	Negative (< 80 IU)	15 (c)	114 (d)	129 (c + d)	Negative predictive value = Predictive value of a negative test = Posttest likelihood or posterior probability of *no* disease = $\frac{d}{c+d} = \frac{114}{129} = 88\%$
		230 (a + c)	130 (b + d)	360 (a + b + c + d)	
		Sensitivity = PiD rate = TP rate = $\frac{a}{a+c} = \frac{215}{230} = 93\%$	Specificity = NiH rate = TN rate = $\frac{d}{b+d} = \frac{114}{130} = 88\%$		Prevalence = pretest likelihood of disease = prior probability of disease $= \frac{a+c}{a+b+c+d} = \frac{230}{360} = 64\%$

So what? Would this really matter? Well, if the CK levels among general admissions with and without myocardial infarction were like those of the coronary care unit patients (that is, if the 80-IU cutoff produced a sensitivity of 93% and a specificity of 88%), the use of the CK test among general hospital admissions would produce the disappointing results shown in Table 4-7.

In this table, the sensitivity is 93% and the specificity is 88%, as before (you can compare them with Table 4-6 if you wish). However, the predictive values have changed dramatically, and now the majority of patients with positive CK tests do *not* have infarcts! The explanation is straightforward, though perhaps not immediately obvious, and can be grasped by comparing the entries in cell *b* of Tables 4-6 and 4-7.

Although specificity (the NiH rate, the TN rate) was the same 88% in both tables, the number of patients who did not have infarcts ($b + d$) rose from 130 in Table 4-6 to 2070 in Table 4-7. Because 12% of these patients wind up in cell *b* (since 88% of them go to cell *d*), cell *b* rose from 16 patients in Table 4-6 to 248 patients in Table 4-7, and thereby exceeded the 215 patients in cell *a* of both tables.*

Although the *fall* in positive predictive value (posttest probability of the target disorder) is the most dramatic effect of a fall in prevalence (pretest probability of the target disorder), you may have noted a concomitant *rise* in negative predictive value (posttest probability of *not* having the target disorder) from 88% in Table 4-6 to 99% in Table 4-7. The explanation for this change is analagous to that for the fall in positive predictive value, and focuses on cell *d*.

Is this fickleness a generalizable phenomenon? Unfortunately, it is. *As prevalence falls, positive predictive value must fall along with it, and negative predictive value must rise.*† After all, positive predictive value is simply the prevalence of the target disorder among patients with positive test results.

Even an excellent symptom, sign, or laboratory test with a sensitivity and a specificity both of 95% will lose positive predictive value and gain negative predictive value as prevalence falls. We have shown this in Table 4-8 for a range of prevalence values.

*The foregoing assumes *no change* in the sensitivity and specificity of the diagnostic test when prevalence changes. However, sensitivity *would* decrease with changes in prevalence if, for example, the infarcts among general hospital admissions were less severe as well as less common. Specificity could fall too if, for example, more noninfarct patients on the general wards had received intramuscular injections (which can produce false-positive CK test results). If sensitivity fell, cell *a* would become smaller, and cell *c* larger, and both predictive values would fall further. Similarly, a fall in specificity would make cell *b* larger and cell *d* smaller, and both predictive values fall. The moral is: when prevalence falls, although sensitivity and specificity *may* change, predictive value *must* change.

†To use our other terms: *As the pretest likelihood or probability of having the target disorder falls, the posttest likelihood or probability of having the target disorder following a positive test must fall along with it, and the posttest likelihood or probability of not having the target disorder following a negative test must rise*; or: *as the prior probablity of having the target disorder falls, the posterior probability of having the target disorder following a positive test must fall along with it, and the posterior probability of not having the target disorder following a negative test must rise.*

Table 4-7. The sensitivity, specificity, and predictive values of the CK test in myocardial infarction among general hospital admissions

		Myocardial infarction			
		Present	Absent		
CK test result	Positive ($\geqslant$ 80 IU)	215 (a)	248 (b)	463 (a + b)	Positive predictive value = Predictive value of a positive test = Posttest likelihood or posterior probability of disease = $\frac{a}{a+b} = \frac{215}{463} = 46\%$
	Negative (< 80 IU)	15 (c)	1822 (d)	1837 (c + d)	Negative predictive value = Predictive value of a negative test = Posttest likelihood or posterior probability of *no* disease = $\frac{d}{c+d} = \frac{1822}{1837} = 99\%$
		(a + c) 230	(b + d) 2070	(a + b + c + d) 2300	Prevalence = pretest likelihood of disease = prior probability of disease = $\frac{a+c}{a+b+c+d} = \frac{230}{2300} = 10\%$
		Sensitivity = PiD rate = TP rate = $\frac{a}{a+c} = \frac{215}{230} = 93\%$	Specificity = NiH rate = TN rate = $\frac{d}{b+d} = \frac{1822}{2070} = 88\%$		

Table 4-8. The effect of prevalence on the predictive value of an excellent sign, symptom, or laboratory test*

Prevalence (Pretest likelihood or prior probability of disease)	99%	95%	90%	80%	70%	60%	50%	40%	30%	20%	10%	5%	1%	0.5%	0.1%
Predictive value of a positive test (Posterior probability of disease following a positive test result)	99.9%	99.7%	99.4%	99%	98%	97%	95%	93%	89%	83%	68%	50%	16%	9%	2%
Predictive value of a negative test (Posterior probability of *no* disease following a negative test result)	16%	50%	68%	83%	89%	93%	95%	97%	98%	99%	99.4%	99.7%	99.9%	99.97%	99.99%
(Posterior probability *of* disease following a negative test result)	84%	50%	32%	17%	11%	7%	5%	3%	2%	1%	0.6%	0.3%	0.1%	0.03%	0.01%

*Both sensitivity and specificity equal 95% in every case.

An examination of Table 4-8 suggests that, as prevalence falls, you appear to learn much more from the *absence* of a sign or symptom or from a negative test result than from the *presence* of a sign or symptom or a positive test. That would be nice if true, and certainly would fit very nicely into the hypothetico-deductive approach to diagnosis, because it would help us shorten our list of hypotheses by demonstrating that some of them are wildly improbable and ought to be dropped.

In light of this latter point, why did we say that it only appears to be true that we learn more from negative than positive diagnostic data at low prevalence? Look at the bottom row of Table 4-8. It is the complement of the row above it, and gives the probability that the patient *has* the target disorder following a negative test result (thus, the last two rows in each column always add to 100%). Now, compare the entries in this last row with those in the top row (the prevalence or pretest probability of the target disorder). In the midportion of the table, they are very far apart. For example, when the pretest probability (prevalence) of the target disorder is 50%, the absence of an excellent sign or symptom or a negative test result drops it by 45% to a posttest probability of the target disorder of only 5%, and a formerly quite plausible diagnostic hypothesis now deserves rejection. However, the drop from pretest to posttest probability following negative diagnostic data becomes progressively smaller as we move toward lower pretest probabilities (prevalence). So when a diagnostic hypothesis is extremely unlikely, say a pretest probability (prevalence) of 5%, the absence of the key sign or symptom or a negative test result drops this by only 4.7% to a posttest probability of .3%, and you have learned very little. That, then, is why we said that it only appears to be true that, at low prevalence (or low pretest probability) of the target disorder you learn more from negative than positive diagnostic data.

What if the sign, symptom, or laboratory test is not excellent? What if it is more typical diagnostic data whose sensitivity (PiD rate, TP rate) is 85% and whose specificity (NiH rate, TN rate) is 90%? We have prepared a graph comparing this situation with that in Table 4-8, and it appears as Figure 4-9.

A comparison of the results from the two different test capabilities depicted in Figure 4-9 confirms (we hope!) your intuition that the change (rise or drop) from pretest to posttest probability of the target disorder is muted (and you learn less) when sensitivity (PiD rate, TP rate) and/or specificity (NiH rate, TN rate) are decreased.

A corollary to the foregoing is that you gain the most from a clinical sign, symptom, or laboratory test (that is, you achieve the largest rise or drop from pretest to posttest probability of the target disorder) when the pretest probability (prevalence or prior probability) of the target disorder is 40% to 60%. This is shown in Figure 4-10.

In the example shown in this figure, sensitivity and specificity of the diagnostic test are 75% and 85%, respectively. Since the dashed line running diagonally across the table represents a completely useless diagnostic test (sensitivity and specificity both equal 50%), the more "bowed" the curves are (that is, the higher the sensitivity and specificity) the greater the change from pretest to posttest probability of the target disorder.

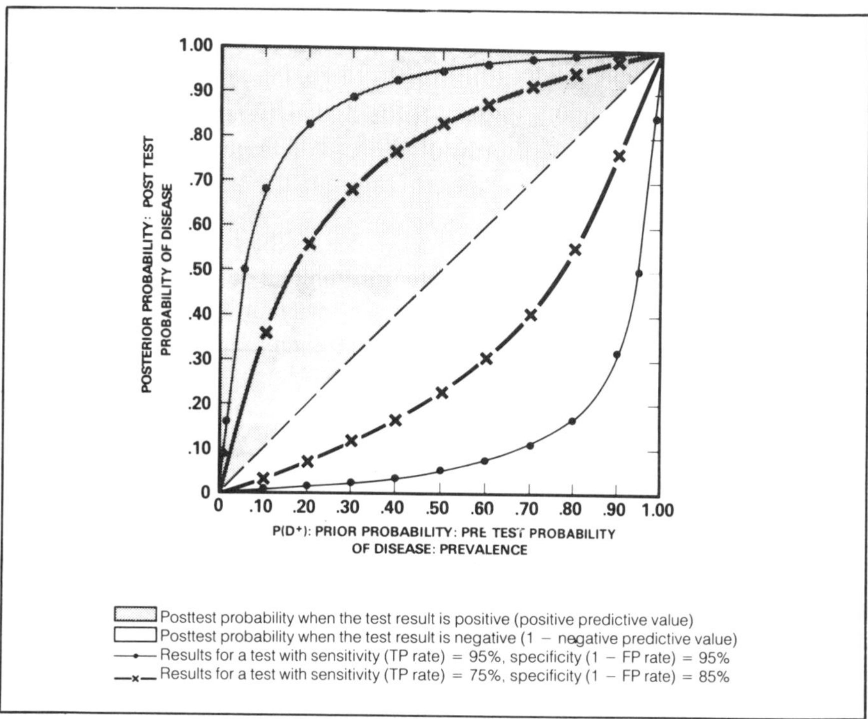

Figure 4-9. The effect of prevalence on the predictive values of a typical diagnostic test.

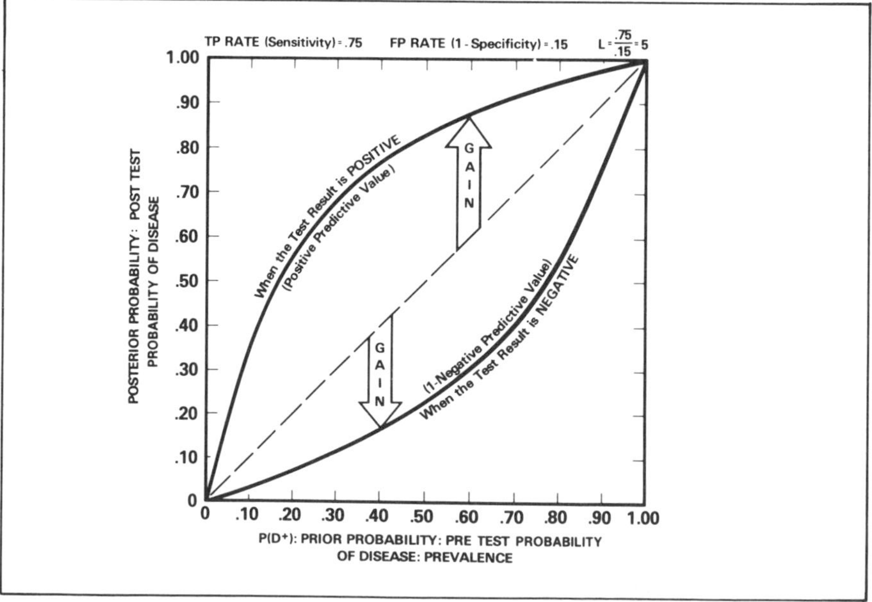

Figure 4-10. The advantages of a pretest likelihood of 40% to 60%.

Moreover, for any diagnostic test the change from pretest to posttest probability of the target disorder is greatest when the pretest probability is 50%. At this level, the presence of the clinical finding or a positive test result virtually clinches the diagnosis and negative diagnostic data effectively eliminate the target disorder from your list of hypotheses. Put another way, a sign, symptom, or laboratory test is of greatest diagnostic use to you when you are in a "50:50" dilemma and cannot decide whether the patient has the target disorder. Thank heaven our tables and formulas converge with our common sense!*

How do you get the pretest probability (prevalence) to 40% to 60%? Getting there has long been one of the mysteries that, because they were difficult to study and articulate, were traditionally called the "art" of medicine. When asked why (on earth!) our teachers had asked the key question of the patient, sought the pathognomonic physical sign, or ordered the definitive laboratory test, most of them mumbled about Osler, "Irish hunches," Avicenna, Willie Sutton, and "clinical judgment."

What has actually happened is the execution of an element of "the science of the art of medicine." These diagnosticians had elicited, without us (or even sometimes them) noticing it, specific points in the patient's history and physical exam that signified a pretest probability of the target disorder in the 40% to 60% range. We will illustrate this with a common diagnostic problem in internal medicine: the ambulatory patient with episodic chest pain. The hypothesis list for such patients usually includes coronary artery disease, and we often consider ordering an exercise electrocardiogram. A positive exercise test will suggest severe coronary artery disease (and we may want to proceed to coronary angiography and aortocoronary bypass), and a negative exercise test will reassure us and the patient and direct our diagnostic effort elsewhere.

Or will it? Table 4-9 summarizes the sensitivity and specificity of the exercise electrocardiogram in coronary artery stenosis (the gold standard for this target disorder was coronary arteriography) [2].

The patients in Table 4-9 had various chest pain syndromes and underwent both exercise electrocardiography and coronary arteriography at a referral center. Using the latter as the gold standard, the exercise ECG had a sensitivity of 60% and a specificity of 91% when 1 mm of ST-segment depression was selected for the cutoff.†

Let us now consider three ambulatory patients with episodic chest pain in whom we are considering ordering an exercise ECG.

*Those who wonder about the common sense of this situation may want to consider whether new information has a greater impact when we are unsure about an issue than when we are almost certain about it.

†Of course, there are newer sorts of exercise tests (but, surprisingly, they haven't been as well evaluated as the older ones) and there's lots more to an exercise ECG than the degree of ST-segment depression, but in the patients who inspired examples B and C these other components were not helpful. Both achieved their age-predicted heart rates at appropriate work loads, their blood pressure responses were normal, neither exhibited any arrhythmias, and both complained of slight anterior neck pain about 2 minutes before the end of their tests that disappeared as soon as they got off the bike.

Table 4-9. The sensitivity and specificity of the exercise ECG in coronary artery stenosis

		70% coronary artery stenosis (by arteriography)		
		Present	Absent	
Exercise ECG	Positive (ST depression ≥1 mm)	137 (a)	11 (b)	148 (a + b)
	Negative (ST depression <1 mm)	90 (c)	112 (d)	202 (c + d)
		a + c 227 Sensitivity = PiD rate = TP rate = $\frac{a}{a+c} = \frac{137}{227} =$ 60%	b + d 123 Specificity = NiH rate = TN rate = $\frac{d}{b+d} = \frac{112}{123} =$ 91%	a + b + c + d 350

Patient A is a 55-year-old mildly hypertensive man with a 4-week history of substernal pressure-pain that radiates to his neck, lower jaw, and down the inner aspect of his left arm. It is precipitated by climbing stairs or walking uphill, and disappears after 3 to 5 minutes of rest. He had a mild episode while undressing for his examination and as his pain was abating you think you heard an S_4 gallop. You decide he has classic angina on effort and consider ordering an exercise ECG to nail down the diagnosis.

Patient B is a 35-year-old man who is otherwise healthy and has no coronary risk factors. He has had "heartburn" for years and now reports a 6-week history of nonexertional, squeezing pain deep to his lower sternum and epigastrium, usually radiating straight through to his back. It is most likely to occur when he lies down after a heavy meal. The remainder of his history and physical exam are negative. You think that his pain is from esophageal spasm and will pursue that diagnosis, but judge that an exercise ECG will rule out significant coronary disease and thus resolve the uncertainty for both of you.

Patient C is a 45-year-old man with a negative past history and no coronary risk factors save a pack-a-day cigarette habit. He reports a 3-week history of precordial and substernal pain, usually fleeting and of a stabbing quality but occasionally as if a heavy weight was on his chest; it is inconsistently related to exertion. On physical exam you find a single costochondral junction that is slightly tender, but pressing on it does not reproduce the patient's pain. You conclude that he may have atypical angina and wonder if an exercise ECG would help.

What are your estimates of the pretest probabilities of significant coronary artery narrowing in each of these patients? Try jotting them down in the margin or, if you are sharing this book with others, on a slip of paper.

As a matter of fact, we do know a fair bit about their pretest probabilities. Based on angiograms or autopsies on several thousand patients with typical and atypical angina and nonanginal pain syndromes [8], their pretest probabilities of significant coronary disease should be: for Patient A, very high (at least 90%); for Patient B, very low (about 5%); and for Patient C, intermediate (about 50%).

How close were your estimates of pretest probability to these published figures? As we pointed out in Chapter 2 on clinical disagreement, clinicians can disagree with one another quite considerably when asked to estimate the probability of specific disorders from patients' symptoms and signs [13]. However, the accuracy of such predictions rises as clinicians gain more experience with the specific target disorder they are attempting to predict [18]. These predictions become even more accurate when the relevant information is organized into tables [9], algorithms [19], or computerized decision trees [7, 18, 35].

There are two messages here. First, if you are already an "expert" in the target disorder you are probably on solid ground in deriving pretest probabilities from clinical data, at least for your own setting. Second, if you are not an expert, then you can either become one, refer your patient to one, or make use of the increasingly common and useful tables of pretest probabilities and algorithms that are found in textbooks and journal articles and, increasingly, computer databases.

There also is a middle ground here. If you are not quite sure of your pretest probability estimate but can confidently specify a range within which it must lie, you can calculate the predictive value or posttest probability for the center point of this range as well as its extremes. In economics, this is called "sensitivity analysis" (not to be confused with the "sensitivity" of a diagnostic test) and permits you to determine how much the posttest probability is affected by uncertainty in the pretest probability. In many other instances uncertainty about the pretest probability of the target disorder can be crucial, and we will provide an example of a sensitivity analysis later. For now, let us return to the exercise ECG example.

Given the estimates from the preceding studies and the sensitivity and specificity of the exercise ECG shown in Table 4-9, how useful will the exercise ECG be in these three patients? Once again, we suggest that you stop reading this and jot down your estimates of the exercise ECG's usefulness in each patient.

We think that the exercise ECG is diagnostically useless in Patients A and B and should not even be carried out in them (at least not for diagnostic purposes). In Patient C, however, we think that the exercise ECG will be extremely valuable. The reasons for our judgments, if not already obvious, should be clear from Table 4-10.

Panel A of Table 4-10 shows us that Patient A's pretest probability of 90% is influenced very little by the results of the exercise ECG, regardless of what they are. We knew the man almost certainly had significant coronary disease before the test; even if it is negative, the probability is still 80% that he has significant

Table 4-10. The usefulness of the exercise ECG in three patients

Panel A: Patient A

Pretest probability = 90%		Coronary disease: Yes	Coronary disease: No		Posttest probability	Change from pretest probability
Exercise ECG	Positive	540 (a)	9 (b)	549	$\frac{a}{a+b} = \frac{540}{549} = 98\%$	+ 8%
	Negative	360 (c)	91 (d)	451	$100\% - \frac{d}{c+d} = 100\% - \frac{91}{451} = 80\%$	− 10%
		900	100	1000	$\frac{a+c}{a+b+c+d} = \frac{900}{1000} = 90\%$	
		$\frac{a}{a+c} = \frac{540}{900} = 60\%$	$\frac{d}{b+d} = \frac{91}{100} = 91\%$			

Panel B: Patient B

Pretest probability = 5%		Coronary disease: Yes	Coronary disease: No		Posttest probability	Change from pretest probability
Exercise ECG	Positive	30 (a)	86 (b)	116	$\frac{a}{a+b} = \frac{30}{116} = 26\%$	+ 21%
	Negative	20 (c)	864 (d)	884	$100\% - \frac{d}{c+d} = 100\% - \frac{864}{884} = 2\%$	− 3%
		50	950	1000	$\frac{a+c}{a+b+c+d} = \frac{50}{1000} = 5\%$	
		$\frac{a}{a+c} = \frac{30}{50} = 60\%$	$\frac{d}{b+d} = \frac{864}{950} = 91\%$			

Table 4-10 (continued)

Panel C: Patient C

Pretest probability = 50%		Coronary disease: Yes	Coronary disease: No		Posttest probability	Change from pretest probability
Exercise ECG	Positive	300 (a)	45 (b)	345	$\frac{a}{a+b} = \frac{300}{345} = 87\%$	+37%
	Negative	200 (c)	455 (d)	655	$100\% - \frac{d}{c+d} = 100\% - \frac{455}{655} = 31\%$	−19%
		500	500	1000	$\frac{a+c}{a+b+c+d} = \frac{500}{1000} = 50\%$	
		$\frac{a}{a+c} = \frac{300}{500} = 60\%$	$\frac{d}{b+d} = \frac{455}{500} = 91\%$			

coronary stenosis.* Patient A does not need an exercise ECG. Rather, the important clinical decision for him is much more likely to be whether we should go directly to coronary angiography (depending on our judgment of the ultimate risks and benefits of finding out whether he is a suitable candidate for one or more bypass grafts).

Patient B does not need an exercise ECG either. We already estimated his pretest probability of significant coronary disease to be only 5%, and *neither* exercise ECG result will alter that likelihood in any important way. Even if his exercise ECG is positive, the odds are still three to one *against* him having significant coronary disease. This is confirmed in panel B of Table 4-10.

It may seem quite cavalier (especially to readers still in subspecialty training) for us to spurn the exercise ECG for Patient B. After all, he did have chest pain (of a sort), and for every 1000 patients like him we will miss 30 who really do have significant coronary heart disease and whose exercise ECGs will be positive (cell *a* of panel B of Table 4-10).

Have we not done these 30 people a disservice by foregoing further testing, especially since the exercise ECG is so safe? The answer lies in weighing the potential good we do the 30 patients who really have significant coronary heart disease and positive exercise ECGs against the potential harm we do to two other groups: first, the 20 people in cell *c* who will be given false-negative clean bills of health (they have had coronary disease but negative exercise ECGs), and second, the 86 people in cell *b* who will receive false-positive, scary labels of severe coronary heart disease when they do not have it. As you will learn in Chapter 5, being told you have a disease (when you do not) is frequently as disabling as actually having it, and almost always more disabling than not knowing that you have a disease (when you do). In our judgment, the harm we do the 86 patients in cell *b* and the 20 in cell *c* outweighs the good we do the 30 in cell *a*, and that is why we would withhold the exercise ECG in such patients. We will come back to this contention, and some ways to resolve it, when we get to the black belt.

However, Patient C can really benefit (at least in a diagnostic way!) from undergoing an exercise ECG, as shown in panel C of Table 4-10. We estimated his pretest probability of significant coronary artery stenosis to be 50%. If his exercise ECG is positive, that probability rises 37%, from 50% to 87%, and we have established his diagnosis. On the other hand, if his exercise ECG is negative, his posttest probability of significant coronary artery stenosis drops 19%, from 50% down to 31%, and we had better consider looking elsewhere for an explanation for his pain.

This latter finding, a posttest probability of 31%, should raise three sorts of uneasy questions in the thoughtful reader. First, recalling our earlier discussion about the uncertainty of our clinical estimates of pretest likelihoods, how "solid"

*Because the posttest probability of *not* having the target disorder after a negative diagnostic test (or negative predictive value) is $(d)/(c + d)$, we subtract the result from 100% to get the posttest probability that the patient *does* have the target disorder *despite* a negative test. Alternatively, we could get the same result by taking $c/(c + d)$.

is this posttest probability of 31%? Second, at what posttest likelihood should we stop the diagnostic process (how low does it have to be to reject the diagnosis, and how high to accept it?). Third, do we really have to quantify our diagnostic uncertainty in this way? Let us take these uneasy questions in order.

First, how accurate is this posttest likelihood of 31% following a negative exercise ECG or, more to the point, how much is it influenced by inaccuracy in our clinical estimate of this patient's pretest probability? To answer this, let us repeat our calculations, using clinically sensible ranges for pretest likelihood taken from the published reports or from our own pretest probabilities we jotted down earlier. The range of published pretest probabilities is furnished by Diamond and Forrester [8], who tell us that the mean (and standard error) for the pretest estimates for individuals such as Patient C are .46(± .018). As it happens, the range enclosed by this mean plus-and-minus-two standard errors will encompass the mean pretest probabilities of 95% of all such samples of such patients (we will not go into the mathematics of this here; the interested reader is referred to any standard textbook of statistics, such as Fleiss [14]). Thus, the pretest probability could be as low as .46 − 2(.018) = .42 or 42% or as high as .46 + 2(.018) = .50 or 50%. This latter pretest probability of 50% formed the starting point for panel C of Table 4-10. If we plug the other extreme figure of .42 into the same diagnostic test, the posttest probability following a negative exercise ECG becomes .24 or 24%, and we have shown this in Table 4-11.

As shown in panel A of Table 4-11, the posttest probability of significant coronary stenosis following a negative exercise ECG is 24%, a bit lower than the result of 31% in panel C of Table 4-10, where the pretest probability was higher, at 50%. Depending on what your "threshold" for further testing or treatment is, this narrow difference between 31% and 24% may or may not make a difference; we will discuss this further when we get to the second uneasy question.

Before we do that, let us consider the common situation in which we do not have such well-researched estimates of pretest probability available. What happens when we have only our own experience to go on, and can narrow the range of plausible pretest probabilities only to somewhere between 30% and 70%? The result is shown in panels B and C of Table 4-11. This sensitivity analysis shows that the exercise ECG provides considerable information even for individuals with pretest probabilities as low as 30% (panel B) or as high as 70% (panel C). In the latter case, however, with a pretest probability of 70%, a negative exercise test hardly rules out coronary disease—the posttest probability remains relatively high at 51%. This posttest probability is over three times that generated for a negative test in a person with a presumed pretest probability of 30%, and we could make a potentially serious mistake in such a case. Rather than end our answer to this first uneasy question on a gloomy note, we will close by reassuring you that experienced clinicians generate far narrower ranges for the pretest probabilities of disorders with which they are familiar than the 30% to 70% we used in this example. Also, useful data bases of pretest probabilities often exist and are becoming easier to find. And even when the pretest probability varied all the way between 30% and 70%, if the exercise test was positive, the clinical diagnosis was essentially confirmed at both ends of the range. One final message of cheer, especially if you found all these calculations tedious: help is on the way! If you stick it out to the brown belt, we will show you how to skip all this computation and convert pretest probabilities to posttest probabilities with a straight-edge and a nomogram.

Our second uneasy question follows from the first: at what posttest probability do we stop the diagnostic process for a given target disorder and either accept it as confirmed or reject it as ruled out? We will answer this one by considering the courses of action open to us when we get back a negative exercise ECG report on Patient C, whose posttest probability as calculated in panel C of Table 4-10 is 31%. We could do four things at this point:

1. We could increase our own sophistication in the interpretation of diagnostic data and see whether his ECG can be interpreted as more than just "negative." For example, if we had a brown belt and could assess his exercise ECG with simple math in our heads, we could recognize that an exercise ECG displaying less than .5 mm of ST-segment depression means that his posttest probability of severe coronary stenosis is, in fact, only 17% (about half of what it appears to be using our green belt). We hope that this eye-opener will show you how much information we toss out when we reduce a wide spectrum of diagnostic test results to the positive/negative dichotomy. We also hope this eye-opener will whet your appetite for the later parts of this chapter.
2. We could go for the gold standard and have Patient C angiographed. This is not a very attractive alternative in terms of discomfort, risk, cost, and the fact (again confirmed in panel C of Table 4-10) that two-thirds of such patients would have negative angiograms.
3. We could apply other noninvasive tests for coronary artery disease in the hope that they would decisively shift the posttest probability further. Suppose, for example, we go on to perform radionuclide angiocardiography* on Patient C and it is negative as well. Can we make use of this information? Yes we can, if we could find information like that shown in Table 4-12.

   In Table 4-12, both tests have been applied to the same patients with (panel I) and without (panel II) coronary artery stenosis. For example, in panel I, where all the patients were shown to have $\geqslant 70\%$ coronary artery stenosis on a subsequent coronary arteriogram, the 276 patients in cell *a* had both positive radionuclide studies and positive exercise ECGs. The 61 patients in cell *c* had negative results for both studies, and patients in the cells noted by *x* had a positive result on one test and a negative result on the other. We can then combine the results of these two panels into a simple (2 × 2) table in two different ways, and this is shown in Table 4-13.

   In panel I of Table 4-13, the two-test combination is called "positive" only if both individual tests are positive, and the combination is called "negative" if either or both individual tests are negative. In panel II of this table, which

*In many centers this second test would be an echocardiogram. The diagnostic principles and calculations are the same, regardless of the second test.

Table 4-11. The usefulness of the exercise ECG for a range of pretest likelihoods

Panel A

Pretest probability = 42%		Coronary stenosis: Present	Coronary stenosis: Absent		Posttest probability	Change from pretest probability
Exercise ECG	Positive	252 (a)	52 (b)	304	$\frac{a}{a+b} = \frac{252}{304} = 83\%$	+41%
	Negative	168 (c)	528 (d)	696	$100\% - \frac{d}{c+d} = 100\% - \frac{528}{696} = 24\%$	−18%
		420	580	1000	$\frac{a+c}{a+b+c+d} = \frac{420}{1000} = 42\%$	
		$\frac{a}{a+c} = \frac{252}{420} = 60\%$	$\frac{d}{b+d} = \frac{528}{580} = 91\%$			

Panel B

Pretest probability = 30%		Coronary stenosis: Present	Coronary stenosis: Absent		Posttest probability	Change from pretest probability
Exercise ECG	Positive	180 (a)	63 (b)	243	$\frac{a}{a+b} = \frac{180}{243} = 74\%$	+44%
	Negative	120 (c)	637 (d)	757	$100\% - \frac{d}{c+d} = 100\% - \frac{637}{757} = 16\%$	−14%
		300	700	1000	$\frac{a+c}{a+b+c+d} = \frac{300}{1000} = 30\%$	
		$\frac{a}{a+c} = \frac{180}{300} = 60\%$	$\frac{d}{b+d} = \frac{637}{700} = 91\%$			

Table 4-11 (continued)

Panel C

Pretest probability = 70%		Coronary stenosis: Present	Coronary stenosis: Absent		Posttest probability	Change from pretest probability
Exercise ECG	Positive	420 (a)	27 (b)	447	$\frac{a}{a+b} = \frac{420}{447} = 94\%$	+24%
	Negative	280 (c)	273 (d)	553	$100\% - \frac{d}{c+d} = 100\% - \frac{273}{553} = 51\%$	−19%
		700	300	1000	$\frac{a+c}{a+b+c+d} = \frac{700}{1000} = 70\%$	
		$\frac{a}{a+c} =$	$\frac{d}{b+d} =$			
		$\frac{420}{700} = 60\%$	$\frac{273}{300} = 91\%$			

Table 4-12. The combination of radionuclide angiocardiography and exercise ECGs in the diagnosis of coronary artery stenosis

Panel I: Patients with ≥70% stenosis

		Radionuclide study		
		Positive	Negative	
Exercise ECG	Positive	276 (a)	23 (x)	299
	Negative	140 (x)	61 (c)	201
		416	84	500

Panel II: Patients with <70% stenosis

		Radionuclide study		
		Positive	Negative	
Exercise ECG	Positive	26 (b)	18 (y)	44
	Negative	164 (y)	292 (d)	456
		190	310	500

makes the most of Patient C's test results (both of which were negative), the two-test combination is called "positive" if either or both tests are positive, but the combination is called "negative" only if both individual tests are negative.

Both Patient C's exercise ECG and his radionuclide angiocardiogram are negative, and his pretest probability of serious coronary stenosis (based on his initial history and physical) was 50%. If we apply panel II of Table 4-13 to his situation, we find a negative predictive value of 83%. His probability of serious coronary stenosis is now 100% − 83% = 17% and we have, indeed, gained something by applying a second diagnostic test. Once again, the facts of the situation and our common sense are in accord.

Before we leave this topic, compare the sensitivities and specificities of panels I and II in Table 4-13. Demanding that both of a pair of diagnostic tests are positive, as in panel I, maximizes specificity and minimizes false-positive "labeling" of innocent patients, but pays the price of lots of false-negative "missed" diagnoses, a shortcoming that can be avoided by demanding that both of a pair of diagnostic tests are negative, as in panel II. This maximizes sensitivity and minimizes false-negative "missed" diagnoses alright, but note how false-positive "labeling" soars in this situation (and would become even higher as the pretest probability or prevalence of coronary ste-

Table 4-13. Two different ways to combine two diagnostic tests

Panel I

	Coronary stenosis: Present	Coronary stenosis: Absent		
Both tests positive	276 (a)	26 (b)	302	Positive predictive value = $\frac{a}{a + b} = \frac{276}{302} = 91\%$
One or both tests negative	224 (c + x)	474 (d + y)	698	Negative predictive value = $\frac{d + y}{(c + x) + (d + y)} = \frac{474}{698} = 68\%$
	500	500	1000	
	Sensitivity = $\frac{a}{a + (c + x)} = \frac{276}{500} = 55\%$	Specificity = $\frac{d + y}{b + (d + y)} = \frac{474}{500} = 95\%$		

Panel II

	Coronary stenosis			
	Present	Absent		
One or both tests positive	439 (a+x)	208 (b+y)	647	Positive predictive value $= \frac{a + x}{(a + x) + (b + y)} = \frac{439}{647} = 68\%$
Both tests negative	61 (c)	292 (d)	353	Negative predictive value $= \frac{d}{c + d} = \frac{292}{353} = 83\%$
	500	500	1000	
	Sensitivity $= \frac{a + x}{(a + x) + c} = \frac{439}{500} = 88\%$	Specificity $= \frac{d}{(b + y) + d} = \frac{292}{500} = 58\%$		

nosis fell). Returning to our main topic, we have identified three strategies for dealing with an equivocal diagnostic situation: become more sophisticated in interpreting the diagnostic test result already at hand, apply the gold standard, or apply a second diagnostic test. The fourth and final strategy simply contrasts the current probability of this diagnosis with the current probabilities for the other diagnosis on the "short list."

4. Finally, we could compare this posttest likelihood of 31% with the probabilities we have assigned to the other diagnostic hypotheses on our short list. If chest wall pain now jumps to the fore with a probability of 65%, we may want to watch and wait.

This last option holds the answer to our second uneasy question: You toss out (or accept) a diagnostic hypothesis when its probability (suitably tempered by considering the harm you will do if you are wrong) is substantially lower (or higher) than the probability of other diagnostic hypotheses on your short list. If the harm you can do by missing a diagnosis is great you will demand a very low probability (< 5%) before you toss it out; that is why even patients with only 10% to 15% pretest probabilities of myocardial infarction still go to the coronary care unit and undergo serial enzyme determinations and daily ECGs. Conversely, if the harm you can do by overdiagnosis is great, you will demand a very high posttest probability (> 95%) before you accept it as established; that is why we insist on tissue diagnosis before we tell patients they have cancer and why we call patients back repeatedly for more blood pressure measurements before we label them hypertensive. When misdiagnosis carries lower penalties we relax, and may reject a diagnostic hypothesis at 40%, or accept it at 60%.

The preceding discussion underscores our third uneasy question: Do we really have to quantify our diagnostic uncertainty in this way?

Only if we want to improve as clinicians. Of course, we deal in uncertainty in everything we do. We cannot be sure about the patient's history, our physical exam, the lab test results, the diagnosis, the patient's prognosis, or whether the treatment will work (even if the patient does take the medicine we have prescribed)! How should we handle this uncertainty? Should we simply deny it, and behave as if uncertainty did not exist? This solution, in addition to being irrational, requires a powerful authoritarian structure to insure that uncertainty, when it does occur, is blamed on inexperience or sloth.

Alternatively, should we acknowledge uncertainty but dress it in nonthreatening words rather than in stark numbers? "Rarely," "doubtful," "often," and "classic" are less threatening to their authors and audience than are 5%, 20%, 60%, and 85%, respectively. One reason for our comfort with words rather than numbers as expressions of uncertainty is the illusion of precision that they impart to our clinical notes and discussions. Although this solution has been criticized for centuries,* its paradoxical nature was only recently revealed by Bryant and Norman [5]. As we pointed out in Chapter 2, when these two investigators gath-

*During the postrevolutionary heyday of the Paris hospitals, Pierre Charles Alexandre Louis called for the abandonment of the terms *often, rarely,* and *many* [1].

ered 30 such terms from diagnostic reports, got 16 clinicians to estimate, to the nearest 5%, the probability of disease corresponding to each of these words, and cajoled them into repeating the whole exercise a week later, two important findings emerged. First, the degree of intraclinician agreement was huge (the correlation between first and second estimates by the same clinician was + .96). Second, the degree of interclinician agreement was dismal. "Doubtful" meant as low as 5% to some clinicians, but as high as 80% to others, and "classic" ranged from a low of 60% all the way to 99%. In fact, 21 of the 30 words exhibited ranges of meaning in excess of 50%. Here, then, is the paradox: *we* know what we mean when we say "doubtful" or "classic," but *nobody else* does! The moral for radiologists (and for any other health professionals who interpret diagnostic data for their colleagues), teachers, and any clinicians who practice in teams is clear: Louis was right, and these terms must be abandoned.

We can no longer ignore this uncertainty, nor can we pass it off as the "art" of medicine. It is time to master the science of the art of medicine and confront this uncertainty. Certainty is a delusion, and uncertainty can, within limits, be quantified to the benefit of the patient. We echo the advice of one of the heroes of Chapter 2, David Spodick: ". . . physicians must be content to end not in certainties, but rather in statistical probabilities. The modern (physician) thus has a right to feel certain, within statistical constraints, but never cocksure. Absolute certainty remains for some theologians—and like-minded physicians." [41].

So there you are. If you want to do it with a simple table:

1. Identify the sensitivity and specificity of the sign, symptom, or diagnostic test you plan to use. Many are already published, and subspecialists worth their salt ought either to know them for their field or to be able to track them down for you. Depending on whether you are considering a sign, a symptom, or a diagnostic laboratory test, you will want to track down a clinical subspecialist, a radiologist, a pathologist, or other expert.
2. Start your table, as shown in the top panel of Table 4-14. Make the grand total $(a + b + c + d) = 1000$.
3. Now, using whatever information you have about the patient *before* you apply this diagnostic test, estimate his or her pretest probability (prevalence) of the target disorder. The next trick is to put appropriate numbers at the bottom of the columns $(a + c)$ and $(b + d)$. The easiest way to do this is to express your pretest probability as a decimal (for example, 33% = .33) and multiply it by 1000, or move the decimal three places to the right (in our example, .33 becomes 330). This result is $(a + c)$, and 1000 minus this result is $(b + d)$.
4. Now you can start to fill in the cells inside the table. Multiply sensitivity (expressed as a decimal) by $(a + c)$ and put the result in cell a. You can then calculate cell c by simple subtraction. This is shown in the second panel of Table 4-14.
5. Similarly, multiply specificity (expressed as a decimal) by $(b + d)$, put the rest in cell d (careful!), and calculate cell b by subtraction. This is shown in the third panel of Table 4-14.

6. Now you can calculate the predictive values (posttest likelihoods, posterior probabilities, as we have been doing throughout this section), and you have your answer. This is shown in the final panel of Table 4-14.

To see whether you have mastered the green belt, try the following example: Suppose you have an alcoholic patient with biopsy-proven portal cirrhosis who, over the course of a few weeks, starts to lose energy, gain weight, and accumulate ascites. He denies alcohol intake and his other signs and symptoms are unchanged. Your differential diagnosis includes hepatoma (you estimate the probability that he has this as 25%), and you order some laboratory tests, including an α-fetoprotein determination.

If this test has a sensitivity of 98% and a specificity of 90% for hepatoma in patients with cirrhosis, what is the posttest probability of this diagnosis in your patient if the test comes back positive? Our answer is in the footnote on page 152.

If you handled the preceding example, you have earned your green belt, and have reached a level of understanding a fair bit beyond the rule-in, rule-out level of the yellow belt. You already can do more than most clinicians, and you may want to stop here, at least for a while.

On the other hand, if you want to go further, take up the blue belt and learn how to handle slightly more complex tables with multiple cutoffs. Along the way, you will find more powerful ways to combine two or more diagnostic tests, will understand how an ROC curve works, and will learn to take advantage of the *degree* of positivity and negativity of diagnostic tests.

Chunk #3 Blue Belt: Doing It with a More Complex Table

Examine Table 4-15. It extends the tables we used for the green belt to several rows, rather than just two. As a result, they retain more of the information that we presented back in Figure 4-1.

Several of the cutoffs in Table 4-15 might look familiar. The cutoff at 40 is the *x* or rule-out (SnNout) cutoff from Figure 4-6, and you met it back when you were getting your yellow belt for "doing it with pictures." The cutoff at 80 is the one we used in the previous section on "doing it with a simple table," and the one at 280 is the *y* or rule-in (SpPin) cutoff, again from Figure 4-6. You will note that the cutoffs need not be evenly spaced (the bottom 3 are 40 IU apart, but there is a jump of 200 to the top one).

Where do we go from here? How do we generate sensitivity and specificity from this more complex table? We do it by creating a series of simple tables, each of which uses a different cutoff from the complex table, as shown in Table 4-16.

The left-hand panel of Table 4-16 simply replicates Table 4-15 and displays the number of patients with and without infarcts who have various levels of CK. The right-hand panels of Table 4-16 display all the simple tables that could be generated from the complex one. Thus, when the cutoff is placed ≥ 280, cell *a* contains the 97 infarct patients whose CK levels were ≥ 280 and cell *c* contains

Table 4-14. Doing it with a simple table

		Target disorder: Present	Target disorder: Absent	
Test	Positive	a	b	
	Negative	c	d	
		a+c Prevalence × 1000		a+b+c+d 1000

		Target disorder: Present	Target disorder: Absent	
Test	Positive	Sensitivity × (a + c) a	b	
	Negative	(a + c) − a c	d	
		a+c	b+d	a+b+c+d

		Target disorder: Present	Target disorder: Absent	
Test	Positive	a	(b + d) − d b	
	Negative	c	d Specificity × (b + d)	
		a+c	b+d	a+b+c+d

		Target disorder: Present	Target disorder: Absent	
Test	Positive	a	b	a+b
	Negative	c	d	c+d

$$\text{Positive predictive value} = \frac{a}{a + b} \qquad \text{Negative predictive value} = \frac{d}{c + d}$$

Table 4-15. Doing it with a more complex table

		Myocardial infarction	
		Present	Absent
CK test result	⩾280	97	1
	80–279	118	15
	40–79	13	26
	1–39	2	88
		230	130

the 133 infarct patients (118 + 13 + 2 = 133) whose CK levels were < 280. And so forth across the remaining panels.

At the bottom of the table we have calculated the sensitivities (PiD rates, TP rates) and specificities (NiH rates, TN rates) for each cutoff. A comparison of these sensitivities and specificities reminds us once again that as one goes up, the other goes down. The extreme right-hand panel simply points out that we can always achieve a sensitivity of 100% if we are willing to drop specificity to zero. As we shall now show you, the gain in predictive value (posttest probability of the target disorder) that follows switching from a simple table to a more complex one may be very great. Consider two patients who enter a coronary care unit with suspected myocardial infarctions, with identical pretest probabilities of 64% as in Table 4-16 where 230/360 = 64%. Suppose that the first patient (A) has a CK of 400 and the second patient (B) a CK of 30. The effect of different cutoffs on the posttest probability of infarction is shown in Table 4-17.

The selection of a cutoff of 280, shown in the top panel of Table 4-17, helped maximize the information gained for Patient A (whose CK was 400). This patient's probability of infarction rose from a pretest value of 64% to a posttest value of 99%, and an infarct is virtually certain. We did not learn much about Patient B (whose CK was 30), though. The change in probability was small, from 64% down to 51%. However, for Patient B we learn more from lower cutoffs, and learn the most from a cutoff of 40, as shown in the bottom panel of Table 4-17. There, Patient B's probability of myocardial infarction falls from 64% down to 2% and we have ruled out this diagnostic hypothesis.

So, this method of doing it with more complex tables permits us to gain more from diagnostic tests than we could with single, simpler tables. This method also helps us understand combinations of tests a bit better, as shown in Tables 4-18 and 4-19.

You may already have realized that Tables 4-18 and 4-19 replicate, using your new understanding, Table 4-13 (all we have done is to express the negative predictive value as its complement, the posttest probability of the target disorder following a negative test result). Once again, the more complex table permits us to achieve a greater pretest to posttest probability change for patients with extreme test results (both tests positive or both tests negative).

Table 4-16. A series of simple tables from one complex table

CK test result		Myocardial infarction: Present	Myocardial infarction: Absent
	≥280	97	1
	80–279	118	15
	40–79	13	26
	1–39	2	88
		230	130

Effect of placing cutoff at various CK levels	a	b	c	d	Sensitivity	Specificity
≥280	97	1	133	129	42%	99%
≥80	215	16	15	114	93%	88%
≥40	228	42	2	88	99%	68%
≥1	230	130	0	0	100%	0%

$$\text{Sensitivity (PiD rate, TP rate)} = \frac{a}{a + c}$$

$$\text{Specificity (NiH rate, TN rate)} = \frac{d}{b + d}$$

Table 4-17. The effect of different cutoffs on the posttest probability of the target disorder

Cutoff at ≥280

		Infarction	
		Present	Absent
CK result	>280	97 (a)	1 (b)
	<280	133 (c)	129 (d)

Posttest probability of infarction

Patient A*: $\frac{a}{a+b} = \frac{97}{98} = 99\%$

Patient B*: $\frac{c}{c+d} = \frac{133}{262} = 51\%$

Cutoff at 80

		Infarction	
		Present	Absent
CK result	≥80	215 (a)	16 (b)
	<80	15 (c)	114 (d)

Posttest probability of infarction

Patient A : $\frac{a}{a+b} = \frac{215}{231} = 93\%$

Patient B : $\frac{c}{c+d} = \frac{15}{129} = 12\%$

Cutoff at 40

		Infarction	
		Present	Absent
CK result	≥40	228 (a)	42 (b)
	<40	2 (c)	88 (d)

Posttest probability of infarction

Patient A : $\frac{a}{a+b} = \frac{228}{270} = 84\%$

Patient B : $\frac{c}{c+d} = \frac{2}{90} = 2\%$

*Patients A's CK = 400 and patient B's CK = 30; the pretest probability of infarction for both patients was 64%.

Table 4-18. A more complex table of two diagnostic tests for coronary artery stenosis

	Target disorder (coronary artery stenosis)	
	Present	Absent
Both positive	276	26
One positive	163	182
Both negative	61	292
	500	500

Sensitivity (PiD rate, TP rate) $= \frac{a}{a + c}$

Specificity (NiH rate, TN rate) $= \frac{d}{b + d}$

Effect of placing cutoff at different levels			
Between one and both positive		Between one and both negative	
276 (a)	26 (b)	439 (a)	208 (b)
224 (c)	474 (d)	61 (c)	292 (d)
55%	95%	88%	58%

Table 4-19. The effect of different combinations of two test results on the posttest probability of coronary artery stenosis*

Cutoff between one and both positive	Coronary artery stenosis: Present	Coronary artery stenosis: Absent		Posttest probability of target disorder
Both tests positive	276 (a)	26 (b)	302	$\frac{a}{a+b} = \frac{276}{302} = 91\%$
One or both tests negative	224 (c)	474 (d)	698	$\frac{c}{c+d} = \frac{224}{698} = 32\%$
	500	500	1000	

Cutoff between one and both negative	Coronary artery stenosis: Present	Coronary artery stenosis: Absent		Posttest probability of target disorder
One or both tests positive	439 (a)	208 (b)	647	$\frac{a}{a+b} = \frac{439}{647} = 68\%$
Both tests negative	61 (c)	292 (d)	353	$\frac{c}{c+d} = \frac{61}{353} = 17\%$
	500	500	1000	

*In both panels, the pretest probability of coronary artery stenosis is 50%.

As you probably have recognized, changes or differences in prevalence (pretest probability of the target disorder) are managed just as they were with the simple tables. Something that you may not have recognized, however, is that you now know a bit about ROC curves!*

Look again at Table 4-16. Along the bottom, we have listed the sensitivity (the PiD rate or TP rate) and specificity (the NiH rate or TN rate) that characterize each cutoff.

The TN rate is, of course, $d/(b + d)$ or (true-negatives)/(false-positives + true-negatives). We could therefore generate a complementary rate, $b/(b + d)$ and call it the false-positive rate or *FP rate*.* And, of course, for any table the FP rate plus the TN rate would sum to 100%. We could therefore add another row to Table 4-16, with FP rates along it, and the result would look like Table 4-20. As expected from realizing that FP rate = (100% − specificity), TP rates and FP rates rise and fall together.

An ROC curve is simply a *graph* of the pairs of TP rates (sensitivity or PiD rates) and FP rates (100% − specificity or 100% − the NiH rate or TN rate) that correspond to each possible cutoff for the diagnostic test result. We have drawn such an ROC curve for CK in myocardial infarction and it appears in Figure 4-11. (For completeness, we have added a point where both the TP rate and the FP rate are zero. To test your understanding so far, what cutoff is this?)†

Figure 4-11 provides a picture of the implications of using different cutoffs, and such ROC curves have some interesting properties. For example, the upper left-hand corner of Figure 4-11 denotes a perfect diagnostic test: a TP rate of 1.00 (all patients with the target disorder are detected: super-SnNout!) and an FP rate of .0 (no one without the target disorder is falsely labeled: super-SpPin!). It

Table 4-20. TP rates and FP rates for different CK cutoffs

	CK cutoff			
	≥280	≥80	≥40	≥1
TP rate (sensitivity, PiD rate)	42%	93%	99%	100%
Specificity (NiH rate, TN rate)	99%	88%	68%	0%
FP rate (100% − specificity)	1%	12%	32%	100%

*There are at least 3 definitions of the false-positive rate in the literature. The one we use here is (1 − specificity) or $b/(b + d)$; a second is (1 − positive predictive value) or $b/(a + b)$; the third determines the proportion of false positives among all patients tested: $b/(a + b + c + d)$ [15]. When reading about false-positive rates, therefore, it would be important to find out which definition was in use.

†The cutoff where the TP rate and FP rate both equal zero lies somewhere beyond the most extremely positive test result. So much for completeness: It makes the curve tidy but adds little to understanding.

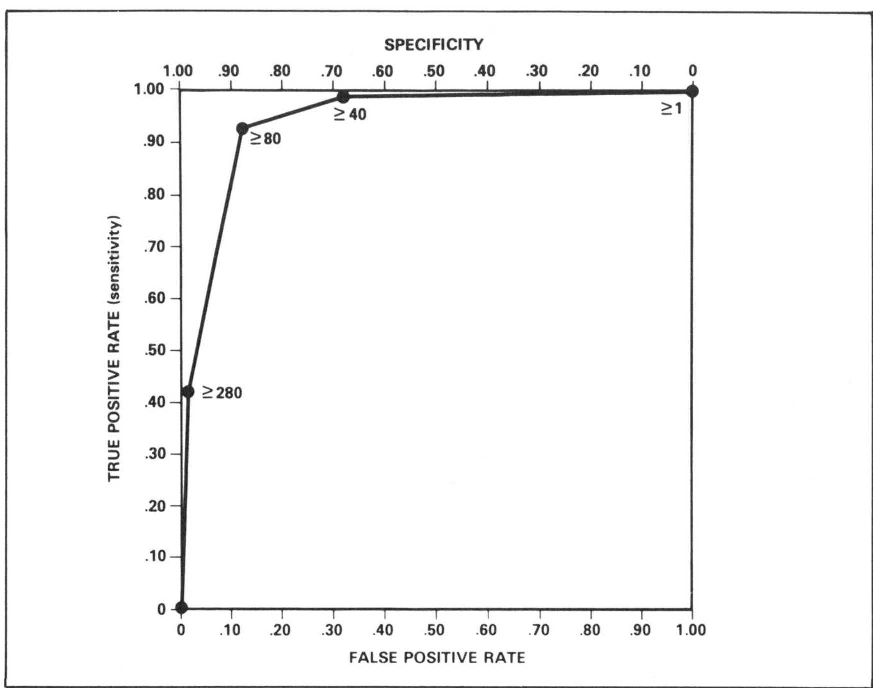

Figure 4-11. An ROC curve for CK values in myocardial infarction.

follows that the point on an ROC curve that is *closest* to this upper left-hand corner is the "best" cutoff in terms of making the fewest mistakes when prevalence is at or around 50% (that is, its use minimizes the sum of false-positives plus false-negatives). You can confirm this by relating Figure 4-11 to Table 4-16. In the former, the closest point to the upper left corner is for the cutoff at 80 CK IU. In Table 4-16 the sum of cells *b* and *c* (that is, the mistakes) for this cutoff is 31; for any other cutoffs in Table 4-16, the sum of cells *b* and *c* is greater than 31. You also may want to look again back at Figure 4-7 and note where the histograms for patients who do and do not have infarcts cross one another. It is at 80 IU and is saying this same thing in a different way.

Finally, one other feature about this upper left-hand corner: It is where (sensitivity + specificity)/2 attains its highest value. Of course, there is much more to picking the correct cutoff than simply minimizing the sum of false-positives plus false-negatives, as you will recall from our earlier discussions. Only if your patient suffered equally from a false-positive and false-negative diagnosis would you seek the upper left-hand cutoff. If false-positive labeling were very harmful, you would select a more leftward (SpPin-ish) cutoff that minimized the false-positive rate. If, on the other hand, false-negative misses were highly dangerous, you would select a (SnNout-ish) cutoff that maximized the true-positive rate.

One last comment about "doing it with a more complex table" and the resulting ROC curves. This strategy can be used to compare the usefulness of two different signs, symptoms, or diagnostic tests for the same target disorder. All you need to do is plot their ROC curves: the one that lies farthest to the "northwest" is the more accurate.*

Well, that is about all we have to say about "doing it with a more complex table." It is especially useful when a diagnostic test produces a wide range of results and when your patient is near one of the extremes, where you can invoke SnNout or SpPin. What you do is:

1. Identify the several cutoffs that could be used.
2. Fill in a complex table along the lines of Table 4-15, showing the numbers of patients at each level who do and do not have the target disorder.
3. Then generate a simple table for each cutoff, as in Table 4-16, and determine its sensitivity and specificity at each of them.
4. Select the cutoff that makes the most sense for your patient's test result and proceed as you did for your green belt.

If you successfully grappled with the foregoing, award yourself a blue belt. If you looked very hard at what was happening, however, we suspect that you noticed that the blue belt is not very useful for patients in the middle zones of test results or for patients with just one positive result from a two-test combination; their posttest probabilities lurch back and forth past 50%, depending on where the cutoff is placed.

You can overcome this problem by taking up the next chunk. It involves some math, but you will find that the clinical application can be done with a simple nomogram or in your head.

Chunk #4 Brown Belt: Doing It with Simple Math in Your Head

Welcome to the brown belt, both those of you who jumped here directly from the yellow belt and those who earned their green and blue belts along the way. The preceding three chunks are all very nice, but we must admit that, with the exception of SpPin and SnNout, they are pretty cumbersome. Do you really want to carry graph paper and scratch pads wherever you go? Well, as it happens, once you have mastered the principles of the yellow belt (or the green belt or the blue belt) you are ready for a great leap forward, and we will show you how to accomplish this here. It involves some more calculations at the start, but once you understand these you should be able to arm yourself with some simple tables (just like the "normal values" tables you probably carry now) and be able to come up with a patient's posttest probability of a target disorder using just a simple nomogram or some mental arithmetic.

We start by generating a new index of how good a diagnostic test is. This new index, which is called a "likelihood ratio," contrasts the proportions of patients with and without the target disorder who display a given level of a diagnostic

*Stated more formally, the sign, symptom, or lab test whose ROC curve encloses (below and to the right) the largest area is the most accurate one.

test result (by "given level" we mean the presence [or absence] of a sign or symptom or any of the levels of a laboratory test result such as those shown in Figure 4-3). As a result, a *likelihood ratio expresses the odds that a given level of a diagnostic test result would be expected in a patient with (as opposed to one without) the target disorder*.

Let's calculate some likelihood ratios and learn their properties. Table 4-21 recapitulates Table 4-4 from the green belt and adds likelihood ratios to it. Because rounding a number like .9348 early in a series of calculations can markedly distort the ultimate answer, we have kept four decimal places in these calculations and then rounded the answers.

The likelihood ratio for a positive test result (CK 80 IU or above) is 7.6, and that means that CK results of this sort are 7.6 times as likely to come from patients *with* infarcts as from patients *without* infarcts. A closer inspection of the proportions that make up this likelihood ratio should evoke recent memories for holders of green or blue belts, for the first proportion ($a/[a + c] = 215/230 = .9348$) is our old friend sensitivity (the PiD rate or TP rate), and the second proportion ($b/[b + d] = 16/130 = .1231$) is 1 − specificity (the FP rate).

The likelihood ratio for a negative test result (CK less than 80 IU) is .07, and that means that CK results of this sort are less than one-tenth as likely to come from patients with infarcts as from patients without infarcts. The proportions that comprise this likelihood ratio for a negative CK test should look familiar as well, for the first one ($c/[a + c] = 15/230 = .0652$) is the complement of sensitivity, the FN rate, and the second one ($d/[b + d] = 114/130 = .8769$ is specificity (the NiH rate or TN rate).

Likelihood ratios possess three properties, the cmbination of which makes the brown belt a very powerful diagnostic strategy. First, because the proportions that make up the likelihood ratio are calculated "vertically" like sensitivity and specificity, likelihood ratios need not change with changes in the prevalence (or pretest probability) of the target disorder. In fact, as you will see shortly, they may be much more stable than even sensitivity or specificity with changes in prevalence. This is because of their second property, the option of calculating likelihood ratios for *several* levels of the sign, symptom, or laboratory test result, rather than just the two levels we have worked with up to now. Table 4-22 shows this second property in action.

Table 4-22 is derived from Table 4-15, and considers four different levels of the CK results. Rather than collapsing these four levels into individual "2 × 2" dichotomies as we did in the blue belt, however, we can preserve all four levels and assign a likelihood ratio to each one. Note how the range of likelihood ratios has dramatically widened from Table 4-21 (a 109-fold range from .07–7.6) to Table 4-22 (a 5500-fold range from .01–55). We have enormously increased the clinical information content of our diagnostic test result! Moreover, we have in a sense come full circle back to "doing it with pictures" and the yellow belt. The top group, with CK results ⩾ 280, corresponds to the rule-in, SpPin, or *y* cutoff of the yellow belt, and the bottom group, with CK results < 40, corresponds to the rule-out, SnNout, or *x* cutoff. While capitalizing on these positive

Table 4-21. How likelihood ratios are generated

		Myocardial infarction				
		Present		Absent		
		Number	Proportion	Number	Proportion	Likelihood ratio
CK test result	Positive (≥ 80 IU)	215 [a]	$\frac{a}{a+c} = \frac{215}{230} = 0.9348$	16 [b]	$\frac{b}{b+d} = \frac{16}{130} = 0.1231$	$\frac{0.9348}{0.1231} = 7.6$
	Negative (< 80 IU)	15 [c]	$\frac{c}{a+c} = \frac{15}{230} = 0.0652$	114 [d]	$\frac{d}{b+d} = \frac{114}{130} = 0.8769$	$\frac{0.0652}{0.8769} = 0.07$
		230 [a+c]		130 [b+d]		

Table 4-22. Likelihood ratios for several levels of a diagnostic test result

		Myocardial infarction				
		Present		Absent		
		Number	Proportion	Number	Proportion	Likelihood ratio
CK test result	⩾280	97	$\frac{97}{230} = 0.4217$	1	$\frac{1}{130} = 0.0077$	$\frac{0.4217}{0.0077} = 55$
	80–279	118	$\frac{118}{230} = 0.5130$	15	$\frac{15}{130} = 0.1154$	$\frac{0.5130}{0.1154} = 4.4$
	40–79	13	$\frac{13}{230} = 0.0565$	26	$\frac{26}{130} = 0.2000$	$\frac{0.0565}{0.2000} = 0.3$
	1–39	2	$\frac{2}{230} = 0.0087$	88	$\frac{88}{130} = 0.6769$	$\frac{0.0087}{0.6769} = 0.01$
		230		130		

features of "doing it with pictures," the likelihood ratio approach also overcomes a major shortcoming of the yellow belt approach: ambiguity over patients in the "no man's land" between the *x* and *y* cutoffs. The likelihood ratio approach subdivides these patients and distinguishes among them very well.

We stated earlier that likelihood ratios are more stable than sensitivity or specificity when prevalence changes. This is because of our previous caution that if the mix (mild versus severe) of patients with the target disorder varies when their prevalence varies, sensitivity and specificity will change as well as predictive values. Because likelihood ratios can be generated for quite narrow "slices" of a diagnostic test result, they will be less susceptible to such changes in the mix of patients with the target disorder.

The third property of the likelihood ratio is the most delightful of all, for it can be used in a very powerful way to shorten a list of diagnostic hypotheses, because:

The pretest odds for the target disorder	×	The likelihood ratio for the diagnostic test result	=	The posttest odds for the target disorder

As a result, if you start from your clinical estimate of the odds* that your patient has a certain target disorder, and then carry out a diagnostic test and apply the likelihood ratio that corresponds to your patient's test result, you can calculate new, posttest odds for the target disorder.

Suppose that you are working up a man with chest pain and you judge that the probability that he has had a myocardial infarction is about 50% (that corresponds to an odds of 50:50 or 1:1). Suppose further that his initial CK result comes back at 180 IU. A quick look at Table 4-22 will confirm that the likelihood ratio for this CK result is 4.4, and you can then apply the third property of likelihood ratios as follows:

The pretest odds for the target disorder	×	The likelihood ratio for the diagnostic test result	=	The posttest odds for the target disorder
1:1	×	4.4	=	4.4:1

The posttest odds can be converted back to a probability of 81%, and your tentative diagnosis is firming up nicely.

This example emphasizes both the diagnostic power of the likelihood ratio strategy and a major drawback to its use. Although it can help us get the most out of the diagnostic tests we use, the need to switch back and forth between probabilities and odds is off-putting at best, and frequently scares clinicians away. We suggest two solutions. The first one (which we first discovered in a letter from Terrance Fagan [12]) uses a nomogram that obviates the need to switch back and forth. The nomogram we use appears in Figure 4-12.

*Punters (and even touts) can avoid confusion by recognizing that these are odds *for* the target disorder, as opposed to the odds we encounter at the greyhound track which are *against* the dog winning the race.

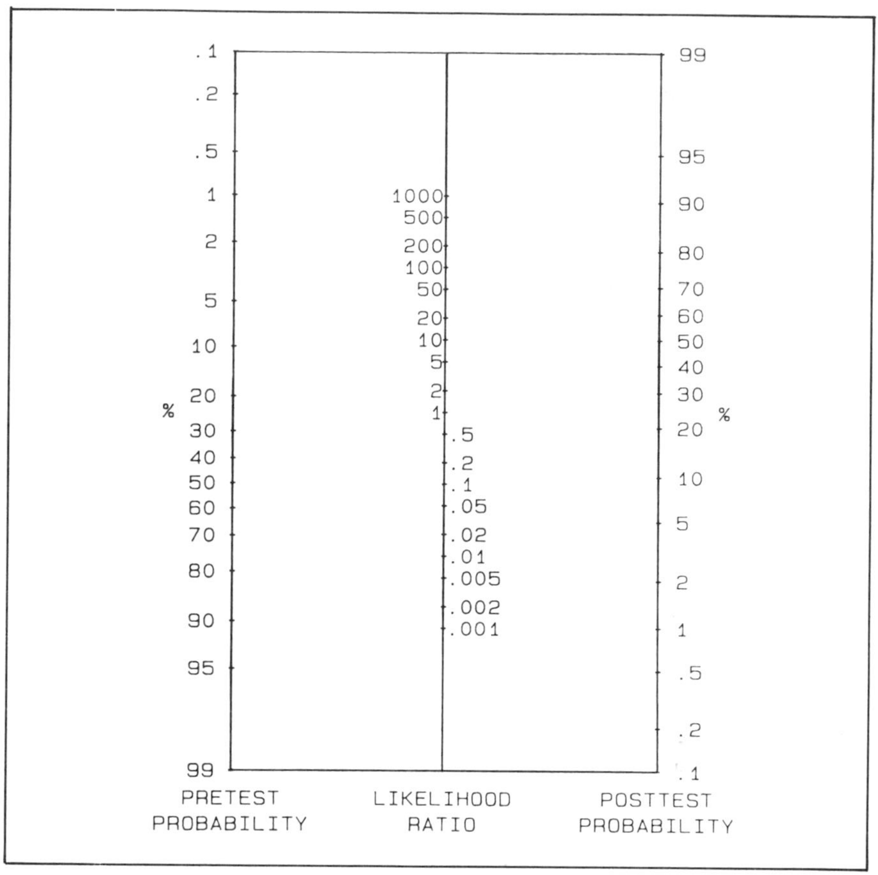

Figure 4-12. A nomogram for applying likelihood ratios. (Adapted from T. J. Fagan. Nomogram for Bayes' theorem. *N. Engl. J. Med.* [Letter] 293:257, 1975.)

In this nomogram, both pretest and posttest odds are already converted to their corresponding probabilities (expressed as percents), and we need not trip over the calculations. Going back to our patient with chest pain, we simply anchor a ruler or other straightedge at the pretest probability of 50% on the left. We then pivot the ruler on this anchor until it also lines up with the likelihood ratio of 4.4 (a bit below 5) in the middle of the nomogram. Sighting along the ruler to the right, we see that the posttest probability is about 80%, and we have done it all with no math or conversions between probabilities and odds. If you find this solution attractive, you might want to photocopy Figure 4-12 and carry it with you.

The second solution to the problem of converting back and forth between odds and probabilities is simply to learn how to do it. If you want to learn how, read on. If not, skip to page 126. To convert from pretest likelihoods (expressed as probabilities) to pretest odds, you simply divide the probability by its complement. That is:

$$\frac{\text{Pretest probability}}{1 - (\text{Pretest probability})} = \text{Pretest odds}$$

Thus, our chest pain patient with the pretest probability of myocardial infarction of 50% has a pretest odds of .50/(1 - .50) = .50/.50 = 1. We have calculated the pretest odds for several clinically relevant pretest probabilities and these appear in Table 4-23.

As you may recall from our patient with the suspected myocardial infarction, the likelihood ratio for his CK results of 180 IU was 4.4, and 1.0 × 4.4 = 4.4, so his posttest odds for having an infarct are 4.4:1. To convert a posttest odds back to a probability, we divide it by itself plus one. That is:

$$\frac{\text{Posttest odds}}{\text{Posttest odds} + 1} = \text{Posttest probability}$$

Thus, our posttest odds of 4.4 is a posttest probability of 4.4/(4.4 + 1) = 4.4/5.4 = .81 or 81%. We have calculated the posttest probabilities for a range of posttest odds and these appear in Table 4-24.

Table 4-23. Converting pretest probabilities to odds

Pretest probability	→ Probability / 1 − probability →	Pretest odds
0.1% or 0.001	0.001/0.999	0.001 : 1
1 % or 0.01	0.01 /0.99	0.01
2 % or 0.02	0.02 /0.98	0.02
3 % or 0.03	0.03 /0.97	0.03
4 % or 0.04	0.04 /0.96	0.04
5 % or 0.05	0.05 /0.95	0.05
10 % or 0.1	0.1 /0.9	0.11
20 % or 0.2	0.2 /0.8	0.25
30 % or 0.3	0.3 /0.7	0.43
40 % or 0.4	0.4 /0.6	0.67
50 % or 0.50	0.5 /0.5	1.0
60 % or 0.6	0.6 /0.4	1.5
70 % or 0.7	0.7 /0.3	2.3
80 % or 0.8	0.8 /0.2	4.0
90 % or 0.9	0.9 /0.1	9.0
95 % or 0.95	0.95 /0.05	19.0
99 % or 0.99	0.99 /0.01	99.0 : 1

Table 4-24. Converting posttest odds to probabilities

Posttest odds	→	Odds / odds + 1	→	Posttest probability
0.001		0.001/1.001		0.001 or 0.1%
0.01		0.01 /1.01		0.01 or 1 %
0.02		0.02 /1.02		0.02 or 2 %
0.03		0.03 /1.03		0.03 or 3 %
0.04		0.04 /1.04		0.04 or 4 %
0.05		0.05 /1.05		0.05 or 5 %
0.1		0.1 /1.1		0.09 or 9 %
0.2		0.2 /1.2		0.17 or 17 %
0.3		0.3 /1.3		0.23 or 23 %
0.4		0.4 /1.4		0.29 or 29 %
0.5		0.5 /1.5		0.33 or 33 %
0.6		0.6 /1.6		0.38 or 38 %
0.7		0.7 /1.7		0.41 or 41 %
0.8		0.8 /1.8		0.44 or 44 %
0.9		0.9 /1.9		0.47 or 47 %
1		1/2		0.5 or 50 %
2		2/3		0.67 or 67 %
3		3/4		0.75 or 75 %
4		4/5		0.8 or 80 %
5		5/6		0.83 or 83 %
10		10/11		0.91 or 91 %
20		20/21		0.95 or 95 %
30		30/31		0.97 or 97 %
40		40/41		0.98 or 98 %
50		50/51		0.98 or 98 %
100		100/101		0.99 or 99 %

Now you are armed with two different ways to use the likelihood-ratio strategy, the nomogram approach and the simple math approach. Use whichever one is more comfortable for you.

As more clinicians recognize the power of this strategy they are requesting information from subspecialists, radiologists, pathologists, and laboratorians on the precise likelihood ratios for the various levels of different signs, symptoms, and laboratory tests. We have started a collection of these and some of them appear in Table 4-25.

Is all of this still a bit mysterious? Is it hard for you to see how we got here in the brown belt from where we were back in the green belt? If so, let's redo a former example with our new strategy. Go back and look at green belt Table 4-6, where the pretest probability of myocardial infarction was 64% and the positive predictive value for a CK test result of 80 or more was 93%. Would we get the same answer with our new strategy?

We can do it with either the nomogram or the conversion back and forth between probabilities and odds. To do the latter, we start by generating the pretest odds from the prevalence of 64%. These odds would be probability/(1 − probability) = 64%/36% = 1.78:1 (a suitable approximation for routine clinical use would be 2:1, but we want to be tidy in this example). Next, we need to generate the likelihood ratio for a CK test result of 80 or more IU, and we can figure that out from Table 4-6 as well. "Sensitivity" is the same as the TP rate, and we see that this is 93%. The FP rate is (100% − specificity) or (100% − 88%) or 12%. Thus, the likelihood ratio is TP rate/FP rate or 93%/12% or 7.75.

If we use our nomogram, we would anchor it at a pretest probability of 64% and rotate it to a likelihood ratio of 7.75. Sighting along to the posttest probability we see that it lies just short of 95%, in good agreement with the positive predictive value of 93%. If we use the simple math approach, we would multiply the pretest odds of myocardial infarction by the likelihood ratio for a CK of 80 or more. This is 1.78 × 7.75 = 13.8:1. Finally, we can convert this posttest odds back to probability by odds/(odds + 1) = 13.8/14.8 = .93. All methods produce the same results and we hope that you will find this reassuring as well as enlightening.

You could have obtained about the same answer with some "rough-and-ready" rounding. The pretest odds of 64%/36% is about 67/33% or 2:1. The likelihood ratio of 93%/12% is about 90%/10% and Table 4-23 shows us this converts to 9:1. The product of the pretest odds and the likelihood ratio then becomes 2 × 9 = 18. Again, Table 4-24 tells you this is between 91% (for 10:1) and 95% (for 20:1), so you can do quite well by rounding off the pretest odds and the likelihood ratio and do it all in your head (at least after a bit of practice).

This little additional example also shows you that you can "do it with simple math in your head" even when diagnostic test results have a single cutoff. If you are told (or can calculate) sensitivity and specificity, you have got the TP rate and (100% − the FP rate) and you are off to the races.

Of course, you are always better off if multiple levels of the diagnostic test result have had their likelihood ratios determined. This is because the *degree* of abnormality in a test result can be taken into account only with multiple levels, each with its own likelihood ratio. The multilevel strategy even allows the creation of a level for the "uninterpretable" test results that are technically inadequate or incapable of being completed.

We hope that you now can see how useful it would be to have the five levels of a diagnostic test result shown in Table 4-26 available for all the symptoms, signs, and laboratory tests we use in striving to explain our patients' illnesses. This particular table is adapted from an overview of 55 studies of the usefulness of serum ferritin in the diagnosis of iron deficiency anemia. Study it and then read on.

If you review the five likelihood ratios that appear in this table, you will see that each one conveys a different message in clarifying the diagnosis of iron deficiency anemia. Noting that the pretest probability of iron deficiency is 809/(809 + 1770) = .31, the top likelihood ratio of 52 permits you to invoke SpPin,

Table 4-25. Likelihood ratios for some symptoms, signs, and laboratory tests

Reference	Target disorders (and gold standard)	Diagnostic data	Results	Likelihood ratio
[8]	>75% Coronary artery stenosis (by angiography or autopsy)	Symptoms of typical angina	Positive history	
			Men	115
			Women	120
[8]	Coronary artery stenosis (by angiography or autopsy)	Symptoms of atypical angina	Positive history	
			Men	14
			Women	15
[6]	Alcohol dependency or abuse (by extensive clinical investigation)	CAGE questions: (cut down, annoy, guilt, eye-opener)*	Yes to 3 or more	250
			Yes to any 2	7
			Yes to any 1	1.3
			No to all 4	0.2
[8]	Coronary artery stenosis (by angiography)	Exercise electrocardiography	Nonsloping ST-segment depression of:	
			>2.5 mm	39
			2–2.49	11
			1.5–1.99	4.2
			1–1.49	2.1
			0.05–0.99	0.92
			<0.05	0.23

[22]	Pancreatic disease (by biopsy, autopsy, or clinical course)	Ultrasound	Definitely abnormal	5.6
			Probably abnormal	2.1
			Possibly abnormal	0.95
			Probably normal	0.43
			Definitely normal	0.32
		CT scan	Definitely abnormal	26
			Probably abnormal	4.8
			Possibly abnormal	0.35
			Probably normal	0.32
			Definitely normal	0.11
[30]	Colorectal cancer (by biopsy or operation)	Carcinoembryonic antigen	>20ng/ml	3.5
			10–19.9	2.3
			5–9.9	1.4
			1–4.9	0.94
			<1	0.46
[4]	Tuberculosis (by culture)	Smears of sputum	Positive	31
			Negative	0.79

[a]See Table 4-5 and accompanying text for details on the CAGE questions.

Table 4-26. Likelihood ratios for five levels of serum ferritin

Level of serum ferritin (μmol/L)	Patients with iron deficiency		Patients free of iron deficiency		Likelihood ratio	Diagnostic level
	Number	Proportion	Number	Proportion		
<15	474	0.5859	20	0.0113	52	Rule-in "SpPin"
15–34	175	0.2163	79	0.0446	4.8	Intermediate high
35–64	82	0.1014	171	0.0966	1.0	Indeterminate
65–94	30	0.0371	168	0.0949	0.39	Intermediate low
⩾95	48	0.0593	1332	0.7525	0.08	Rule-out "SnNout"

since it produces a posttest probability of iron deficiency anemia of over 95%. The second level generates an "intermediate high"* likelihood ratio of 4.8, which is greater than 1.0, but not by much, shifting the posttest probability to not quite 70%, and indicating that you'll have to seek other evidence, perhaps even a bone marrow examination. The third level generates an "indeterminate" likelihood ratio close to 1.0 and does not shift the pretest probability much at all, telling you that you knew as much before the test as you do after it. The fourth level generates an "intermediate low" likelihood ratio of .39 which is less than 1.0, but again not by much, shifting the posttest probability down, but not decisively so (to about 15%), once again suggesting that you will have to seek additional evidence. Finally, the bottom level generates another powerful likelihood ratio (.08) that is close to zero and permits you to invoke SnNout because it produces a posttest probability of less than 4%, ruling out iron deficiency anemia.

We predict that more and more diagnostic data will be presented in this form and have summarized some examples of them, plus some two-level diagnostic data, in Table 4-25.

Once again, the enormous power of a careful history is apparent in this table. And now we can exploit much more of the range of responses to the CAGE questions, identifying levels for SpPin (yes to three or all four questions) and indeterminacy (yes to any one of them). The example of ultrasound for pancreatic disease provides us with three lessons: First, the uncertainties that inhabit the real world of diagnostic imaging can be captured by the brown belt; second, the individual expressions of uncertainty used there really do convey different diagnostic information; and, third, the "possibly abnormal" reading really is the indeterminate hedge (likelihood ratio of .95) we've often suspected! This ex-

*We are using names for these three middle zones suggested by David Simel [38].

ample also reminds us that we might want to consider the accuracy of individual local components of an image (e.g., are there metastases in the liver?) as well as the overall global reading (e.g., is this abdominal ultrasound normal?) [3].

Now that you are getting comfortable at "doing it with simple math in your head" we will let you in on a secret: you have been applying a modification of "Bayes' theorem," an approach to diagnosis that is usually presented with all sorts of scary symbols and complex formulas. We will not show any of these symbols or formulas here because you do not need them!

The distinction between pretest probabilities, on the one hand, and likelihood ratios, on the other, underscores an issue raised in the previous two chapters. As you will recall, one strategy for minimizing clinical disagreement and error is by "blinding" the assessment of raw diagnostic data. A strong case can therefore be made that those who interpret x rays, cardiograms, biopsies, and the like should, at least on their initial interpretations, generate likelihood ratios for those target disorders that might produce such an image or tracing, but with *no other knowledge about the patient*. These likelihood ratios can then be applied, by the diagnostician who ordered the test, to the appropriate pretest likelihoods and the relevant posttest likelihoods generated [37].

This "blind" approach may resolve the diagnostic problem on the first pass and, at any rate, will avoid most of the biases we described in Chapter 2. On the other hand, a knowledge of the diagnostic hypotheses under consideration may be crucial to the execution of the proper views, special stains, or other variations in diagnostic testing that are required for certain target disorders. In the latter case, negotiation between the diagnostician and laboratorian is essential. At any rate, keeping considerations of pretest probabilities and likelihood ratios separate will both reduce clinical disagreement or error and sharpen our diagnostic power.

Now let's move to a final advantage of "doing it with likelihood ratios," the ability to carry out *sequences* of diagnostic tests. The reason that you can do this so easily with this strategy is that the *post*test odds or probability for one test becomes the *pre*test odds or probability for a second, independent diagnostic test.

As usual, we shall show you how to do this with an example. Say that a 45-year-old woman calls your office receptionist with a 1-month history of intermittent chest pain, and is given an early appointment to see you. Like a good (i.e., typical) hypothetico-deductive diagnostician, as soon as you hear her chief complaint you form a mental "short list" of possible explanations, consisting of:

1. Something in the chest wall, possibly related to emotional stress
2. Something in the esophagus or upper gastrointestinal tract
3. Coronary heart disease
4. Something else (that is, none of the above)

Now, when this 45-year-old woman walks through your door, her pretest probability of coronary heart disease is only about 1% (so, her pretest odds are

.01/(1 − .01) = .01/.99 = .01:1). As you talk with her about her pain, however, it becomes clear that it is substernal, more heavy than painful, radiates down her left inner arm, is brought on by physical effort, and is relieved by 4 to 6 minutes of rest. She has, in fact, typical angina, and the likelihood ratio for coronary heart disease in the presence of this symptom is huge, at over 100. So, this first diagnostic test, a careful history, produces a very large change in her likelihood of coronary artery disease:

Pretest odds × likelihood ratio = posttest odds

and in this case:

.01 × 100 = 1:1

This posttest odds can be converted to a probability of 50% by calculation (odds/[odds + 1] = 1/2 = 50%) or by consulting Table 4-24. Alternatively, you could have done it all with the nomogram in Figure 4-12.

Having boosted her posttest probability of coronary artery disease to the range (40%–60%) where most diagnostic tests can be most helpful, you decide to suggest an exercise ECG. She agrees, undergoes the test, and exhibits 2.2 mm of ST-segment depression. Reference to Table 4-25 confirms that this degree of depression has a likelihood ratio of 11:1 (or, to make doing it in your head easier, a rough-and-ready ratio of 10:1).

So, your sequence now looks like this:

The pretest odds for the target disorder	×	The likelihood ratio for the diagnostic test result	=	The posttest odds for the target disorder
From the history: .01	×	100	=	1
From the exercise ECG: 1	×	10	=	10:1

With your post(two)test odds 10:1, your posttest probability is now 10/11 or 91%, and your hypothesis of coronary artery disease is confirmed.* You could, of course, do the same thing with the nomogram of Figure 4-12. Just be careful when you take the posttest probability following the first test and reanchor it as the pretest probability for the second test.

This example has an additional moral. Look at the relative size of the likelihood ratios for a brief, immediate, relatively cheap history and a much longer, delayed, and relatively expensive exercise electrocardiogram. There is no contest. Likelihood ratios for key points of the history and physical examination, both for this and for most other target disorders, are mammoth and dwarf those derived from most excursions through high technology.

*Note also that if she had exhibited less than .5 mm of depression the appropriate likelihood ratio would be .23 and 1 × .23 = .23:1 = 19%. Almost any result of her exercise ECG would have been enormously useful clinically.

Any time we combine several diagnostic tests into a sequence, whether by likelihood ratios or any other strategy, we run the risk of generating a distorted posttest probability at the end of the sequence. As usual, this is best shown with an example.

Suppose that a patient with a pretest probability of 20% for serious (that is, ⩾ 70%) coronary artery stenosis undergoes both exercise electrocardiography and radionuclide angiocardiography and has positive results for both. If the likelihood ratios for positive exercise tests and positive radionuclide studies, when considered individually, are 6.80 and 2.19, respectively, what is this patient's posttest probability of serious coronary stenosis after both tests? Why not try working this out for yourself? Jot down your answer here (or on some scratch paper if you are sharing this book). A hint: You ought to look at Table 4-27 (which is a reworked Table 4-12) when you are finished.

We calculated this one by four different strategies. Three of these strategies utilized key information from Table 4-27 and came up with a posttest likelihood of 73% (rounded from 72.6%). We hope that you got this answer, too. The fourth way simply combined the likelihood ratios for each test as presented in the text and came up with a different answer, 79% (rounded from 78.8%). We hope that you did *not* get this fourth answer, because it is wrong, and although it is not off by much, it represents an *overestimation* of the patient's posttest probability that we had better explain (especially if we plan to put together a chain of several diagnostic tests, rather than just two of them).

This fourth, incorrect answer could be derived using either the nomogram or a hand calculator. Using the nomogram, we would anchor the straightedge at a pretest probability of 20%, rotate it to the likelihood for the positive exercise test of 6.8, and follow the edge along to a posttest probability of a bit more than 60%. This becomes the pretest probability for the second test, the radionuclide angiocardiogram, so we go back to the left side of the nomogram and start over again, anchoring our straightedge a bit above 60%. Rotating it to the likelihood for the positive radionuclide angiocardiogram of 2.19, we can follow along to the posttest probability of almost 80%.

Why is this answer wrong? It is wrong because it assumes that the patient's result on one of the two tests (say, the exercise test) bears no relationship to that patient's result on the other of the two tests (the radionuclide angiocardiogram); that is, it assumes that the two tests are *independent*. Put more concretely, this incorrect fourth approach and its answer assumes that the radionuclide study is no *more* (or less) likely to be positive when the exercise ECG is positive than when the exercise ECG is negative.

A study of Table 4-27 reveals that this is not the case. The two diagnostic tests are not independent in panel A (where all patients have ⩾ 70% coronary artery stenosis), because the radionuclide study (summarized to the right of the 2 × 2 table) is, in fact, much more likely to be positive (sensitivity of radionuclide study = 92.3%) when the exercise ECG is positive than when the exercise ECG is negative (sensitivity of radionuclide study = 69.7%).

The two diagnostic tests are not independent in panel B (where all patients have < 70% stenosis) either. The radionuclide study is much more likely to be

Table 4-27. The combination of radionuclide angiocardiography and exercise ECGs in the diagnosis of coronary artery stenosis

Panel A: Patients with ≥70% stenosis

		Radionuclide study (RS)			Sensitivity of radionuclide study (TP rate)	
		Positive	Negative			
Exercise ECG (EECG)	Positive	276	23	299	When EECG ⊕	$\frac{276}{299} = 92.3\%$
	Negative	140	61	201	When EECG ⊖	$\frac{140}{201} = 69.7\%$
		416	84	500	Overall	$\frac{416}{500} = 83.2\%$
Sensitivity of exercise ECG (TP rate)		When RS ⊕	When RS ⊖	Overall		
		$\frac{276}{416} = 66.3\%$	$\frac{23}{84} = 27.4\%$	$\frac{299}{500} = 59.8\%$		

Panel B: Patients with <70% stenosis

		Radionuclide study (RS)			Specificity of radionuclide study (1 − FP rate)	
		Positive	Negative			
Exercise ECG (EECG)	Positive	26	18	44	When EECG ⊕	$\frac{18}{44} = 40.9\%$
	Negative	164	292	456	When EECG ⊖	$\frac{292}{456} = 64.0\%$
		190	310	500	Overall	$\frac{310}{500} = 62.0\%$
		Specificity of exercise ECG (1 − FP rate)				
		When RS ⊕	When RS ⊖	Overall		
		$\frac{164}{190} = 86.3\%$	$\frac{292}{310} = 94.2\%$	$\frac{456}{500} = 91.2\%$		

negative (specificity of the radionuclide study = 64.0%) when the exercise ECG is negative than when the exercise ECG is positive (specificity of the radionuclide study = 40.9%).

So, patients who are positive on one of these tests are likely to be positive on the other one as well, and patients who are negative on one test are likely to be negative on the other one as well. The test results are *dependent*, and we have decided to call the sort of dependence shown in Table 4-27 *concordance*.

How did we get the three other answers, all of which used Table 4-27 one way or another? The first way simply reorganized the information in Table 4-27 into a single table, as shown in Table 4-28 (which some of us met before as Table 4-13).

Panel A of Table 4-27 provides information on 500 patients with coronary stenosis ≥ 70%; 276 had positive results for both tests and therefore go in cell *a* of Table 4-28, with all the rest going into cell *c*. Panel B of Table 4-27 provides information on 500 patients with coronary stenosis < 70%; only 26 had positive results for both tests and therefore go in cell *b* of Table 4-28, and all the rest go into cell *d*. We can then calculate the likelihood ratio for having both tests positive *from data that take into account the concordance between these two tests*, and it comes out to 10.6. We could now use the nomogram as before, anchoring our straightedge at 20%, rotating it to a likelihood ratio of just above 10, and sighting along to a posttest probability of just over 70%.

The second and third ways to answer this question calculated likelihood ratios for the second test, *given* the result of the first test, and also used information from Table 4-27. The generation of these likelihood ratios is shown in Table 4-29.

The results of Table 4-29 agree with our intuition, don't they? The likelihood ratio for a positive result of either test is *lower* when the other test has already produced a positive result. We can use these results with our nomogram. Anchoring our straightedge at 20%, we rotate it to the likelihood ratio of a positive

Table 4-28. When both of two convergent tests for coronary stenosis are positive

	Coronary stenosis		
	Present (panel A)	Absent (panel B)	Likelihood ratio
Both tests positive	276 (55.2%) [a]	26 (5.2%) [b]	$\frac{0.552}{0.052} = 10.6$
One or both tests negative	[c] 23 + 140 + 61 = 224 (44.8%)	[d] 18 + 164 + 292 = 474 (94.8%)	$\frac{0.448}{0.948} = 0.47$
	500 (100%)	500 (100%)	

Table 4-29. Likelihood ratios for the second of a pair of diagnostic tests, given the results for the first test

	Likelihood ratios (L.R.) when the test result is positive	
	Exercise ECG	Radionuclide study
As an independent test	$\frac{0.598}{(1 - 0.912)} = 6.80$	$\frac{0.832}{(1 - 0.620)} = 2.19$
When other test positive	$\frac{0.663}{(1 - 0.863)} = 4.84$	$\frac{0.923}{(1 - 0.409)} = 1.56$

Pretest #1 likelihood × first test's L.R. (as an independent test) = posttest #1 likelihood
||
Pretest #2 likelihood × second test's L.R. (given the results of the first test)
= posttest #2 likelihood

exercise ECG of 6.80 (since we are *not* yet taking the radionuclide study result into account, we use the likelihood ratio for a positive exercise ECG when considered as an independent test) and sight along it for a posttest probability of just over 60%. Reanchoring at a pretest probability of just over 60%, we rotate the straightedge to the likelihood ratio for a positive radionuclide study, *given that the exercise ECG already was positive*, of 1.56. Sighting along our straightedge we now find a posttest probability of just over 70%.

Would we get a similar result if we started with the positive radionuclide study (as an independent test) and then incorporated the positive exercise ECG, using the likelihood ratio for the latter that applied when the radionuclide study was positive? Why not try it and see?

Some quick calculations will, in fact, show us that all three answers that use Table 4-27 in some way are equivalent:

1. What is the likelihood ratio for both positive tests generated from Table 4-28? It is 10.6.
2. What is the likelihood ratio for both positive tests in Table 4-29 when the exercise ECG is handled as an independent test and the radionuclide study takes the exercise ECG result into account? It is 6.80 × 1.56 = 10.6!
3. What is the likelihood ratio for both positive tests in Table 4-29 when the radionuclide study is treated as an independent test and the exercise ECG takes the radionuclide study result into account? It is 2.19 × 4.84 = 10.6!

Two final questions about independence and convergence will put the foregoing into a practical frame of reference. First, does convergence really matter? In the example we worked through, all our extra effort resulted in exposing an overestimation of the posttest probability by only 6% (or a proportional overestimation of 6%/73% = .08). In fact, convergence is not often a problem with short chains of two or three diagnostic tests, but may produce clinically significant distortions with longer chains. Of course, convergence is a potential problem no matter what strategy we use to evaluate diagnostic data, and seasoned clinicians often handle it well on an intuitive basis. All that we have done here, once again, is look for the science of the art of medicine and see how it can be used to generate a solution to a common problem.

The second practical question about convergence is: How do you decide when it is important? The best way to decide is to find data like those in Table 4-27 that actually tell you whether and how much convergence is going on. Articles presenting these sorts of data are increasing and a famous one presented the "Pozen score," which identified the independent contributions of four elements of the history and three aspects of the initial electrocardiogram to the diagnosis of new coronary ischemic events among patients presenting to emergency room with chest pain [35]. Until such reports become the norm, you will have to rely on your own experience; when you find that your "high posttest probability" diagnoses are wrong, you should stop and think. Assuming that you are using the nomogram correctly and are not making computation errors, and assuming that your clinical skills and your local diagnostic facilities are of reasonable quality, when your "high posttest probability" diagnoses are wrong you have either overestimated these patients' pretest probabilities or have used falsely inflated likelihood ratios. If your pretest probabilities are on firm ground (that is, in agreement with published reports of high quality) you should examine your likelihood ratios for distortion through the effects of unrecognized convergence. Once again, a search of the relevant literature will be in order.

Enough of the problems that arise when we use the likelihood-ratio approach. They are universal problems that affect us regardless of how we approach diagnostic data, and the likelihood-ratio strategy simply exposes them for recognition and study. It instructs as well as informs those who use it, and we predict that likelihood ratios will soon replace sensitivity, specificity, and all that.

Doing it with likelihood ratios fits nicely with our clinical views about utility, too. By making the most out of the entire range of diagnostic test results (several levels, each with its own likelihood ratio, rather than a single cutoff and a single ratio) and by permitting us to keep track of the likelihood that a patient has the target disorder at each point along the diagnostic sequence, we can carry patients to extremely high or extremely low likelihoods. One very useful result of this is to sharply reduce the numbers of ultimately false-positive patients (who suffer the slings of labeling and the arrows of needless therapy) and the ultimately false-negative patients (who miss their chance for diagnosis and, possibly, efficacious therapy).

In summary, to interpret signs, symptoms, and laboratory tests with the likelihood ratio strategy:

1. For target disorders that are important in your practice, seek out (in the literature or from the clinical or laboratory experts who ought to know) likelihood ratios for: (a) key symptoms and signs; (b) several levels (rather than just the positive and negative) of diagnostic test results; and (c) combinations of diagnostic tests (so you can decide whether convergence is likely to be a major issue).

2. Identify, where feasible, logical sequences of diagnostic tests.
3. Estimate the pretest likelihood of the target disorder for an individual patient, and, using either the nomogram or the conversion formulas, apply the likelihood ratio that corresponds to the first diagnostic test result.
4. Remembering that the resulting posttest odds or probability from the first test becomes the pretest odds or probability for the next diagnostic test, repeat the process for all the pertinent symptoms, signs, and laboratory studies that pertain to your target disorder, correcting for convergence as necessary.

And that is it. If you can use this strategy, award yourself a brown belt and recognize that you are now far more sophisticated in interpreting diagnostic tests than the great majority of your teachers.

About all that is left now are some rather complex strategies that combine diagnosis and therapy, quantify our as yet nonquantified ideas about utility, and necessitate at least a hand calculator to carry out. Because they help us to deal with difficult diagnostic situations, they can be extremely useful in every field of medicine. If you want to learn about them, proceed to the black belt.

Chunk #5 Black Belt: Doing It with a Hand Calculator

Most diagnostic decisions can be made with one of the previous chunks. If you are lucky, the symptom, sign, or laboratory result you elicit will be pathognomonic for the target disorder (that is, its specificity is 100%), and all you will need is a yellow belt ("doing it with pictures"). In other diagnostic situations you will be able to use your green, blue, or brown belts to employ sequences of signs, symptoms, or laboratory tests to raise the pretest likelihood for the final diagnostic test into the 40% to 60% range where that final test can either make the diagnosis or effectively rule it out.

In many diagnostic situations the price your patient pays for your misdiagnosis is much higher in one direction (e.g., a false-positive diagnosis of a relentless, untreatable target disorder in a patient who does not have it) than in the other (e.g., a false-negative clean bill of health in a patient who does have the relentless and untreatable target disorder). You can, in such cases, select a cutoff that minimizes the harm done by reducing false-positives to or near zero.

Occasional diagnostic decisions are not so easy, however, and may not be resolvable with what you have learned so far. False-positives and false-negatives both may suffer to the same degree, and the diagnostic test you are considering may be risky or painful. And it is sometimes impossible to keep all these considerations in mind simultaneously, and clinical discussions of such dilemmas may become nonproductive wrangles.

This final chunk will introduce the rudiments of a diagnostic strategy for coping with these rare but perplexing diagnostic problems. The strategy is called *decision analysis* and can be defined in a clinical context as a method of describing complex clinical problems in an explicit fashion, identifying the available courses of action (both diagnostic and management), assessing the probability and value (or utility) of all possible outcomes, and then making a simple calcu-

Table 4-30. Exercise electrocardiography results when the pretest probability of significant coronary artery stenosis is 5%

		>70% Coronary stenosis		
		Present	Absent	
Exercise ECG	Positive	30 (a)	86 (b)	116 (a+b)
	Negative	20 (c)	864 (d)	884 (c+d)
		50 (a+c)	950 (b+d)	1000 (Σ)

lation to select the optimal course of action. In trying to understand this strategy we have learned most from the writings of Barbara McNeil, Stephen Pauker, Jerome Kassirer, William Schwartz, and Alan Detsky [10, 25, 29, 32, 33, 37] tempered by cautionary notes from David Ransohoff, Alvan Feinstein, and James Dolan [11, 36], and explored in some detail in a book edited by Milton Weinstein and Harvey Fineberg [42]. For reasons that we'll explain later, we don't consider ourselves at all talented in applying this strategy, so serious students of this field should run, not walk, to the journal *Medical Decision Making*.

As described by Stephen Pauker and Jerome Kassirer [24], the application of decision analysis involves six steps and, as usual, we will introduce them with an example. Because some of you may be smarting still over our decision to forego an exercise ECG on Patient B in panel B of Table 4-11, let us reconsider him.

As you may recall, this was a 35-year-old man with "heartburn" for several years, no coronary risk factors, and a 6-week history of nonexertional, squeezing chest pain deep to his lower sternum and epigastrium, usually radiating straight through to his back and most likely to occur when he lies down after a heavy meal. He has a negative physical exam, and you place esophageal spasm at the top of your diagnostic hypotheses, judging his probability for significant coronary artery stenosis at 5%.

The sensitivity and specificity of the exercise electrocardiogram are 60% and 91%, respectively, and Table 4-30 summarizes the results of such testing among patients in whom the prevalence (pretest probability) of significant coronary artery stenosis is 5%.

There are six steps of decision analysis that apply to this diagnostic problem.

STEP 1. CREATE A "DECISION TREE" OR MAP OF ALL THE PERTINENT COURSES OF ACTION AND THEIR CONSEQUENCES

In the present case, we could send him for an exercise ECG or withhold it. If we withhold it, we will fail to diagnose significant coronary stenosis 5% of the

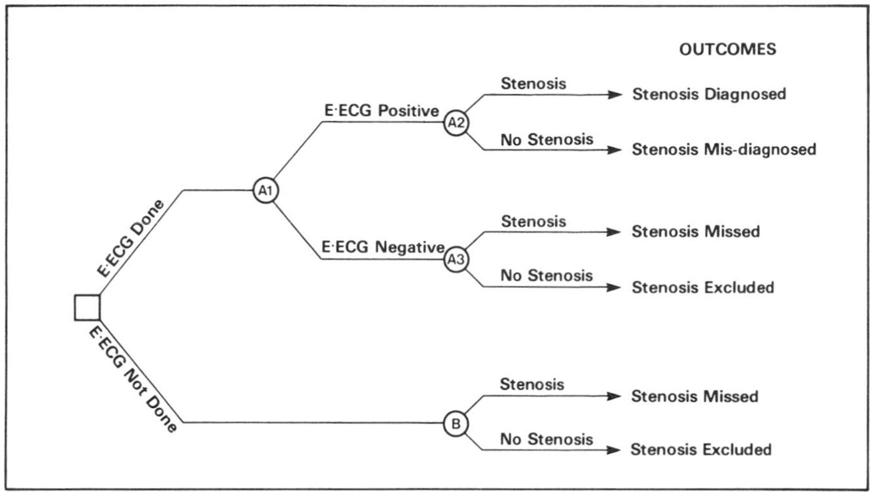

Figure 4-13. A decision tree for exercise electrocardiography.

time, but will be correct in discarding this diagnostic hypothesis 95% of the time. If we send him for an exercise ECG, it can come back positive or negative. Referring to Table 4-27, if it comes back positive, it could be a true-positive (cell *a*: he does have significant coronary stenosis) or a false-positive (cell *b*: he would be labeled with a disease he does not have). If the exercise ECG comes back negative, it could be a true-negative (cell *d*: we have correctly ruled out significant coronary stenosis) or a false-negative (cell *c*: we have missed significant stenosis). These courses of action and their consequences are shown in the decision tree in Figure 4-13.

This decision tree maps out the options and outcomes we have just discussed. In this (and other) decision trees, the boxes denote clinical choices between different courses of action (decision nodes), and the circles (chance nodes) denote chance events (tests are positive or negative; patients do or do not have the target disorder). We can now go to the next step.

STEP 2. ASSIGN PROBABILITIES TO THE BRANCHES THAT SPROUT FROM EACH "CHANCE NODE"

In this example, we can assign probabilities for all the nodes by carefully examining Table 4-31. The branches from chance node B simply reflect the prevalence of significant stenosis ($[a + c]/\Sigma = .05$) and its complement. Those sprouting from chance node A1 are the proportions of such patients who will have positive ($[a + b]/\Sigma = 116/1000 = .12$) and negative ($[c + d]/\Sigma = 884/1000 = .88$) test results. The branches sprouting from chance node A2 are the proportions of those patients with positive exercise ECGs who do ($a/[a + b] = 30/116 = .26$) and do not ($b/[a + b] = 86/116 = .74$) have significant stenosis, and those sprouting from chance node A3 the proportions of patients with negative tests who do ($c/[c + d] = 20/884 = .02$) and do not ($d/[c + d) = 864/884 = .98$) have significant stenosis. These probabilities have been

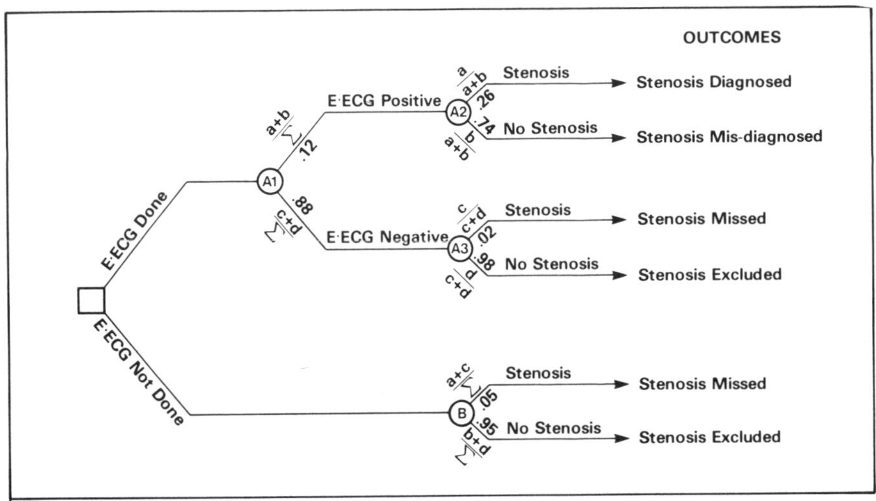

Figure 4-14. A budding decision tree for exercise electrocardiography.

added to our decision tree and the result is shown in Figure 4-14. We are now ready for the third step of decision analysis.

STEP 3. ASSIGN UTILITIES TO EACH OF THE POTENTIAL OUTCOMES SHOWN ON THE DECISION TREE

Clinicians, patients, and even hospital administrators agree that some health outcomes are better than others. The product of their quality of life and quantity of life makes them preferable to other outcomes, and in decision analysis we refer to this product of quality × quantity as "utility" (although you may prefer to think of it as "value" or "worth"). Of course, we already think in these terms in making most of our clinical decisions. All that decision analysis requires is for us to do our best to *quantify* the utilities of the different outcomes of the decision tree on a common scale.

The easiest way to start this process is to *rank* the outcomes from best to worst. In our example, we believe that you would agree with the following ranking:

Best
1. *Stenosis excluded:* The patient is free of serious stenosis, and has not been labeled.
2. *Stenosis misdiagnosed:* The patient is free of serious stenosis, but has been labeled and must suffer that knowledge and the risks of any subsequent therapy.
3. *Stenosis diagnosed:* The patient has serious stenosis and knows it, but can benefit from efficacious therapy.

Worst
4. *Stenosis missed:* The patient has serious stenosis, but it has been missed and he will not receive efficacious therapy.

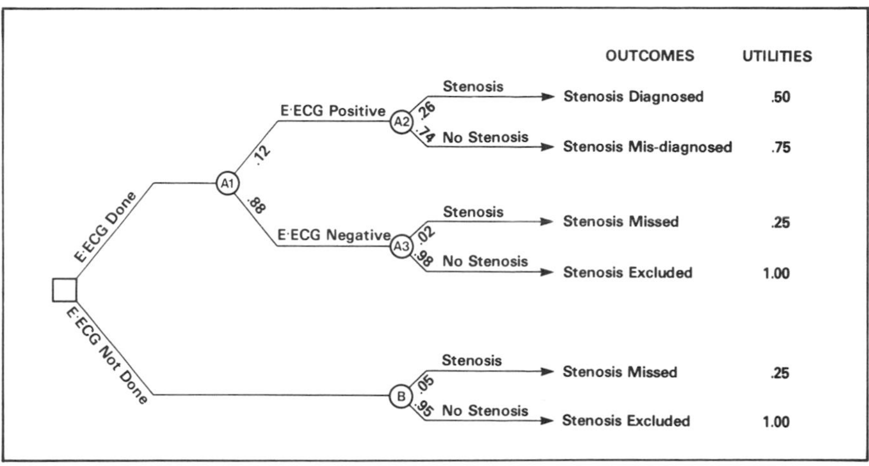

Figure 4-15. A blooming decision tree for exercise electrocardiography.

After ranking the outcomes we proceed to assign numerical values to them, and this is where decision analysis gets tough, *not* because it is artificial (for we are constantly assigning utilities whenever we deal with patients) but because it forces us to be explicit in assigning these utilities.

In ideal circumstances we can go to the clinical literature and track down data on both the quantity (survival rates) and quality (morbidity, disability, etc.) of life for the outcomes at the end of the tree and the two subsequent examples in this chunk will do that. Better still, we could determine these utilities from the patient's perspective and make the decision analysis serve the patient. For purposes of this initial example, let us short-cut this process and accept that the utilities we developed looked like this:

1. Stenosis excluded = 1.00
2. Stenosis misdiagnosed = .75
3. Stenosis diagnosed = .50
4. Stenosis missed = .25

We have added these utilities to our decision tree, and it now looks like Figure 4-15. Now we are ready for the next step, and here is where the math comes in.

STEP 4. COMBINE THE PROBABILITIES AND UTILITIES FOR EACH NODE ON THE DECISION TREE

This is done from right to left by a process of multiplication and addition known as "folding back." At node A2, this consists of multiplying the probability of *stenosis diagnosed* by its utility (.26 × .50 = .130) and the probability of *stenosis misdiagnosed* by its utility (.74 × .75 = .555), and then adding these products (.130 + .555 = .685) and assigning this "expected utility" to node A2. For node A3 the corresponding products are, for *stenosis missed*, (.02 ×

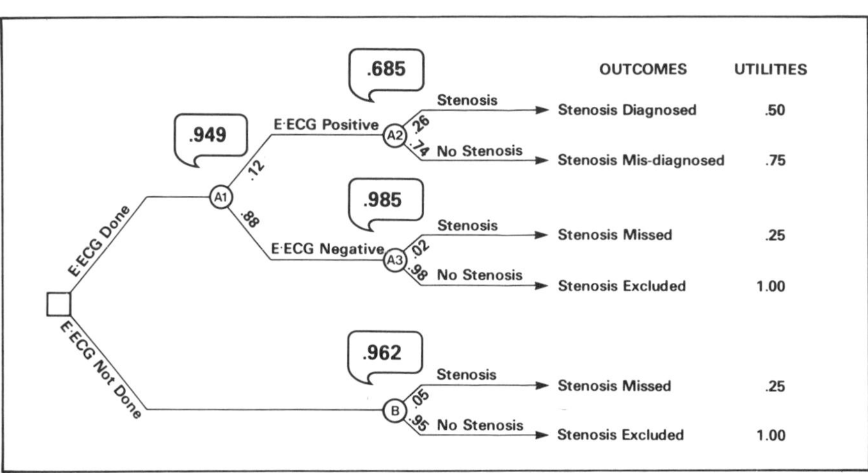

Figure 4-16. A fruit-bearing decision tree for exercise electrocardiography.

.25 = .005) and for *stenosis excluded*, (.98 × 1.00 = .980), and their sum (.005 + .980 = .985) is assigned to node A3.

We can carry this folding back one step further by multiplying the expected utility for node A2 by the probability assigned the upper branch sprouting from node A1 (.685 × .12 = .082), multiplying the expected utility for node A3 by the probability assigned the lower branch sprouting from node A1 (.985 × .88 = .867), and adding these two products (.082 + .867 = .949). This sum, .949, is the expected utility for the entire decision to send patients like this for exercise ECGs.

The expected utility for the decision *not* to send such patients for exercise ECGs is the sum of the products of the probabilities and utilities associated with node B. For *stenosis missed* this is (.05 × .25 = .012) and for *stenosis excluded* (.95 × 1.0 = .950); their sum is (.012 + .950 = .962) and .962 is the expected utility for node B. All of this folding back has been added as balloons to our decision tree and the result is shown in Figure 4-16.

STEP 5. PICK THE DECISION THAT LEADS TO THE HIGHEST EXPECTED UTILITY

In our example, the decision *to* send such patients for exercise ECGs leads to an expected utility of .949, whereas the decision *not to* send such patients for exercise ECGs leads to an expected utility of .962; and so such patients are better off if we do not subject them to exercise electrocardiography.

We are not finished yet, however, for there is one more vital step.

STEP 6. TEST YOUR DECISION FOR ITS VULNERABILITY TO CLINICALLY SENSIBLE CHANGES IN PROBABILITIES AND UTILITIES

Would we still reject exercise electrocardiography if the patient's pretest likelihood was 10% rather than 5%? If the utility for the outcome of *stenosis misdi-*

agnosed was .90 rather than .75? If we included a small (.01%) but awful (utility = .0%) risk of dying during an exercise electrocardiogram?*

No decision analysis is complete until you have tested it to see whether it resists credible changes in probabilities and utilities. If it does, the preferred course of action is clearly reinforced. If, on the other hand, credible changes in probabilities or utilities switch the decision, or if the expected utilities for the alternative courses of action become so close to each other that their difference is judged trivial, you are in a toss-up situation in which it makes no difference what you do.

Clinicians with wide experience in applying decision analysis to tough clinical problems have documented that one-sixth of them wind up as toss-ups [24]. Since this strategy is usually reserved for really tough decisions, this relatively high rate of toss-ups should not surprise us. For our part, we are more impressed by the ability of decision analysis to handle five-sixths of tough decisions than by its failure to resolve the one-sixth that are unresolvable. We have used decision analysis on our own in-patient services whenever we were in a diagnostic or management quandary and found published data we judged to be of sufficient quality to plug in. By our count, this amounts to one decision analysis per 80 admissions to a busy secondary-level medical service.

The preceding example provides the basic steps in decision analysis, and should help you set it up and apply it in various diagnostic situations. As you can see, it is most helpful in deciding *whether* to carry out a diagnostic test, and a hand calculator (or slide rule or abacus) can take most of the pain and time out of the calculations.

We will close this section with two more examples that extend the decision analysis approach. The first one permits you to define the specific pretest likelihoods at which your diagnostic and treatment decisions should switch, and the second provides a more sophisticated view of utilities.

The "threshold" approach uses decision analysis to assist decisions about whether to carry out diagnostic tests (and be guided by them) on the one hand, or whether to make therapeutic decisions without them. This strategy, suggested by Stephen Pauker and Jerome Kassirer [33], identifies two pretest likelihoods and, thereby, three clinical decisions, as shown in Figure 4-17.

In this figure we see that if the clinician judges the pretest likelihood to be less than cutoff A (called the "test threshold"), the patient is unlikely to have the target disorder and neither result of the diagnostic test would appreciably alter this likelihood; accordingly, we should neither treat nor even test the patient. Similarly, if the pretest likelihood is judged to be greater than cutoff B

*You may want to crank these through and decide for yourself. When we calculated them, they came out like this:

	Node A	*Node B*	*Decision*
Prevalence 10%	.918	.925	Do not send
Utility for stenosis misdiagnosed = .90	.962	.962	Toss up!
Small risk of dying during exercise ECG	Can only fall	Unchanged	Do not send

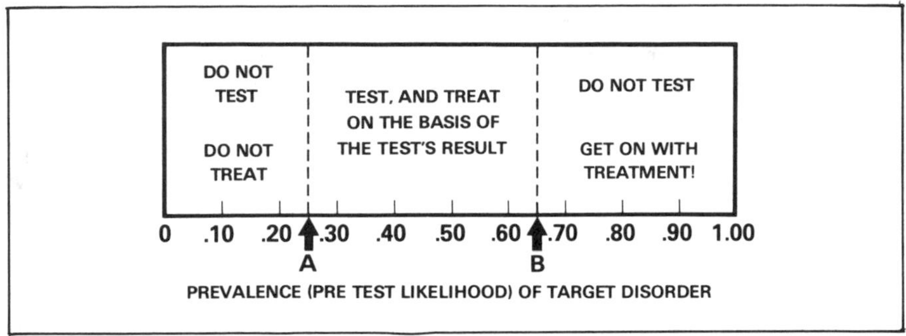

Figure 4-17. Pretest likelihood of disease and decisions whether to test or treat.

(called the "test-treatment threshold"), we ought to assume that the patient has the target disorder and get on with treatment. It is only when the pretest likelihood is judged to fall *between* cutoffs A and B that we should test, and then treat, the patient on the basis of this test result.

Stephen Pauker and Jerome Kassirer developed a strategy for defining cutoffs A and B, based both on the accuracy of the relevant diagnostic test and also on the utility of the management of patients with and without the target disorder. They begin by defining their terms:

Benefit of appropriate Rx = average gain in utility (benefits minus risks) among patients with the target disorder who are rightly treated

Risk of inappropriate Rx = average loss in utility among patients who do not have the target disorder and are wrongly treated. Risk of the diagnostic test = average loss in utility from serious complications of the diagnostic procedure

They then showed that the prevalence (pretest likelihood or prior probability) of the target disorder that corresponds to cutoff A is:

Cutoff A = Test threshold

$$= \frac{\text{(FP rate)(risk of inappropriate Rx)} + \text{(risk of the diagnostic test)}}{\text{(FP rate)(risk of inappropriate Rx)} + \text{(TP rate)(benefit of appropriate Rx)}}$$

and cutoff B is:

Cutoff B = Test-treatment threshold

$$= \frac{\text{(TN rate)(risk of inappropriate Rx)} - \text{(risk of the diagnostic test)}}{\text{(TN rate)(risk of inappropriate Rx)} + \text{(FN rate)(benefit of appropriate Rx)}}$$

To show how this procedure works, they present a 60-year-old man with epigastric pain, hematemesis, and a barium meal showing a 2-cm ulcer on the greater curvature of his stomach. His clinicians judge the likelihood that he has gastric cancer to be .10, and must decide whether to gastroscope him. In this patient, then, the target disorder is stomach cancer, the treatment for which is surgery, and the relevant diagnostic test is gastroscopy (and brush cytology). The options are:

1. Consider the ulcer to be benign, do not gastroscope, and do not operate.
2. Gastroscope, and operate if the results are positive.
3. Consider the ulcer to be malignant, do not gastroscope, and operate at once.

The utility measure they selected was mortality. Reviews of the pertinent literature indicated an average 33% gain in the relative survival rates of gastric cancer patients operated early (with local disease) versus later (with regional involvement), and this was taken as the gain in utility for the "benefit of appropriate Rx." The surgical mortality for laparotomy in a 60-year-old man was judged to be 2%, and this was selected as the loss in utility for the "risk of inappropriate Rx." Finally, .005% of patients undergoing gastroscopy die as a result of the diagnostic test and this became the "risk of the diagnostic test."

The sensitivity and specificity of gastroscopy plus brush cytology for gastric cancer were judged to be 96% and 98%, respectively.

The factors could then be summarized:

Benefit of appropriate Rx = .33
Risk of inappropriate Rx = .02
Risk of the diagnostic test = .00005
TP rate = .96
FP rate = .02
FN rate = .04
TN rate = .98

From the foregoing, the cutoffs could be calculated:

Cutoff A = Test Threshold

$$= \frac{\text{(FP rate)(risk of inappropriate Rx)} + \text{(risk of the diagnostic test)}}{\text{(FP rate)(risk of inappropriate Rx)} + \text{(TP rate)(benefit of appropriate Rx)}}$$

$$= \frac{(.02)(.02) + (.00005)}{(.02)(.02) + (.96)(.33)} = \frac{(.0004) + (.00005)}{(.0004) + (.3168)}$$

$$= \frac{.00045}{.31720} = .0014$$

Cutoff B = Test-treatment threshold

$$= \frac{\text{(TN rate)(risk of inappropriate Rx)} - \text{(risk of the diagnostic test)}}{\text{(TN rate)(risk of inappropriate Rx)} + \text{(FN rate)(benefit of appropriate Rx)}}$$

$$= \frac{(.98)(0.02) - (.00005)}{(.98)(.02) + (.04)(.33)} = \frac{(.0196) - (.00005)}{(.0196) + (.0132)}$$

$$= \frac{.01955}{.0328} = .60$$

The extremely low value for cutoff A (test threshold) indicates that if the clinicians caring for such a patient had even the slightest suspicion of gastric cancer, the option of ignoring it and forgetting about gastroscopy was simply not on. On the other hand, if these clinicians judged that the pretest likelihood for stomach cancer exceeded .60 at cutoff B (the test-treatment threshold) they need not bother with gastroscopy, but should go directly to surgery. Since the clinicians caring for the patient in this example judged that the pretest likelihood of gastric cancer was .10, a point that lies between cutoffs A and B, the appropriate option is to proceed to gastroscopy and be guided by its result.

The foregoing is an elaborate analysis, but in our judgment approaches of this sort will help us and our patients derive the greatest benefit from diagnostic tests that are risky or not widely available. Moreover, Paul Glasziou has described a simple method for carrying out the foregoing test with a knowledge of its likelihood ratios and the nomogram we presented back in Figure 4-12 [16]:

1. Decide on the treatment threshold, above which you would decide to treat and below which you would hold off. Anchor a straight edge at this point on the posttest probability scale.
2. Rotate the straight edge until it lines up with the likelihood ratio for a positive test. Its projection to the pretest probability scale defines the test threshold.
3. Repeat step 2, but this time rotate the straight edge until it lines up with the likelihood ratio for a negative test. Its projection to the pretest probability scale defines the test-treatment threshold.*

The final example raises our sophistication in thinking about survival by pointing out that the immediate future is more important to patients (that is, it has a higher utility) than the distant future. Although we all probably acknowledge that this is so, it has a major effect on some of our diagnostic decisions, as shown by Barbara McNeil and Stephen Pauker [29].

When McNeil interviewed patients with bronchogenic carcinoma and determined their utilities for both short-term and long-term survival, it was docu-

*To test your understanding of this rapid method, suppose that your treatment threshold was low, at 25%, and the diagnostic test possessed likelihood ratios of 4 when positive, and .67 when negative. You should generate a test threshold of about 8% and a test-treatment threshold of about 33%.

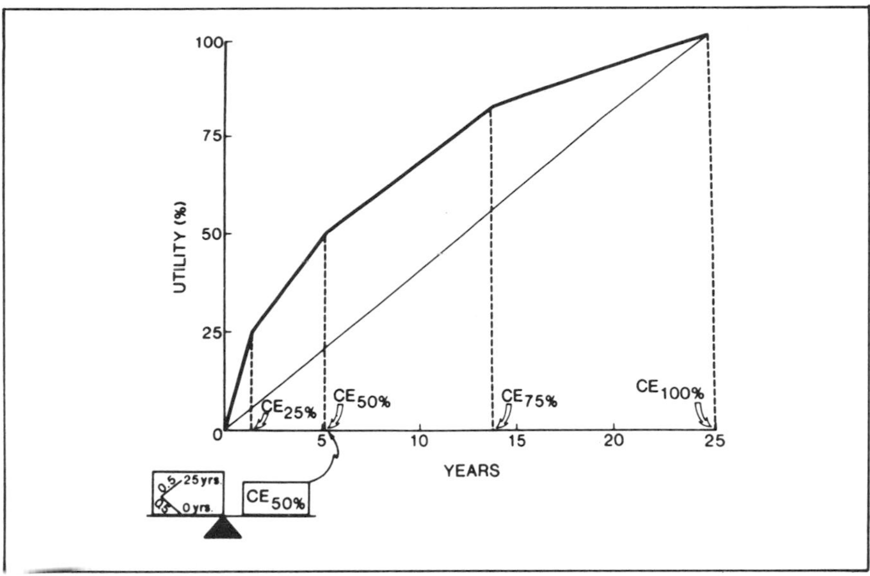

Figure 4-18. The utility of short-term versus long-term survival for patients with bronchogenic carcinoma. (From B. J. McNeil and S. G. Pauker. The patient's role in assessing the value of diagnosis tests. *Radiology* 132:605, 1979.)

mented that they considered the former much more valuable. This is shown in Figure 4-18.

The vertical axis in this figure is utility and the horizontal axis depicts guaranteed life spans of 0 (death now) to 25 years (the average life-expectancy of the youngest study patient if he were cured of his lung cancer). These patients were shown a series of gambles, such as that displayed in the left lower corner of Figure 4-18, and were asked to identify the period of guaranteed survival (as CEs or "certainty equivalents") that was, in their judgment, equivalent to the 50–50 chance of total cure from immediate surgery (which would give them the 25-year life expectancy) or of death during or shortly after their operation. By varying the duration of life expectancy following a surgical cure, it became possible to construct the upper curve shown here. If short-term and long-term survival had similar utility, these patients' utilities would have lain along the straight line, but this was not the case. These patients preferred short-term survival over long-term survival and their utilities rose above the 45-degree diagonal and then fell back again; that is, they were averse to the risk of early death from surgery, despite its efficacy.

What do these results have to do with diagnostic tests? They cast new light on the question of whether to apply diagnostic tests for inoperability to patients with bronchogenic carcinoma. These additional diagnostic tests, although expensive, could identify the 20% of lung-cancer patients who already have occult metastases at the time of diagnosis and cannot, as a result, benefit from surgery.

This situation was subjected to decision analysis to contrast immediate surgery for all versus preliminary diagnostic testing for occult metastases and surgery only for those with negative tests. If the first year after diagnosis was no more or less valuable than year 5, the resulting utilities would call for us *never* to execute diagnostic tests for inoperability unless the sensitivity and specificity of these tests exceeded 99%.

However, because surgery is associated with a perioperative mortality of 10%, and because this wipes out early, more highly valued years in order to maximize later, less valued years, the utilities must be altered to reflect this "aversion" to the risk of early operative death. When this is done, the resulting expected utilities would call for us *always* to carry out diagnostic tests for inoperability, even if the sensitivity of these tests were as low as 50% (if specificity were maintained at 90%).

This final example should convince you (if you were not already) that the measurement of utilities is difficult. It is not as if we are not doing this all the time anyway; it is simply that, by making this utility-setting explicit, we reveal how complex this judgment really is.

That is how to use decision analysis in making diagnostic decisions. We will meet it again when we consider alternative strategies for deciding which treatment to apply once a diagnosis is made. In summary, to do it with more complex math:

1. Create a "decision tree" or map of all the pertinent courses of action and their consequences.
2. Assign probabilities to the branches that sprout from each "chance node."
3. Assign utilities to each of the potential outcomes shown on the decision tree.
4. Combine the probabilities and utilities for each node on the decision tree.
5. Pick the decision that leads to the highest expected utility.
6. Test your decision for its sensitivity to clinically sensible changes in probabilities and utilities.

Well, that is it. If you grasped what you have read here and can begin to apply it to difficult clinical decisions, award yourself a black belt. You have come a long way from "doing it with pictures" and are now able to extract the maximum diagnostic information that can be provided from signs, symptoms, and laboratory investigations without resorting to a computer.

References

1. Ackerknecht, E. H. *Therapeutics From the Primitives to the 20th Century.* New York: Hafner, 1973. P. 105.
2. Bartel, H. G., Behar, V. S., Peter, R. H., et al. Graded exercise stress tests in angiographically documented coronary heart disease. *Circulation* 49: 348, 1974.
3. Black, W. C., and Dwyer, A. J. Local versus global measures of accuracy: An important distinction for diagnostic imaging. *Med. Decis. Making.* 10: 266, 1990.
4. Boyd, J. C., and Marr, J. J. Decreasing reliability of acid-fast smear techniques for detection of tuberculosis. *Ann. Intern. Med.* 82: 489, 1975.
5. Bryant, G. D., and Norman, G. R. Expressions of probability: Words and numbers. *N. Engl. J. Med.* (Letter) 302: 411, 1980.

6. Bush, B., Shaw, S., Cleary, P., et al. Screening for alcohol abuse using the CAGE questionnaire. *Am. J. Med.* 82: 231, 1987.
7. DeDombal, F. T., Leaper, D. J., Horrocks, J. C., et al. Human and computer-aided diagnosis of abdominal pain: Further report with emphasis on performance of clinicians. *Br. Med. J.* 1: 376, 1974.
8. Diamond, G. A., and Forrester, J. S. Analysis of probability as an aid in the clinical diagnosis of coronary artery disease. *N. Engl. J. Med.* 300: 1350, 1979.
9. Diamond, G. A., Forrester, J. S., Hirsch, M., et al. Application of conditional probability analysis to the clinical diagnosis of coronary artery disease. *J. Clin. Invest.* 65: 1210, 1980.
10. Detsky, A. S. Decision analysis: what's the prognosis? *Ann. Intern. Med.* 106: 321, 1987.
11. Dolan, J. G. Can decision analysis adequately represent clinical problems? *J. Clin. Epidemiol.* 43: 277, 1990.
12. Fagan, T. J. Nomogram for Bayes' Theorem. *N. Engl. J. Med.* (Letter) 293: 257, 1975.
13. Feightner, J. W., Norman, G. R., and Haynes, R. B. The reliability of likelihood estimates by physicians. *Clin. Res.* 30: 298, 1982.
14. Fleiss, J. L. *Statistical Methods for Rates and Proportions.*New York: Wiley, 1973.
15. Germanson T. Screening for HIV: Can we afford the confusion of the false positive rate? *J. Clin. Epidemiol.* 42: 1235, 1989.
16. Glasziou, P. Threshold analysis via the Bayes nomogram. *Medical Decision Making* 11: 61, 1991.
17. Griner, P. F., Panzer, R. J., and Greenland, P. *Clinical Diagnosis and the Laboratory.* Chicago: Yearbook, 1986. P. 323
18. Goldman, L., Waternaux, C., Garfield, F., et al. Impact of a cardiology data bank on physicians' prognostic estimates. *Arch. Intern. Med.* 141: 1631, 1981.
19. Goldman, L., Weinberg, M., Weisberg, M., et al. A computer-derived protocol to aid in the diagnosis of emergency room patients with acute chest pain. *N. Engl. J. Med.* 307: 588, 1982.
20. Guyatt, G. H., Patterson, C., Ali, M., et al. Diagnosis of iron-deficiency anemia in the elderly. *Amer. J. Med.* 88: 205, 1990.
21. Hawkins, B. R., Dawkins, R. L., Christiansen, F. T., and Zilko, P. J. Use of the B27 test in the diagnosis of anklyosing spondylitis: A statistical evaluation. *Arthritis and Rheum.* 24: 743, 1981.
22. Hessel, S. J., Siegelman, S. S., McNeil, B. J., et al. A prospective evaluation of computed tomography and ultrasound of the pancreas. *Radiology* 143: 129, 1982.
23. Hull, R., Hirsh, J., Sackett, D. L., et al. Replacement of venography in suspected venous thrombosis by impedance plethysmography and ^{125}I-fibrinogen leg scanning. *Ann. Intern. Med.* 94: 12, 1981.
24. Kassirer, J. P., and Pauker, S. G. The toss-up. *N. Engl. J. Med.* 305: 1467, 1981.
25. Kassirer J. P., Moskowitz, A. J., Lau, J., and Pauker, S. G. Decision analysis: A progress report. *Ann. Intern. Med.* 106: 275, 1987.
26. Levin, B. E. The clinical significance of spontaneous pulsations of the retinal vein. *Arch. Neurol.* 35: 37, 1978.
27. Levy, D. E., Bates, D., Caronna, J. J., et al. Prognosis in nontraumatic coma. *Ann. Intern. Med.* 94: 293, 1981.
28. Marton, K. J., Sax, H. C., Jr., Wasson, J., et al. The clinical value of the upper gastrointestinal tract roentgenogram series. *Arch. Intern. Med.* 140: 191, 1980.
29. McNeil, B. J., and Pauker, S. G. The patient's role in assessing the value of diagnostic tests. *Radiology* 132: 605, 1979.
30. National Cancer Institute of Canada and American Cancer Society (NCI/ACS). A collaborative study of a test for carcinoembryonic antigen (CEA) in the sera of patients with carcinoma of the colon and rectum. *Can. Med. Assoc. J.* 107: 25, 1972.

31. Newman, G. F., Rerych, M. T., Upton, D. C., and Jones, R. H. Comparison of electrocardiographic and left ventricular function changes during exercise. *Circulation* 62: 1204, 1980.
32. Pauker, S. G., and Kassirer, J. P. Clinical application of decision analysis: A detailed illustration. *Semin. Nucl. Med.* 302: 1109, 1980.
33. Pauker, S. G., and Kassirer, J. P. The threshold approach to clinical decision making. *N. Engl. J. Med.* 302: 1109, 1980.
34. Pozen, M. W., D'Agostino, R., Mitchell, J., et al. The usefulness of a predictive instrument to reduce inappropriate admissions to a coronary care unit. *Ann. Intern. Med.* 92: 238, 1980.
35. Pozen, M. W., D'Agostino, R. B., Selker, H. P., et al. A predictive instrument to improve coronary-care-unit admission practices in acute ischemic heart disease. *N. Engl. J. Med.* 310: 1273, 1984.
36. Ransohoff, D. F., and Feinstein, A. R. Is decision analysis useful in clinical medicine? *Yale J. Biol. Med.* 29: 165, 1976.
37. Schwartz, W. B., Wolfe, H. J., and Pauker, S. G. Pathology and probabilities: A new approach to interpreting and reporting biopsies. *N. Engl. J. Med.* 305: 917, 1981.
38. Simel, D. L., Feussner, J. R., Delong, E. R., and Matchar, D.B. Intermediate, indeterminate, and uninterpretable diagnostic test results. *Med. Decis. Making.* 7: 107, 1987.
39. Singer, J. Value of clinical signs in diagnosis of deep vein thrombosis. *Lancet* 1: 1186, 1980.
40. Smith, A. F. Diagnostic value of serum-creatine-kinase in a coronary care unit. *Lancet* 2: 178, 1967.
41. Spodick, D. H. On experts and expertise: The effect of variability in observer performance. *Am. J. Cardiol.* 36: 592, 1975.
42. Weinstein, M. and Fineberg, H. *Clinical Decision Analysis.* Toronto: Saunders, 1980.

*The table for your cirrhotic with the positive α-fetoprotein test should look like this:

		Hepatoma			
		Yes	No		
AFP test result	Positive	245 (a)	75 (b)	320 (a+b)	⊕ PV = 77%
	Negative	5 (c)	675 (d)	680 (c+d)	⊖ PV = 99%
		250 (a+c)	750 (b+d)	1000 (a+b+c+d)	

Your patient's likelihood of hepatoma is now 77%

5

Early Diagnosis

Up to now, this book has focused on the diagnosis of symptomatic disease. However, this section on diagnosis would be incomplete without a final chapter on the early diagnosis of presymptomatic disease. This cornerstone of clinical preventive medicine is often misunderstood and, although its application often can be of enormous benefit to patients, it is frequently oversold. However, the application of a clinical epidemiologic point of view to the concepts and evidence concerning early diagnosis can dispel much of the current confusion and cut through the rhetoric. Once again, this "basic science for clinical medicine" can help us become more effective clinicians. And because early diagnosis entails major issues in therapy as well as diagnosis, its discussion provides a useful bridge between the first two sections of this book.

The Strategies and Objectives of Early Diagnosis

Early diagnosis is sought through two different strategies. First, members of the general public can be invited to undergo tests of various sorts in order to separate them into those with higher and lower probabilities of disease (the former group are then urged to seek medical attention for definitive diagnosis). This form of early diagnosis is called *screening*, and is epitomized by the "Healthorama" booth at the county fair, where passersby are exhorted to submit their arms for blood pressure measurement, their breath for respiratory function, their blood for lipids and their urine for glucose. The combination of several disparate tests in this fashion constitutes *multiphasic screening*.

Other forms of screening are both compulsory and aimed at specific individuals, as when immigrants submit to testing for tuberculosis or airline pilots to periodic electrocardiograms. Many physicians carry out a particular form of screening in which patients are invited to make appointments for a series of screening tests plus a general history and physical examination. These *periodic health examinations* may include extensive, expensive maneuvers such as sigmoidoscopy and stress electrocardiography, especially when performed on senior executives.

The second strategy of early diagnosis relies on the fact that almost everyone sees a physician once in awhile (for example, 75% of Canadians see a physician at least once a year, and 90% see one at least once every 5 years). As a result, clinicians need not call for volunteers but can simply seek early diagnosis when patients come to them for unrelated, intercurrent illnesses. This strategy is called *case finding* and it is exemplified by testing for hyperlipidemia in a 50-year-old who complains of sinusitis, checking the vision and hearing of a septuagenerian who presents with an upper-respiratory infection, and measuring the blood pressure of every adult patient who walks into the office for any reason.

It should be obvious by now that the targets for early diagnosis are not just disease entities such as tuberculosis and cancer. These targets include the predictors or "risk factors" for disease; thus, screening, case finding, and especially periodic health examinations often include questions about alcohol and tobacco use and measurements of blood lipids, glucose, height and weight, and the like.

Although the focus of this chapter is early diagnosis for the sake of the patient, it should be noted that screening and case finding often are executed with other objectives. For example, considerable screening is carried out in order to protect economic wagers; this is what the "life insurance physical" is all about. When you buy life insurance you are betting the company that you are going to die and it is betting you that you won't (at least not until you have paid up your policy). The company may insist that you undergo a physical examination in order to protect its side of the bet; the examination focuses on predictors of early demise (hypertension, diabetes, obesity and the like) and the company reserves the right, based on your results, to refuse to bet with you. Note that the insurance company's objective here is not to maintain or improve your health; it simply wants to win more bets than it loses.

Another reason for screening also places a low priority on health benefits to those screened, and this objective applies when prospective immigrants or teachers are screened for tuberculosis, and crane operators for uncontrolled hypertension. The goal here is the protection of others from tubercle bacilli or falling objects, and this objective is served by denying immigration or employment; treatment of positive screenees is a secondary priority.

A third reason to carry out periodic health examinations, or even case finding, is to establish "baselines" of what patients' electrocardiograms, blood chemistries, and so on are like when they are well; indeed, some clinicians advocate that patients ought to carry copies of these in their wallets and purses. Then, when something does go wrong, the clinician in attendance will have these earlier findings for comparison. Rigorous evaluation of the effects of such baseline information on the outcomes of subsequent illnesses is rare and, as we will show you shortly, continuing skepticism is in order about their worth.

At any rate, this chapter is not directed toward the use of screening, periodic health examinations, or case finding for benefit of life insurance companies, employers, or clinicians. Rather, the focus here is the use of these strategies to benefit patients, especially through the early diagnosis of asymptomatic disease.

Case finding covers a much larger proportion of the population than screening, since screening is carried out only sporadically and rarely captures more than 5 or 10% of eligible citizens. Moreover, because case finding is executed at the same site as definitive diagnosis and therapy, the problem of linking those who "screen positive" to a source of care is obviated. Case finding is better than periodic health examinations as well. Because in many regions the great majority of individuals visit a physician at least once a year, coverage is much more complete, and the busy clinicians can include a bit of "preventive medicine" in every visit rather than trying to squeeze appointments for periodic health examinations into an already overcrowded appointment schedule. Finally, decisions about what to include in case finding have tended to be hardheaded and related to payoffs for patients. Decisions about what to include in periodic health exams, on the other hand, have tended to be influenced more by what it is technically possible to do *to* patients than by what it is clinically possible to do *for* them. It is for these reasons that the Canadian Task Force on the Periodic Health Examination recommended the abandonment of the Periodic Health Examination and its replacement by case finding [4].

Early Diagnosis and the Natural History of Disease

Regardless of the strategy selected, the objective of early diagnosis is constant: the early detection of presymptomatic disease. This notion of early diagnosis presupposes an orderly biology or "natural history" of disease, divided into the four stages depicted in Figure 5-1.

1. *Biologic onset.* The disease begins with that initial interaction between man, causal factors, and the rest of the environment labelled "biologic onset." We cannot detect the presence of disease at this point in its natural history, but it is there. For some diseases biologic onset occurs at conception, and in many others it probably precedes the later stages by decades.
2. *Early diagnosis possible.* With the passage of time, and although the affected individual remains free of any symptoms, the mechanisms of disease produce structural or functional changes such that, if we applied the correct test, we could achieve the early diagnosis of the disease. At this point, early diagnosis becomes possible by means of screening, case finding, or a periodic health examination.
3. *Usual clinical diagnosis.* In the absence of intervention or spontaneous disappearance, the disease progresses to the point where symptoms appear and the affected individual becomes ill and seeks clinical help. This is the point of "usual clinical diagnosis."
4. *Outcome.* Finally, the disease runs its course and arrives at its "outcome" of recovery, permanent disability, or death.

It is this orderly progression from biologic onset, to the point where early diagnosis is possible, to the time of usual diagnosis, and ultimately to its out-

Figure 5-1. The natural history of disease.

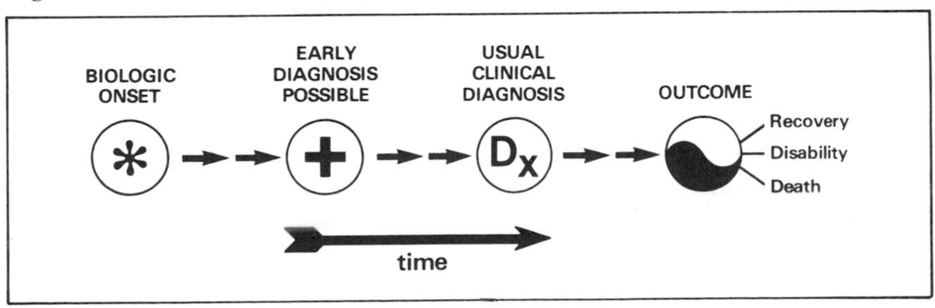

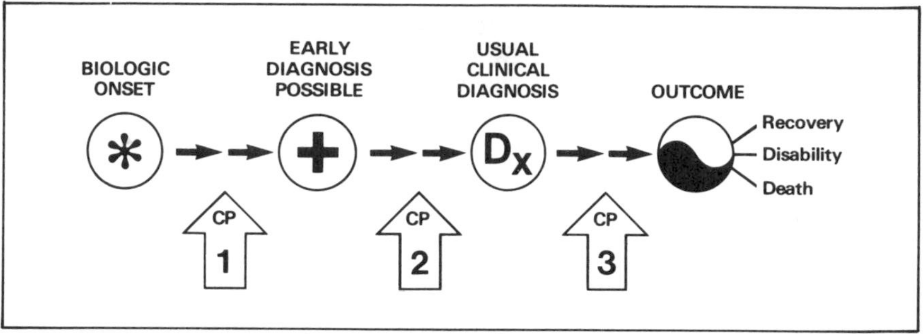

Figure 5-2. Critical points in the natural history of disease. CP = critical point.

come that renders a disease vulnerable to assault through screening, case finding, and the periodic health examination. This orderly progression is not enough, however, because another assumption underlies attempts at early diagnosis. This element was described by Hutchison in 1960 [14] and consists of a "critical point" in the natural history of a disease, *before which therapy is either more effective or easier to apply than afterward.* Now, a disease may have several critical points (arguably pulmonary tuberculosis) or may have none (arguably several cancers), and the location of these critical points along its natural history is crucial to the value of early diagnosis, as shown in Figure 5-2.

If a disease's only critical point were in position 1, between biologic onset and the time that early diagnosis became possible, we can see how screening or case finding would be too late to be of help; the critical point is already passed by the time that detection becomes possible. Similarly, if a disease's only critical point were at position 3, between the time of usual clinical diagnosis and disease outcome, early detection is a waste of time. In this case it would be less trouble all around to wait until symptomatic patients sought clinical help.

It is only when a disease possesses a critical point at position 2, between the time that early diagnosis becomes possible and the time of usual clinical diagnosis, that screening and case finding hold any promise of improving the outcomes of those who have the target disorder.

Admissible Evidence

How do we tell whether a disease has a critical point at position 2 and its detection is worth our critical effort? Unfortunately, the only way to tell for sure is to track down a properly executed randomized trial in which individuals were randomly allocated (by a system analogous to tossing a coin) to receive or not receive the screening or case-finding maneuver. The best standard therapy would have been provided to the experimental patients detected early and to any other patients (experimental or control) detected at the usual time of diagnosis. All patients in both groups would then have been followed up to see whether they succumbed to the target disease.

For example, a group of clinicians and methodologists led by Sam Shapiro [19] randomly allocated over 60,000 New York women (who were enrolled in the Health Insurance Plan [H.I.P.] of Greater New York) to receive or not receive invitations for annual mammography (two views) plus clinical breast examination. These annual examinations were offered for 4 years, and their yield is summarized in Table 5-1.

The potential benefits of mammography, clinical breast examination, and their combination looked promising in terms of the relatively low percent of cases with axillary node metastases at operation. The proof of the pudding, however, was whether deaths from breast cancer were reduced through early diagnosis, and this is shown in Table 5-2 [18, 19].

No benefit could be confirmed among women under age 50, but striking reductions in breast cancer mortality were observed at age 50 and beyond (the mortality from other causes of death was identical, confirming that randomization had produced comparable groups of experimental and control women). This landmark randomized trial (confirmed by additional subsequent trials) demonstrated that a critical point does, in fact, exist in the natural history of breast cancer and that it is located between the point where early diagnosis is possible and the time of usual clinical diagnosis.

Two randomized trials have tested whether multiphasic approaches to early diagnosis are beneficial, and both concluded that they are not. In the first trial [13], Walter Holland, Michael D'Souza, and Anthony Swan at St. Thomas's Hospital Medical School randomly allocated almost 7000 patients from two London general practices to receive or not receive periodic health examinations (that included histories, physical examinations, chest x rays and ECGs, pulmonary function tests, and tests on their blood and feces). Five years later these investigators could demonstrate no beneficial effects on mortality, self-perceived health, risk factors, or absenteeism. All they found was an increase in subsequent visits to the doctor in the screened group.

A short time later, and on the other side of the world, Timothy Durbridge and his colleagues conducted the previously noted randomized trial of hospital admission screening [6]. They randomly allocated about 1500 admissions to an Australian hospital into three groups. One group underwent about 40 tests on admission to the hospital, and the results were given to their clinicians. The second group underwent all the same tests, but the results were not reported. The third group were not screened on admission at all. These investigators were not able to demonstrate any benefit of admission screening in terms of mortality, morbidity, time to diagnosis, levels of nursing care required during their hospitalization, or in the satisfaction of either the patients or their clinicians. Once again, however, they did find that screening led to higher total costs for medical care. So it appears that although automating the clinical laboratory and cranking out batteries of test results may make the laboratory more efficient, it makes looking after patients less efficient.

The several breast cancer screening trials represent the best current evidence that any early diagnostic maneuvers are of any help to cancer patients. Another

Table 5-1. Breast cancers diagnosed early in the H.I.P. study

		Age at diagnosis				Percentage with positive axillary nodes
		40–49	50–59	60 +	Total	
Mode of early diagnosis	Only by mammography	6 (19%)	27 (42%)	11 (31%)	44 (33%)	16%
	Only by clinical exam	19 (62%)	26 (40%)	14 (38%)	59 (45%)	19%
	Detected by both modes	6 (19%)	12 (18%)	11 (31%)	29 (22%)	41%
		31 (100%)	65 (100%)	36 (100%)	132 (100%)	

Data modified from S. Shapiro. Evidence of screening for breast cancer from a randomized trial. *Cancer* (Suppl.) 39:2772, 1977.

Table 5-2. Some results of the H.I.P. randomized trial of early diagnosis in breast cancer

	Deaths per 10,000 women per year				
	From breast cancer				
	40–49	50–59	60–69	From all other causes	From cardiovascular disease
Control women	2.4	5.0	5.0	54	25
Experimental women	2.5	2.3	3.4	54	24

Data modified from S. Shapiro. Personal communication, 1976; and Evidence of screening for breast cancer from a randomized trial. *Cancer* (Suppl.) 39:2772, 1977.

trial [1] tested whether 6-monthly chest x rays would benefit lung cancer victims and documented no decrease in mortality in the x-rayed group; by the time a lung cancer is visible on a chest x ray, any critical point in its natural history has already been passed. Subsequent randomized trials tested whether adding sputum cytology to periodic chest x rays would be beneficial, and they were negative as well [7]. Finally, several trials are underway which will determine whether periodic stool testing for occult blood can reduce mortality from colorectal cancer [5, 10]. By these means, crucial knowledge about the clinical benefits of early detection strategies is coming to hand.

Inadmissible Evidence

Isn't this insistence on randomized trials overly pedantic and does it not represent another example of the classic failure of academics to realize what is going on in the front lines of clinical medicine? After all, all clinicians who have had any real experience *know* that early diagnosis works, and each of us accumulates several patients who have done extremely well after having their cancer diagnosed in an early, presymptomatic stage. Common sense tells us that early diagnosis works.

Unfortunately, making clinical judgments about the value of early diagnosis is one of the tasks in which our common sense leads us astray. It goes back to the faulty synthesis of correct observations into incorrect inferences that we discussed back in the chapter on the clinical examination (Chap. 2). In fact, our clinical observations *are* correct: patients whose cancers are diagnosed early do have better 5-year survivals than other patients diagnosed in later, symptomatic stages. It is our inference that these observations prove the value of early diagnosis that is faulty; in fact, *early diagnosis will always appear to improve survival, even when therapy is worthless!*

There are three reasons for this paradox. First, the patients and other people who volunteer for screening and periodic health examinations appear to be healthier before they start. This can be demonstrated by going back to the H.I.P trial we discussed a bit earlier. A reexamination of the right-hand columns of Table 5-2 confirms the effectiveness of the randomization: the overall experimental and control groups were identical for causes of death for which they were not screened, and deaths from other causes and from cardiovascular disease were identical.

Now, only about two-thirds of experimental women responded to their invitation to attend for mammography and clinical breast examination, and the other third refused. This provided an opportunity to compare those who volunteered with those who refused for causes of death for which they were never screened. The results are shown in Table 5-3 [18, 19].

In Table 5.3 we see that the subset of experimental women who volunteered for breast cancer screening experienced only about *half* the mortality from other causes exhibited by those women who refused; the volunteers fared far better for diseases for which they were never screened and never (on this basis) treated! Volunteers for screening are generally a strange and healthy lot, and we cannot generalize from them to our other patients.

The next reason that early diagnosis will always appear to improve survival, even when therapy is worthless, arises from the way that we measure survival after cancer is detected. This is usually done as shown in Figure 5-3.

Here we see 5 years of follow-up of a group of cancer patients identified at the time of usual clinical diagnosis, 10% of whom die each year, yielding a 5-year survival of 50%. If we diagnosed a group of such patients at age 45, half of them would be alive at age 50.

Now, suppose that we developed a screening test that could detect this cancer one year earlier, before such patients developed symptoms. Suppose further that the treatment of this cancer was no more effective when applied early than when applied at the time of usual clinical diagnosis. If we carry out the standard (but incorrect) comparison of our old and new results, we are likely to make the mistake shown in Figure 5-4.

The old results are expressed in a solid line as before, with zero-time the time of "usual clinical diagnosis." When the new results are charted, however, a zero-time corresponding to the 1-year previous "early diagnosis" is used and

Table 5-3. More results of the H.I.P. trial

		Deaths per 10,000 women per year	
		From all causes	From cardiovascular causes
Control women		54	25
Experimental women	Volunteered	42	17
	Refused	77	38

Data modified from S. Shapiro. Personal communication, 1976; and Evidence of screening for breast cancer from a randomized trial. *Cancer* (Suppl.) 39:2772, 1977.

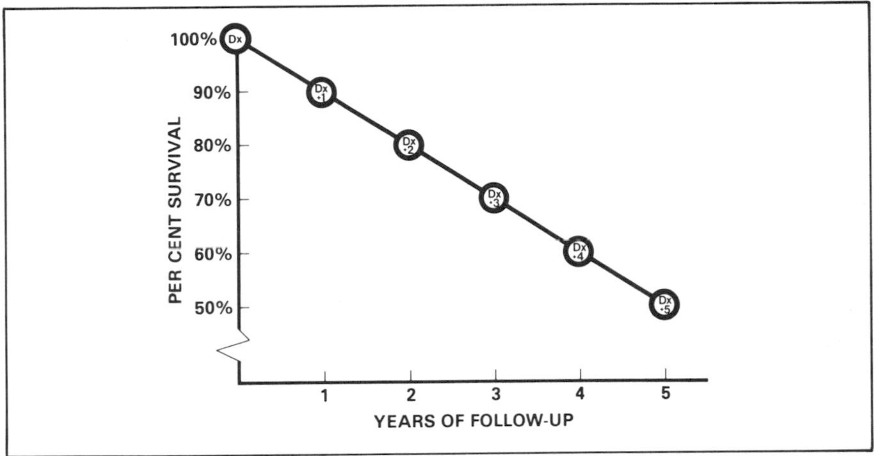

Figure 5-3. Survival following the detection of cancer at the time of usual clinical diagnosis.

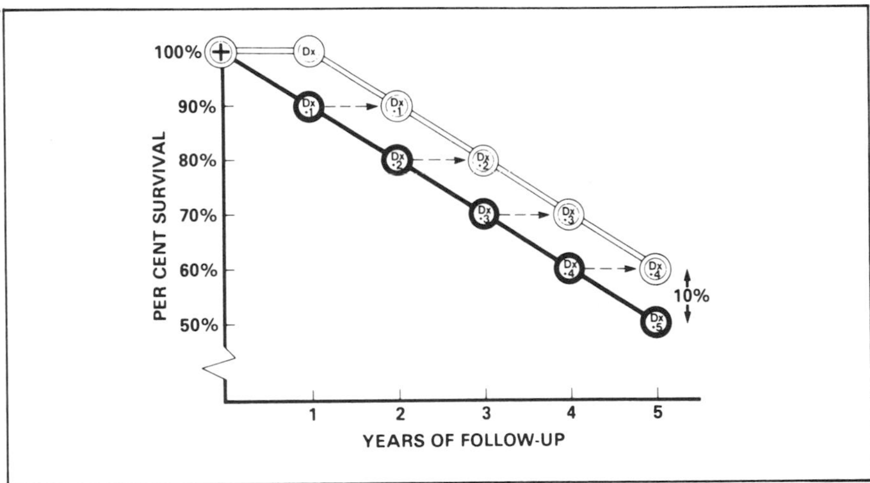

Figure 5-4. Failure to correct for "zero-time shift" in assessing the value of early diagnosis.

the resulting survival curve, illustrated by the open line, is shifted 1 year to the right. As a result of this "zero-time shift," even when therapy is worthless a 10% improvement in 5-year survival is guaranteed.

This apparent improvement in 5-year survival is fictitious, however, for all we have done is to shift the starting point for the five-year survival measurement 1 year backward, from the time of usual clinical diagnosis—the "Dx" sign—to the " + " sign of early diagnosis. Our group of 45-year-old cancer patients are simply diagnosed 1 year earlier, at age 44. Only half of them will be alive at age 50, as before, and we have given them not an extra year forward of life but an

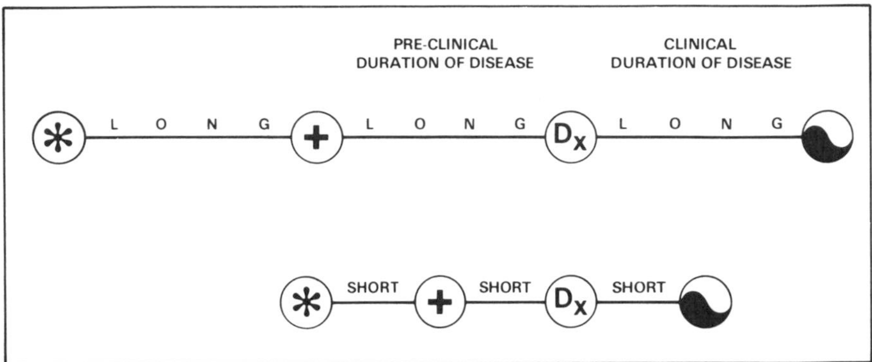

Figure 5-5. The relation between the preclinical and clinical duration of disease.

extra year backward of disease!* This is a key issue, and we will come back to it again later.

The final reason why early diagnosis will appear to improve survival, even when therapy is worthless, has to do with fast and slow growing tumors and is illustrated in Figure 5-5.

Occasionally, after we have diagnosed a cancer of the lung, stomach, or colon we go back to earlier radiographs and discover, to our dismay and chagrin, that the cancer was already there on the previous study. Usually it was too small or indistinct to have been diagnosable on the earlier film, but its location and configuration are enough to convince us that it was there. Studies of such cases and their subsequent clinical courses have taught us that some cancers grow very quickly and others, even of the same organ, grow much more slowly [9, 22]. These fast or slow growth rates tend to operate throughout the natural history of a given patient's disease, as shown in Figure 5-5. Patients with long preclinical durations of disease tend to have long clinical durations of disease, and those with short preclinical durations tend to have short and rapidly fatal clinical durations.

Although this relationship between the preclinical and clinical durations of disease may characterize most diseases, its effect on the assessment of early diagnosis was ignored until it was pointed out by Manning Feinleib and Marvin Zelen in 1969 [8]. This effect is illustrated in Figure 5-6.

Once again, patients detected through early diagnosis (depicted by the vertical staff topped by the "+" sign) will have longer survival than those detected at the time of usual clinical diagnosis, even when therapy is worthless. This is because the slow growing tumors are detectable longer than the fast growing ones and will, therefore, be preferentially identified by any early diagnosis strategy. The fast growing tumors, with their shorter survival, will be left for routine diagnosis, and the comparison distorted.† Note here that even correcting for

*This "zero-time shift" is also commonly referred to as "lead-time bias."

†The preferential detection of slow growing tumors is often called "length-time bias."

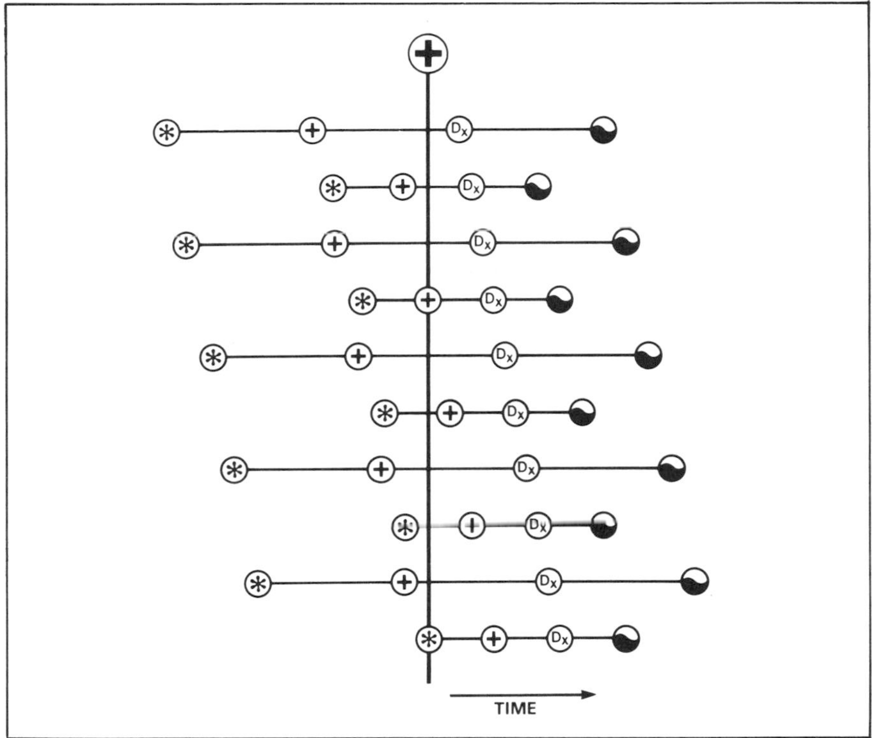

Figure 5-6. Preclinical duration of disease and the likelihood of early diagnosis.

"zero-time shift" will fail to overcome this pitfall in assessing the value of early diagnosis.

In summary, there are three reasons why common clinical inferences about the value of early diagnosis are inadmissible: the volunteer effect, the zero-time shift problem (lead-time bias), and the preferential detection of slowly progressive disease (length-time bias). As a result of these three factors, early diagnosis will always appear to improve survival, even when therapy is worthless. Accordingly, we must insist on evidence from proper randomized trials of early diagnostic maneuvers before we act.

The Hazards of Inappropriate Early Diagnosis

Some readers may still regard our insistence on evidence from randomized trials as excessively rigorous. After all, it will take several years to carry out the necessary randomized trials, and in the meanwhile countless patients will lose their chance for early diagnosis.

We believe that a firm stand requiring hard evidence from randomized trials is correct, both for the reasons already given and for two more: the implied pledge to the patient who undergoes early diagnosis, and the potential for doing harm to the early diagnosed patient.

Consider first our implied (and frequently stated) pledge to symptomatic patients when they seek us out and ask us for help. Although we promise to do our best for them, we do *not* guarantee them better health (in fact, clinicians who do provide such guarantees are often labeled quacks and charlatans). We diagnose and treat these symptomatic patients as best we can, realizing that standard therapies for their conditions may never have been validated and may not even work, and that even the validated ones will not work for everyone. Their symptoms and their call for help force us to act, often on the basis of incomplete evidence about the value of what we are about to do.

Now consider our implied (but almost never stated) pledge to the symptom-free citizens whom we solicit for screening or periodic health examination. The tables are reversed: we are seeking them out. They feel fine, but we are asking them to come for tests and possibly extensive, prolonged therapy. Surely in this case our implied promise to them is better health; not that their subsequent treatment *may* work but that it *does* work; not that we will simply do our best but that we will make them healthier. When we impose ourselves on the public in this fashion, we require very firm evidence that our early diagnosis and subsequent therapy will do more good than harm.

This last comment introduces the second reason for demanding hard evidence for the benefit of early diagnosis: the potential for doing harm to the early diagnosed patient. Advocates of screening and periodic health examinations sometimes act as if there were only two possible outcomes of these undertakings: on the one hand, positive benefit and, on the other, no effect. What is often ignored is the third possible outcome: harm.

This harm can be of two sorts. First, the diagnosis can be wrong. The risk of making a false-positive diagnosis becomes huge when we are looking for rare disorders in symptomless patients. An example of this is shown in Table 5-4.

Although the sensitivity (PiD rate, TP rate) and specificity (NiH rate, TN rate) of the B27 test for ankylosing spondylitis are excellent (90% and 95%, respectively), this disorder is so rare that, of every 100 individuals with a negative family history but a positive B27 test, 98 do *not* have ankylosing spondylitis (in fact, this is probably a low estimate of the extent of misdiagnosis; the pretest probability of this disorder is probably closer to .05%, which means that 99 of 100 individuals with positive B27 tests are misdiagnosed) [11, 21]. We are left with lots of individuals with positive tests but no symptoms, and most of them do not have the target disorder. The best way to resolve this sort of dilemma is to stay out of it in the first place.

Second, the treatment initiated as a result of early diagnosis may, in fact, do more harm than good. A catastrophic example is provided by a widespread treatment for hyperlipidemia. Most periodic health examinations in the 1960s and 1970s included measurements of blood lipids, and both screening and case finding for hyperlipidemia were very popular, especially in the United States. When elevated serum cholesterol was found on these examinations, dietary advice was usually offered and, if the elevation persisted, drug therapy with clofibrate often was initiated to bring the cholesterol level down. As a result, it was not unusual

Table 5-4. The B27 test in the early diagnosis of ankylosing spondylitis

		Ankylosing spondylitis: Yes	Ankylosing spondylitis: No		
B27 test	Positive	90 (a)	510 (b)	600 (a+b)	Positive predictive value = Posttest likelihood or posterior probability of disease = $\frac{a}{a+b} = \frac{90}{600} = 15\%$
	Negative	10 (c)	9390 (d)	9400 (c+d)	Negative predictive value = Posttest likelihood or posterior probability of *no* disease = $\frac{d}{c+d} = \frac{9390}{9400} = 99.9\%$
		100 (a+c)	9900 (b+d)	10,000 (a+b+c+d)	
		Sensitivity = $\frac{a}{a+c} = \frac{90}{100} = 90\%$	Specificity = $\frac{d}{b+d} = \frac{9390}{9900} = 95\%$		Prevalence = Pretest likelihood = Prior probability of disease = $\frac{a+c}{a+b+c+d} = \frac{100}{10{,}000} = 1\%$

to find ostensibly healthy, asymptomatic, middle-aged men taking this drug as a result of having undergone a "cholesterol count."

It had been known for some time that clofibrate could lower serum cholesterol levels, and so it was assumed that lowering this "risk factor" with this drug had to be beneficial. However, it was only after this lipid screening and risk factor modification had been going on for several years that a proper randomized trial of clofibrate was carried out in healthy middle-aged men with hypercholesterolemia.* The results were shocking: mortality in clofibrate-treated men was 17% *higher* than among men on placebos, and this excess mortality continued for four years following withdrawal of the drug [23].

Extrapolation of these results to the United States where most of this screening and treatment took place provided a somber lesson. It was estimated that the detection of hyperlipidemia and its treatment with clofibrate led to the deaths of over 5000 asymptomatic Americans [16]. Unless we are willing to permit a future recurrence of a catastrophe of this magnitude, we must insist on sound evidence from randomized trials that early diagnosis and specific forms of therapy do more good than harm *before* we solicit our patients and the public to submit to them.

The third sort of harm that can come from early diagnosis is the damage done when we tell someone who feels well that they are sick. This phenomenon, which we shall call "labeling," is well known in social psychology but only now becoming recognized by most clinical disciplines.

Consider what happens when we tell a symptomless steelworker for the first time that he has hypertension [12, 20]. His absenteeism from work due to illness, which was previously indistinguishable from that of his normotensive coworkers, doubles in the next year and remains high. He is not sick more often, but when he develops minor illnesses he stays away roughly twice as long, treating himself as if he were quite fragile (or, in social psychological terms, he "adopts the sick role"). His psychological well-being declines and he is less satisfied with his work and his marriage. His income suffers, and he perceives himself as not advancing as rapidly as his workmates.

There are a couple of additional surprises in our follow-up of such patients. We cannot pass off their subsequent behavior as simply representing the side effects of antihypertensive drugs, for these same changes occur in men who are only labeled but never treated. Moreover, teaching these men about their disease and its treatment (which, as you will learn later in this book, does nothing for their compliance with their antihypertensive drug regimens) tends to accentuate the effects of labeling.

Other investigators have, with some exceptions, confirmed these observations in hypertensives elsewhere [15], and even more dramatic effects of labeling are seen with other diagnoses. As you may recall from our earlier chapter on the clinical examination, normal children who were misdiagnosed as having organic heart disease show as much deterioration in physical and social function as chil-

*This trial was a forerunner of the later, positive trials of other approaches to lowering serum cholesterol.

dren who really do have damaged hearts. More recently, a randomized trial of the Denver Developmental Screening Test revealed that children who screened positive and received counselling and referral to all sorts of health professionals and agencies fared no better in their future academic, cognitive, or developmental performance than children whose positive screening results were never revealed [3]. Moreover, the labeled children's parents were far more likely to worry about their school performance, and teachers tended to report more behavioral problems among them.

Labeling happens all the time. We accept it as inevitable when it results from routine diagnosis among symptomatic patients; after all, they come to us asking for it. When labeling occurs through early diagnosis, however, we must consider it in its own right. The screenee has no symptoms and is not asking to be labeled. We must decide whether we really ought to take away someone's health through early diagnosis by labeling him or her with a disease that requires intervention.

This labeling of ostensibly healthy individuals as diseased happens every time we achieve an early diagnosis, regardless of whether the subsequent therapy is effective, worthless, or harmful. When therapy is effective, both we and the patient are usually willing to live with the label, for the ultimate outcome is worth it. If, however, the therapy is worthless or no more effective when applied early than when applied later among symptomatic patients, we have needlessly taken away "healthy" time from our patients and have merely made them sick longer. Moreover, when therapy is harmful we have both robbed our patients of healthy months or years, and have needlessly exposed them to damaging interventions.

Our final set of comments about the hazards of inappropriate early diagnosis steps away from our usual focus on individual patients and looks at populations, professional credibility, and the search for useful new knowledge [17]. The decision to case-find in an individual patient, even when the associated treatment is unproven, costs relatively little and limits the human risk of side effects and toxicity should the remedy later be shown to be useless or harmful. However, this opportunity for waste and harm is progressively magnified when an untested procedure is applied throughout a practice (as universal case finding or as part of a periodic health examination scheme) or in the town at large (as a screening program).

In addition, the widespread implementation of untested methods of early diagnosis renders their subsequent rigorous evaluation much more difficult and less decisive; indeed it may even become impossible to correct the original error. Moreover, research into alternative strategies is discouraged in the interim.

How to Decide When to Seek an Early Diagnosis

This chapter could close with a list of early diagnoses worth pursuing. Instead, we will end it with some guides that clinicians can use to decide when, and on which patients, they should attempt the early diagnosis of presymptomatic disease. We have adopted the strategy of showing you how to decide for yourself, rather than simply telling you which screening tests to do, for two reasons. First, any specific advice could be out of date by the time this book is published.

Table 5-5. How to decide when to seek an early diagnosis

1. Does early diagnosis really lead to improved clinical outcomes (in terms of survival, function, and quality of life)?
2. Can you manage the additional clinical time required to confirm the diagnosis and provide long-term care for those who screen positive?
3. Will the patients in whom an early diagnosis is achieved comply with your subsequent recommendations and treatment regimens?
4. Has the effectiveness of individual components of a periodic health examination or multiphasic screening program been demonstrated prior to their combination?
5. Does the burden of disability from the target disease warrant action?
6. Are the cost, accuracy, and acceptability of the screening test adequate for your purpose?

Important randomized trials are still underway to determine the value of testing stools for occult blood, and of treating certain forms of elevated blood pressure. Their results will render obsolete any set of recommendations we might make.

The second reason returns to the basic objective of this book: helping clinicians make better clinical decisions by showing them how to critically appraise clinical articles. We want to show you how to decide whether to apply a particular maneuver for early diagnosis. To tell you *which* tests to use would defeat the purpose of the book.

When deciding whether to carry out a given test for the early diagnosis of presymptomatic disease, you should ask yourself the questions* that are listed in Table 5-5.

DOES EARLY DIAGNOSIS REALLY LEAD TO IMPROVED CLINICAL OUTCOMES (IN TERMS OF SURVIVAL, FUNCTION, AND QUALITY OF LIFE)?

As you have learned earlier, the therapy for the condition must favorably alter its natural history, not simply by advancing the time at which diagnosis occurs, but by improving survival, function, quality of life or all three. The modification of "risk factors" is not sufficient evidence of effectiveness, nor is the fact that the proposed therapy is widely accepted. Claims for therapeutic benefit must withstand close scrutiny and experimental evidence from randomized trials is a prerequisite.†

You need to be sure that, on average, the long-term beneficial effects of therapy outweigh the long-term detrimental effects of the treatment regimen and labeling of patients as diseased.

*A related set of questions has been developed by David Cadman, Larry Chambers, and William Feldman for use in deciding whether to launch a community-wide screening program [2].
†Detailed guides for scrutinizing the results of randomized trials are presented in Chapter 7.

CAN YOU MANAGE THE ADDITIONAL CLINICAL TIME REQUIRED TO CONFIRM THE DIAGNOSIS AND PROVIDE LONG-TERM CARE FOR THOSE WHO SCREEN POSITIVE?

Increased demands on your time start, not end, with early diagnosis and you need to be sure that you have enough of it. Large numbers of labeled but untreated hypertensives attest to the size of this problem.

WILL THE PATIENTS IN WHOM AN EARLY DIAGNOSIS IS ACHIEVED COMPLY WITH YOUR SUBSEQUENT RECOMMENDATIONS AND TREATMENT REGIMENS?

If patients will not take their medicine, all the foregoing screening and diagnosis, however elegantly they were conceived and executed, are nullified. Once again, all that you have left is a labeled patient.

This question may best be answered on an individual patient-by-patient basis, and we know many clinicians who say they would withhold early diagnostic tests from patients with past histories of noncompliance.*

HAVE THE EFFECTIVENESS OF INDIVIDUAL COMPONENTS OF A PERIODIC HEALTH EXAMINATION OR MULTIPHASIC SCREENING PROGRAM BEEN DEMONSTRATED PRIOR TO THEIR COMBINATION?

The appropriateness of a mix of tests must consider whether differences in the distributions of two diseases render the combination of their respective screening tests nonsensical. It was this consideration that led the Canadian Task Force on the Periodic Health Examination to propose quite different "health protection packages" for patients of different age, sex, and social status [4].

DOES THE BURDEN OF DISABILITY FROM THE TARGET DISEASE WARRANT ACTION?

The disease you are searching for should be either so common or so awful as to warrant all the work and expense of detecting it in its presymptomatic state.

ARE THE COST, ACCURACY AND ACCEPTABILITY OF THE SCREENING TEST ADEQUATE FOR YOUR PURPOSE?

After acquiring one or more "belts" in the previous chapter, this question may appear easy to answer. There is an additional twist, however, because in early diagnosis these tests are applied to asymptomatic people with generally very low pretest likelihoods (or prior probabilities) of disease. Accordingly, you may have to juggle the cutoff for a positive test or, better still, make full use of the likelihood ratios for different levels of the test result if you are to avoid both missing cases who could benefit, on the one hand, and avoiding unnecessary labeling, on the other.

*We have devoted Chapter 8 to some practical clinical aspects of compliance.

References

1. Brett, G. Z. The value of lung cancer detection by six-monthly chest radiographs. *Thorax* 23: 414, 1968.
2. Cadman, D., Chambers, L. W., Feldman, W., and Sackett, D. L. Assessing the effectiveness of community screening programs. *J.A.M.A.* 251: 1580, 1984.
3. Cadman, D., Chambers, L. W., Walter, S. D., et al. Evaluation of public health preschool child developmental screening: The process and outcomes of a community program. *Am. J. Pub. Health* 77: 45, 1987.
4. Canadian Task Force on the Periodic Health Examination. The periodic health examination. *Can. Med. Assoc. J.* 121: 1193, 1979.
5. Chamberlain, J. Is screening for colorectal cancer worthwhile? *Br. J. Cancer* 62: 1, 1990.
6. Durbridge, T. C., Edwards, F., Edwards, R. G., and Atkinson, M. An evaluation of multiphasic screening on admission to hospital. Précis of a report to the National Health and Medical Research Council. *Med. J. Aust.* 1: 703, 1976.
7. Eddy, D. M. Screening for lung cancer. *Ann. Intern. Med.* 111: 232, 1989.
8. Feinleib, M., and Zelen, M. Some pitfalls in the evaluation of screening programs. *Arch. Environ. Health* 19: 412, 1969.
9. Feinstein, A. R., Schimpf, C. B., and Hull, E. W. A reappraisal of the staging and therapy for patients with cancer of the rectum. *Arch. Intern. Med.* 135: 1441, 1975.
10. Gilbertson, V. A., Church, T. R., Grewe, F. J., et al. The design of a study to assess occult-blood screening for colon cancer. *J. Chron. Dis.* 33: 107, 1980.
11. Hawkins, B. R., Dawkins, R. L., Christiansen, F. T., and Zilko, P. J. Use of the B27 test in the diagnosis of anklyosing spondylitis: A statistical evaluation. *Arthritis and Rheum.* 24: 743, 1981.
12. Haynes, R. B., Sackett, D. L., Taylor, D. W., et al. Increased absenteeism from work after detection and labeling of hypertensive patients. *N. Engl. J. Med.* 299: 741, 1978.
13. Holland, W. W., D'Souza, M. D., and Swan, A. V. Is mass screening justified? *T. Soc. Geneesk* 56: 22, 1978.
14. Hutchison, G. B. Evaluation of preventive services. *J. Chron. Dis.* 11: 497, 1960.
15. Macdonald, L. A., Sackett, D. L., Haynes, R. B., and Taylor, D. W. Labelling in hypertension: A review of the behavioral and psychological consequences. *J. Chron. Dis.* 37: 933, 1984.
16. Round the World: Clofibrate. Correspondents Report. *Lancet* 1: 771, 1981.
17. Sackett, D. L., and Holland, W. W. Controversy in the detection of disease. *Lancet* 1: 357, 1975.
18. Shapiro, S. Personal communication, 1976.
19. Shapiro, S. Evidence of screening for breast cancer from a randomized trial. *Cancer* (Suppl.) 39: 2772, 1977.
20. Taylor, D. W., Haynes, R. B., Sackett, D. L., and Gibson, E. S. Long-term follow-up of absenteeism among working men following the detection and treatment of their hypertension. *Clin. Invest. Med.* 4: 173, 1981.
21. van der Linden, S. M., Valkenburg, H. A., de Jongh, B. M., and Cats, A. The risk of developing ankylosing spondylitis in HLA-B27 positive individuals. *Arth. Rheum.* 27: 241, 1984.
22. Weiss, W., Boucot, K. R., and Cooper, D. A. Growth rate in the detection and prognosis of bronchogenic carcinoma. *J.A.M.A.* 198: 1246, 1966.
23. World Health Organization. Trial on primary prevention of ischaemic heart disease using clofibrate to lower serum cholesterol: Mortality followup. Report of the Committee of Principal Investigators. *Lancet* 2: 379, 1980.

II

Management

6

Making a Prognosis

Having applied the strategies and tactics of the foregoing section and arrived at a diagnosis that explains the patient's illness, we now confront two new questions:

1. What do we tell the patient? Should we keep mum, reassure him that his illness is trivial, or advise him to make out his will?
2. What do we do for the patient? Should we reassure him and leave him alone, simply watch and wait, or treat him as soon as possible?

The answers to these questions depend, in a crucial way, on our understanding of the time course of the interactions between our patient, the causal factors for his disease, and the rest of his environment, beginning with the biologic onset of disease and ending with his recovery, death, or arrival at some other physical, social, and emotional state. In the previous chapter, we named this time course the *natural history of disease*. Of special interest to us now is a subset of the natural history that begins when the diagnosis is made, and this subset is often called the *clinical course* of disease.

In deciding what to tell, and do for, the patient we will be extrapolating from what we know about the likely clinical course of the patient's disease in order to make judgments about the patient's *prognosis* —the relative probabilities that he will develop each of the alternative outcomes of the natural history of his disease.

Suppose, for example, that you discover a symptomless subcutaneous lipoma on the back of an anxious steelworker who has come to you for insomnia and dyspepsia, which began after being laid off by the mill. Aware of the benign clinical course of such lumps and alert to the potential dangers of labeling the patient as having a "tumor," you probably will decide to tell him nothing, at least until his current problem is resolved, and simply will make a note to check the lipoma at a subsequent visit to confirm its innocence.

Suppose, on the other hand, the biopsy of a mass discovered on rectal examination of an otherwise robust 62-year-old waitress with recent rectal bleeding reveals a well-differentiated carcinoma. Aware of the serious prognosis and alert to the potential benefit of prompt surgical evaluation, you will inform the patient of her condition and arrange an early referral.

The preceding examples are pretty clear cut, and your response to them may be so "automatic" that no conscious considerations of their prognoses would even take place. In other cases, however, prognosis is by no means clear and you will have to do some careful thinking.

Suppose, for example, you detect 10 to 15 degrees of scoliosis in an otherwise healthy 12-year-old student who has come for her preschool examination. Do you tell her and her parents (and, if so, what do you say?), refer her to an "orthopod," or what? Suppose a fit, 32-year-old engineer passes (and loses) his first ever urinary stone and has a normal history, physical, urinalysis, and serum calcium. Do you execute a "stone workup" now or wait to see whether he has a recurrence? Suppose you have finally controlled a 37-year-old accountant's left-sided ulcerative colitis that had troubled him since he was 32. Should you now recommend a prophylactic colectomy to obviate the risk of subsequent cancer?

In these latter examples it is not obvious what you should tell, or do for, the patient and you must develop some strategies for making these tougher prognoses. Two such strategies are worth discussing here. First, you can rely on an "expert opinion," either by looking it up in a textbook or by consulting the appropriate specialist. This strategy certainly appears to make sense for the "once-in-a-lifetime" cases that you are unlikely to encounter again, and you can save your precious reading time for pursuing other, more common problems. However, as we shall soon find out, experts often disagree with one another, and frequently err when they try to extrapolate from their setting and experience (usually based on tertiary care) to other settings. Moreover, most textbooks fail to describe the settings and experiences that form the bases for their statements about prognosis.

The second strategy for making a prognosis is to "read up" on a case and find out for yourself what the clinical literature has to say about its clinical course and prognosis. Of course, you may feel that you are just too busy to traipse after the clinical literature, and that you can and should rely on expert opinions for every prognostic question that crops up in your practice. But if this is your view, couldn't you be replaced by a less expensive clinician and a set of algorithms?

Or you may prefer to rely on your "clinical experience" and simply recall similar patients you have seen before and what happened to them. Many times this strategy is very useful, especially when the illness is a quite common one. However, there are two drawbacks to this approach that limit its usefulness. First, our memories are not nearly so accurate as we may think. Our estimates of our prior experience tend to place undue weight on our most recent or most spectacular patients [14]. Second, even if we have accurately recorded and recalled the prognostic outcomes of our prior patients, we need to have seen a very large number of them before we can have much confidence in our prognostic statements about them. Suppose, for example, that we had seen a new case of urinary stone every month for 4 years, and had been able to keep track of every one of them for at least 2 years thereafter. Suppose further that 5 of these 48 patients had a recurrence of stone colic, for a recurrence of 5/48 or 10%. How confident can we be that, based on our clinical experience, the recurrence rate of symptomatic urinary calculi is "about 10%"? As it happens, not very confident. In fact, to be 95% sure that our estimate of such patients' prognoses encompasses the true recurrence rate, we would have to quote an interval of recurrences all the way from 1% to 19%.* Thus, our individual clinical

*For those who want to know how this was calculated, the 95% "confidence interval" for a

experiences often do not include enough cases to permit us to make confident predictions about prognosis, and we therefore must track down larger collections of such patients as they are described in the clinical literature.

And even the literature may not help us narrow these confidence limits very much. For example, we recently were debating whether to anticoagulate a patient with nonvalvular atrial fibrillation in order to reduce her risk of embolic stroke, and one of our clinical clerks had tracked down an article which reported a subgroup of 30 similar patients, none of whom were anticoagulated and none of whom had gone on to stroke. How confident can we be that this 0/30 really means 0% and excludes stroke risks of the magnitude that we might want to treat? Because the formula in the footnote doesn't work for extreme proportions like 0% or 100%, we generated Table 6-1 to help you answer this sort of question.

As you can see from Table 6-1, the 95% confidence limits on a stroke rate of 0% among 30 patients goes all the way up to 10%. This table also tells us that confidence limits remain pretty wide until the number of patients in the report reaches at least 40, and that very narrow confidence limits are not achieved until very large numbers of patients are in the report.

Let's return to the patients who opened the chapter. Using the search strategies described in Chapter 11, you should unearth several articles on each of their problems in short order. The initial scanning of these papers probably will generate more heat than light, for you almost certainly will find that they disagree on basic elements of the prognosis of the diseases they are describing. For example, the published spontaneous recovery rates for scoliosis vary *sevenfold* [8]; the risks of recurrence over the ten years following a first urinary stone range from 20% [7] (in which case you might well decide to forego a stone workup after a first bout of colic) to almost 100% [1] (in which case you might as well do it now); and published rates of cancer risk in left-sided ulcerative colitis vary from that seen in the general population [3] to nearly 10% [5].

With this much inconsistency in the clinical journals, how are we to use them sensibly in making clinical decisions about the clinical course and prognosis of human illness? As it happens most of the inconsistencies among the published studies of clinical course and prognosis are due to the different ways (many of them wrong) that their authors selected and followed the patients. Nonetheless, the requirements for the proper study of clinical course and prognosis are relatively straightforward, involve the sort of "applied common sense" we have called upon throughout this book, and can be translated into a brief set of standards or readers' guides that can be applied quickly to published articles. The six guides for reading such articles can be posed as questions and are listed in Table 6-2; once again, because they focus on how the clinical study was carried out they are applied to the Patients and Methods section of the article [2].

---

proportion like 10% is that proportion minus and plus twice its standard error. Since the standard error of a proportion (let's call it p) that is based on a total sample of n patients is: $p\sqrt{p(1-p)/n}$, the standard error of our 10%, based on 48 patients, is: $\sqrt{.10(.90)/48} = .043$, or 4.3%. Thus, $10\% - 2(4.3\%) = 1.4\%$ and $10\% + 2(4.3\%) = 18.6\%$.

Table 6-1. 95% Confidence limits on extreme results

If the denominator is:	And the % is 0%, the true % could be as *high* as:	And the % is 100%, the true % could be as *low* as:
1	95%	5%
2	78%	22%
3	63%	37%
4	53%	47%
5	45%	55%
6	39%	61%
7	35%	65%
8	31%	69%
9	28%	72%
10	26%	74%
15	18%	82%
20	14%	86%
25	11%	89%
30	10%	90%
35	8%	92%
40	7%	93%
45	6%	94%
50	6%	94%
55	5%	95%
60	5%	95%
65	5%	95%
70	4%	96%
75	4%	96%
80	4%	96%
85	3%	97%
90	3%	97%
95	3%	97%
100	3%	97%
150	2%	98%
300	1%	99%

Table 6-2. Guides for reading articles to learn the clinical course and prognosis of disease

1. Was an "inception cohort" assembled?
2. Was the referral pattern described?
3. Was complete follow-up achieved?
4. Were objective outcome criteria developed and used?
5. Was the outcome assessment "blind"?
6. Was adjustment for extraneous prognostic factors carried out?

From the Department of Clinical Epidemiology and Biostatistics, McMaster University, Hamilton, Ontario. How to read clinical journals: III. To learn the clinical course and prognosis of disease. *Can. Med. Assoc. J.* 124:869, 1981.

Was an "Inception Cohort" Assembled?

Patients should have been identified at an early and uniform point (inception) in the course of their disease (such as when they first developed unambiguous symptoms or received their first definitive therapy), so that those who succumbed or completely recovered are included with those whose disease persisted.

Many studies of prognosis are done backwards. For example, several studies of the risk of stone recurrence ask *currently* symptomatic patients if they have had stones *previously*, failing to realize that recurrent stone formers (with positive past histories) have multiple chances to be included in such studies, but patients without recurrences (with negative past histories) have only one chance of being included; no wonder recurrence rates vary all over the map! Similarly, in one study of cancer risk in ulcerative colitis, the stimulus for including several patients in the study was their development of cancer [5]. Clearly they had not been followed since the inception of their ulcerative colitis, and since colitis patients who remained cancer-free could not be entered through this mechanism, the apparent risk of cancer in ulcerative colitis patients had to become spuriously elevated [10].

The failure to start a study of clinical course and prognosis with an inception cohort has an unpredictable effect on its results. In most cases, the effect would be to make prognosis appear gloomier than it really is. However, distortion in the opposite direction also can occur. Suppose we wanted to learn more about the prognosis of patients following a myocardial infarction and read an article about a collection of such patients that had been assembled in a coronary care unit. Such a study could not, of course, include myocardial infarction patients who died before they could get to the coronary care unit. Because these early deaths constitute more than half of those who will die within the first year of their myocardial infarction, a study confined to coronary care unit patients would paint a falsely rosy prognosis.

Clearly the failure to assemble a proper inception cohort of patients who are at an early and uniform point in the course of their disease usually constitutes a fatal flaw in studies of prognosis. The application of this guide to an article can increase your efficiency in reading the clinical literature: If an article's authors failed to assemble an inception cohort, discard it early and go on to something else. In this way, you can focus your precious reading time on the most valid and useful articles.

What if none of the articles are based on an inception cohort? What then? Our choices are three: We can abandon the search and retreat to expert opinion; second, we can decide whether the failure to assemble an inception cohort is likely to distort the prognosis in a more favorable (or less favorable) direction and recognize that its result is overly optimistic (or pessimistic); finally, we can consider whether our management decision is affected by clinically sensible upward or downward revisions of the reported prognosis and act accordingly.

Was the Referral Pattern Described?

The pathways by which patients entered the study sample should be described. It must be possible for you, the reader, to be able to tell whether the results apply to patients in your practice. Did they come from a primary care center; were all hospitals in a defined region scoured for cases; or were they assembled in a tertiary care center that attracted the hopeless, wealthy, or bizarre? It is in the assembly of patients that studies of the course and prognosis of disease often flounder, for it is here that four types of bias are most pervasive [9].

Because a major clinical center's reputation results in part from its particular expertise in a specialized area of clinical medicine, it will be referred problem cases likely to benefit from this expertise (*centripetal bias*) and its experts may preferentially admit and keep track of these cases over other, less challenging or less interesting ones (*popularity bias*). In any event, the selection that occurs at each stage of the referral process can generate patient samples at tertiary care centers that are much different from those found in the general population (*referral filter bias*). Finally, patients differ in their financial and geographic access to the clinical technology that identifies them as eligible for studies of the course and prognosis of disease; if this degree of access is linked to the risk of a specific outcome (such as would occur, for example, if wealthier patients whose depression was more likely to respond to drugs had greater access to dexamethasone suppression testing than poorer patients with worse prognoses), the resulting *diagnostic access bias* will distort the conclusion of the study.

For example, the prognosis of febrile seizures is of enormous importance to patients, clinicians, and parents alike. Are they almost always innocuous or are they harbingers of later nonfebrile fits? Should clinicians reassure and observe, or should they label these children as epileptic and start them on anticonvulsants? A key element of this clinical decision is the rate at which children with uncomplicated febrile convulsions go on to have nonfebrile seizures. Clinicians who seek the answer to this question in the clinical literature cannot be blamed for coming away highly confused. As shown in Figure 6-1, the published risks for subsequent nonfebrile seizures following febrile convulsions vary almost 40-fold, from 1.5% to 58.2% [4].

In Figure 6.1 we have charted the rates of subsequent nonfebrile seizures (along with their 95% confidence intervals) reported in studies of children between 7 months and 7 years of age whose first seizures were accompanied by fever but were not regarded as symptomatic of any acute neurologic illness. As nearly as we can tell, each of these studies was based on an inception cohort; nonetheless, their results vary tremendously.

However, when these studies are segregated by a second sampling factor, the *source* (sampling frame) from which patients were selected, an important second principle emerges. The 10 studies shown at the left of Figure 6-1 and depicted by solid boxes all took place at specialty clinics or hospitals. They enrolled children referred to them with febrile convulsions and followed these children for the subsequent occurrence of nonfebrile seizures. Their results vary almost tenfold from 6% to 58.2%.

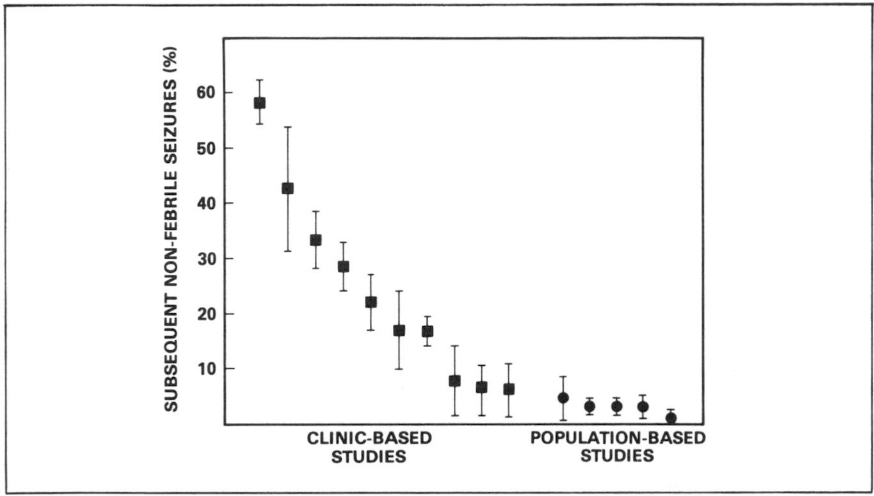

Figure 6-1. The risk of nonfebrile seizures following febrile convulsions. ■ = studies from specialty clinics and hospitals; ● = studies from general populations. (Adapted from J. H. Ellenberg and K. B. Nelson. Sample selection and the natural history of disease. Studies of febrile seizures. *J.A.M.A.* 243:1337, 1980.)

On the other hand, the five studies on the right-hand side of Figure 6-1, depicted by solid circles, all used geographic or population-based sampling frames. Thus, they scoured all the potential information sources for an entire region: all regional hospital and referral clinic records, the office records of primary care clinicians, and even the results of periodic inquiries of the eligible families themselves. When investigations followed these population-based inception cohorts forward, very similar (and much lower) rates of subsequent nonfebrile seizures were documented (4.6%; 3%; 3%; 3%; 1.5%), whose 95% confidence intervals overlapped. A similar pattern was observed for recurrences of febrile seizures; clinic-based studies reported rates anywhere from 12% to 75%, whereas the population-based rates were all clustered between 29% and 35%.

These systematic differences in the results of population-based and specialty clinic-based studies of the clinical course and prognosis of febrile seizures are explainable on clinically sensible grounds: the more severe or prolonged the febrile seizure, the more likely the child will be referred to a hospital or to a specialty clinic. Thus, the hospital- or clinic-based study samples became progressively affected by this overrepresentation of children with relatively poor prognoses.

The preceding is an example of the "referral-filter" bias in which "the selection that occurs at each stage in the referral process can generate patient samples that are much different from those found in the general population" [10]. In this particular case, referral was influenced by disease severity, and because a clinical center's reputation usually results from its particular expertise in a specialized area of clinical medicine, it will be referred problem cases likely to benefit from its special competence. Although this usually makes for excellent clinical care, it often, as we have seen, cripples that center's ability to generalize from its studies of the clinical course and prognosis of its referrals.

Sampling biases can distort both the timing and the rates of important prognostic outcomes [6]. Despite this serious drawback, the study of inception cohorts at tertiary care centers yields useful information to other clinicians who work in such settings. Clinicians who see febrile seizures in tertiary care should base their prognostic statements on the left side, not the right side, of Figure 6-1.* Moreover, studies in tertiary care can provide useful information on the potential importance of prognostic subgroups as long as sampling biases affect each of the prognostic subgroups equally, but this equality may be difficult to show and risky to assume.

These sampling biases are largely responsible for the chaos that characterizes most discussions of the course and prognosis of human disease when experiences in tertiary care are extrapolated to primary care, and these pitfalls are not casually avoided. Short of the Framingham-type of study, in which a large population of individuals is assembled and closely followed for decades, the sampling approach worth looking for is the one that has systematically gathered eligible cases from *all* the clinical facilities in a given catchment area through the careful review of old clinical records or, better still, through continuing surveillance for new cases.

In summary, an understanding of how the patients were assembled for the study, plus additional information about their age, sex, severity, comorbidity, and so on, will help you decide whether they resemble your own patients enough for you to apply the results of their follow-up in your own practice.

Was Complete Follow-up Achieved?

All members of the inception cohort should be accounted for at the end of the follow-up period, and their clinical status should be known. This is because patients do not disappear from a study for trivial reasons. Rather, they leave the study because they refuse therapy or recover or die or retire to the sunbelt or simply grow tired of being followed. All of these reasons are linked to important prognostic outcomes and, if you are to use the results of the article in making prognostic judgments about your own patients, you deserve to know how *all* the members of the inception cohort fared.

For example, of a cohort of 186 patients treated in Birmingham, England, for neurosis, a vigorous follow-up study eventually tracked down 180 [12]. The death rate among the three-fifths who were easily traced was only 3%. However, the death rate among the remaining 66 patients who were tougher to trace was nine times as great, at 27%!

Of course, it is difficult for the authors to achieve perfection; they are bound to lose a few members of their inception cohort. There are, though, some rough rules of thumb that you can apply here. We would suggest the following steps:

*But these clinicians had better be careful what they teach primary care residents about this!

1. Identify the prognostic outcome of greatest relevance to you and your patient.
2. See if you can reconstruct the fraction from which the risk (or rate) of this outcome was generated. That is, see if you can construct a fraction whose numerator contains all the patients who developed the prognostic outcome and whose denominator contains all the patients, both with and without that outcome.
3. Now, take the number of patients who were "lost to follow-up":
   a. Add this number to *both* the numerator *and* the denominator of the fraction you worked out in step 2 and recalculate the rate. This will give you the "highest" result that would apply if *all* lost patients had developed the prognostic outcome.
   b. Repeat step 3a, but this time add the number of lost patients *just* to the denominator of the fraction you worked out in step 2 and recalculate the rate. This will give you the "lowest" result that would apply if *none* of the lost patients developed the prognostic outcome.
4. Now, compare the "highest" and "lowest" results. Are they close enough that your decision about what to tell (and do to) the patient would be the same, regardless of which of them were true? If so, thank your (and the authors'!) lucky stars and proceed. If, however, your decision about how to manage the patient would be quite different if the highest or lowest result applied, you ought to put the article aside and look for something better.

Let's work through an example to show how this works and to make an additional point. Suppose that a study of prognosis achieves a 92% follow-up of 71 patients (that is, 6 patients are lost to follow-up, leaving 65 patients for the analysis). Suppose further that 39 of these 65 patients experience a relapse during their follow-up, for a relapse rate of 39/65 = 60%. We would determine the "highest" result by adding the 6 lost patients *both* to the numerator and the denominator, thus: (39 + 6)/(65 + 6) = 45/71 = 63%; we would determine the "lowest" result by adding the 6 lost patients *just* to the denominator, thus: 39/(65 + 6) = 39/71 = 55%. Because the highest relapse rate of 63% and the lowest relapse rate of 55% are close together, our decision about how to manage our patient probably would not change, regardless of what happened to the patients who were lost to the study.

Suppose, on the other hand, the case-fatality rate observed during this same study was 1/65 or 1.5%. The "highest" result assumes that all lost patients died and becomes: (1 + 6)/(65 + 6) = 7/71 = 10%. The "lowest" result assumes that all losts lived and becomes: 1/(65 + 6) = 1/71 = 1.4%. The highest case fatality is seven times the lowest and might, indeed, influence at least what we tell (if not what we do for) the patient. In this case, we might want to look further for a more accurate and precise estimate of the case-fatality rate for this disease.

The additional point revealed in this example is that the *lower* the risk of a prognostic outcome, the *greater* the potential effect of patients who are lost to follow-up.

Were Objective Outcome Criteria Developed and Used?

The prognostic outcomes should be stated in explicit, objective terms so that you, as the reader of the subsequent report, will be able to relate them to your own practice. Suppose that you came upon an article about the prognosis of patients with transient ischemic attack. If the article describes the risk of "subsequent stroke" without presenting the explicit, objective criteria for what constituted a "stroke," you are in a quandary. Are these "strokes" limited to severe derangements of sensation or motor power such that their victims require assistance in dressing, feeding, and toileting? Or, are the majority of these "strokes" merely transient or trivial changes in sensation or in deep or superficial reflexes? The implications of these different definitions for counseling patients or initiating therapy are whopping.

Not only should an article describe explicit, objective outcome criteria; it should provide reassurance that these criteria were applied in a consistent manner. As you will recall from Chapter 2, even experienced clinicians will disagree with themselves and other clinicians about key manifestations of disease. As a result, what is a mild stroke to one clinician is merely a normal variant to another, and a patient's apparent prognosis will be determined not by biology but by the luck of the draw in who is selected to perform the final examination. All of this brings us to the next guide.

Was the Outcome Assessment "Blind"?

The examination for important prognostic outcomes should have been carried out by clinicians who were "blind" to the other features of these patients. This is essential if two additional sources of bias are to be avoided. First, the clinician who knows that a patient possesses a prognostic factor of presumed importance may carry out more frequent or more detailed searches for the relevant prognostic outcome (*diagnostic-suspicion bias*). Second, pathologists and others who interpret diagnostic specimens can have their judgments dramatically influenced by prior knowledge of the clinical features of the case (*expectation bias*).

The expectation bias should be familiar to readers of Chapter 2, for it appeared prominently there (remember the tonsils?). In order to reduce expectation bias, many clinical centers recognize the need, even in routine practice, for an initial "blind" assessment of diagnostic tests such as electrocardiograms and radiographs [13]. Thus, in a published report about prognosis, the diagnostic-suspicion bias should have been avoided by subjecting *all* patients to the *same* diagnostic studies, ideally at prescribed intervals and, by all means, at the end of the study.

What about the outcome of death? Surely, blindness is not a prerequisite for assessing so "rigor"ous an outcome. Although reporting the *fact* of death is an unambiguous task (and need not, therefore, be blind), assigning a *cause* of death is subject to both diagnostic-suspicion and expectation biases and should, therefore, have been done blindly.

Was Adjustment for Extraneous Prognostic Factors Carried Out?

Suppose you wanted to know whether the duration of your ulcerative colitis patient's disease was an important determinant of the risk of developing cancer. To get a clear-cut answer to this question, you would like to be sure that there would be no interference from other factors that might both accompany disease duration and affect prognosis (such as an earlier age at onset, more courses of a wider range of drugs, and so on). The failure to meet this standard can result in assigning causal roles to factors that are merely "markers" for other factors of real importance.

Of course, it is usually impossible for the clinical reader to become sufficiently familiar with the mathematical tap dancing used to adjust for extraneous prognostic factors to be able to tell whether, for example, the authors should have used a discriminant function analysis rather than a stepwise multiple logistic regression; this is one of those situations in which you must (and usually can) rely on the journal to have had the article previously reviewed and approved by a thoughtful biostatistician. However, the article is much less likely to have undergone any sophisticated methodologic review if no adjustment for extraneous prognostic factors was attempted, and the reader is therefore left with the responsibility to decide *whether* an adjustment procedure was required (but not *how well* it was executed).

We can give you two rough "rules of thumb" to apply to the "predictive models" that often emerge from these multivariate adjustments. First, if the article concludes that some constellation of symptoms, signs, and laboratory results accurately predicts a certain prognosis, you should demand evidence that the authors have confirmed the constellation's predictive power in a second, independent sample of patients (the test sample), because the multivariate approaches used here will fail to distinguish important prognostic factors from unimportant idiosyncracies of the particular patient sample (the training sample) to which they are applied. You want to be sure that the constellation works among test sample patients as well as training sample patients before you apply it to patients in your own practice.

The second rough rule of thumb has to do with the numbers of patients that should have been included in the training and test samples. Although there are sophisticated methods for determining appropriate sample sizes in these situations, you should look for at least 10 patients for every prognostic factor the authors studied. Thus, a study of whether some combination of blood pressure, blood glucose, initial level of consciousness, walking ability, position sense, tendon reflexes, and muscle power had an effect on the prognosis of patients with stroke should have included at least 10 patients for each of these 7 factors, or at least 70 patients in all, to really tease them apart and to generate results that are likely to be both true and clinically useful.

This section has presented six guides that a busy clinician can apply to an article on the clinical course and prognosis of disease. Their application should have two results: first, many if not most of the prognosis articles you come across can be discarded early on, increasing the efficiency with which you spend your precious reading time. This will be particularly so if you rigorously apply the first guide (was an inception cohort assembled?), for most of the faulty studies of clinical course and prognosis fail this initial test.

The second result of applying these guides is that the articles that do pass muster will provide you with prognostic information that is valid, consistent, and applicable in your own clinical practice. As you work your way through the disorders you most commonly encounter in your practice, you gradually will accumulate a very useful body of prognostic information that will permit you to decide, with considerable confidence, what to tell (and do to) an ever larger proportion of the patients you encounter.

But what about the disorders for which "good data" are still missing (when this book was written, this case still applied to the risk of progression in mild scoliosis and to the risk of cancer in ulcerative colitis)? What should you do then? We would suggest these three courses of action.

First, if the clinical situation warrants, you can inform the patient that the answer to his prognosis is not clear but that its limits can be specified. Second, to the extent that you can influence the development of proper clinical research, you can emphasize to clinical researchers the need for a valid answer to this practical clinical problem. Finally, you can dispel any illusions that your colleagues and students may have that the particular prognostic issue has been resolved. To paraphrase Josh Billings: "It ain't what we don't know that gets us (and our patients!) into trouble. It's what we do know that ain't so!" [11].

If you decide that the patient's illness is sufficiently serious to warrant intervention and you need to do something, the next challenge is: do what? Chapter 7 will take up this question and will help you select that intervention that is most likely to do more good than harm.

References

1. Coe, F. L., Keck, J., and Norton, E. R. The natural history of calcium urolithiasis. *J.A.M.A.* 238: 1519, 1977.
2. Department of Clinical Epidemiology and Biostatistics, McMaster University, Hamilton, Ontario. How to read clinical journals: III. To learn the clinical course and prognosis of disease. *Can. Med. Assoc. J.* 124: 869, 1981.
3. Ekbom, A., Helmick, C., Zack, M., and Adami, H. Ulcerative colitis and colorectal cancer: A population-based study. *N. Engl. J. Med.* 323: 1228, 1990.
4. Ellenberg, J. H., and Nelson, K. B. Sample selection and the natural history of disease. Studies of febrile seizures. *J.A.M.A.* 243: 1337, 1980.
5. Greenstein, A. J., Sachar, D. B., Smith, H., et al. Cancer in universal and left-sided ulcerative colitis: Factors determining risk. *Gastroenterology* 77: 290, 1979.
6. Melton, L. J., III. Selection bias in the referral of patients and the natural history of surgical conditions. *Mayo Clin. Proc.* 60: 880, 1985.
7. Recurrent renal calculi. *Br. Med. J.* 282: 5, 1981.
8. Rogala, E. J., Drummond, D. S., and Gurr, J. Scoliosis: Incidence and natural history. A prospective epidemiological study. *J. Bone Joint Surg. (Am.)* 60: 173, 1978.
9. Sackett, D. L. Biases in analytic research. *J. Chron. Dis.* 32: 51, 1979.
10. Sackett, D. L., and Whelan, G. Cancer risk in ulcerative colitis: Scientific requirements for the study of prognosis (editorial). *Gastroenterology* 78: 1632, 1980.
11. Shaw, H. W. *Josh Billings: Hiz Saying.* London: Hotten, 1869.

12. Sims, A. C. P. Importance of a high tracing-rate in long-term medical follow-up studies. *Lancet* 2: 433, 1973.
13. Spodick, D. H. On experts and expertise: The effect of variability in observer performance. *Am. J. Cardiol.* 36: 592, 1975.
14. Tversky, A., and Kahneman, D. Judgment under uncertainty: Heuristics and biases. *Science* 185: 1224, 1974.

7

Deciding on the Best Therapy

This chapter analyzes the three principal decisions that determine the rational treatment of any patient:

1. *Identifying the ultimate objective of treatment.* Is the ultimate objective to achieve cure, palliation, symptomatic relief, or what?
2. *Selecting the specific treatment.* Does the patient require any treatment at all? What sorts of evidence, from what sources, should determine the choice of the specific treatment to be used to reach this goal?
3. *Specifying the treatment target.* How will you know when to stop treatment, change its intensity, or switch to some other treatment?

For example, when considering a patient with symptomless but moderately severe essential hypertension (fifth-phase diastolic blood pressure 110 mm Hg), you might make these three decisions as follows:

1. *Ultimate objective of treatment.* To prevent (further) target organ damage to the brain, eye, heart, kidney, and large vessels that would cause disability or untimely death.
2. *Choice of specific treatment.* On the basis of randomized clinical trials of active agents versus placebo, antihypertensive drugs.
3. *Treatment target.* A fifth-phase diastolic blood pressure (right arm, sitting) of less than 90 mm Hg, or as close to that as tolerable in the face of drug side effects.

These three primary decisions, when consciously carried out and conscientiously noted in the clinical record, can lead to consistent, coherent patient management, even when responsibility is shared by several clinicians or a whole team. The failure to make and record these decisions, on the other hand, can lead to management chaos. When the ultimate objective of treatment is unclear or unspecified, the specific treatments selected may, in fact, defeat or postpone its achievement. This brand of management chaos sometimes disrupts the care of the terminally ill. That the ultimate objective of the treatment of such patients is palliative (e.g., eliminate pain and preserve dignity) is usually acknowledged, but this acknowledgement often fails to be clearly documented in the clinical record. As a result, management becomes chaotic when the patient spikes a fever, even if he remains quite comfortable, and especially when the responsible clinician is off duty. X rays are taken, white cells are counted and differentiated; blood, orifices and excreta are cultured; and antibiotics are injected. In short, the dying patient is pestered, hurt, and robbed of dignity. Even more spectacular chaos reigns when the patient's heart stops.

When we fail to make the second principal decision rationally and our selection of specific treatments is based on authoritarian advice or our conviction that such therapy *seems* to work or *ought* to work (as opposed to hard evidence that it *does* work), not only may worthless treatment be applied; sometimes it is downright harmful. Today's therapy, when derived by induction from biologic facts or uncontrolled clinical experience, may become tomorrow's bad joke; some of us are even old enough to recall chuckling over our ancestors' naive acceptance of blood-letting as we hooked our ulcer patients up to gastric freezing machines.

Finally, if we fail to confront the third primary decision and don't identify the precise targets of treatment, how will we know when to stop, shift, or change our therapy?

What you have just read may give you the impression that, as long as we identify the three principal decisions, deciding on the best therapy is a straightforward affair. It isn't. This is because there are two additional elements that profoundly affect these three primary decisions. The first additional element is the scarcity of high-quality evidence on the risks and benefits of specific treatments. As a result, we not only must critically assess the validity and applicability of the available evidence, but also must extrapolate beyond what is known to be true for other patients to what is likely be true for our patient. The science of this art of assessment and extrapolation is young but boisterous, and comprises much of this chapter and Chapter 11, Tracking Down the Evidence to Solve Clinical Problems, and Chapter 13, How to Read Reviews and Economic Analyses.

The second additional element that profoundly affects the three primary treatment decisions is the major role that patients can (and, for many of our readers, must) play in making these decisions. Since any decision about the ultimate objective of treatment is made for the sake of the patient, most clinicians involve, and even defer to, the patient's wishes (or those of an impaired patient's family) in this decision. And when assessing the risks and benefits of specific treatments, the patient's perspective on these risks and benefits (especially as they involve trade-offs between the quantity and quality of life) may be not only useful but crucial. As you'll see shortly, that's what the "N-of-1" trial is all about. Finally, as we shall show you in Chapter 8 on compliance, involving patients in identifying and monitoring the achievement of the treatment targets and objectives may have a beneficial effect on their compliance with the treatment regimen.

As with other elements of the critical assessment and extrapolation of clinical evidence, the science of the art of determining and incorporating our patients' preferences and "utilities" into our treatment decisions is still in its infancy [14, 40]. Nonetheless, we and our patients can benefit from learning about it, and a later portion of this chapter will show how "decision analysis" can help us integrate both of these elements.

Deciding on the Ultimate Objective of Treatment

The following six objectives, singly or in combination, comprise the ultimate objectives of treatment:

1. *Cure* (e.g., kill the microbe, cut out the tumor, desensitize the phobic patient)
2. *Prevent a recurrence* (e.g., give prophylactic antibiotics following recovery from acute rheumatic fever, or major tranquilizers following discharge for schizophrenia)
3. *Limit structural or functional deterioration* (e.g., reconstruct, rehabilitate)
4. *Prevent the later complication* (e.g., give diuretics to symptomless hypertensives and aspirin to threatened strokes)
5. *Relieve the current distress* (e.g., replace the hormone, provide emotional support or counseling, give painkillers, antidepressants and antiinflammatory drugs)
6. *Deliver reassurance* (e.g., "unlabel" the misdiagnosed, transmit the truly favorable prognosis)
7. *Allow to die with comfort and dignity* (e.g., cancel further diagnostic testing and focus on the relief of current symptoms and the preservation of self-esteem).

In deciding which of the these objectives to pursue, we believe that it is useful to consider the same three elements of a sickness that we introduced in the opening chapter of this book [67]:

1. *The disease or target disorder* The anatomic, biochemical, physiologic, or psychologic derangement whose etiology (if known), maladaptive mechanisms, presentation, prognosis, and management we read about in medical texts
2. *The illness* The signs, symptoms, and behaviors exhibited by the patient as a result of, and responding to, the target disorder
3. *The predicament* The social, psychological, and economic fashion in which the patient is situated in the environment.

The need to correctly assess the *disease* element is self-evident. Clinicians are chagrined and patients usually are punished when disease is wrongly diagnosed and, as a result, incorrectly treated (a special case, the diagnosis of nondisease, will be taken up later). With the growth of disease-specific therapy, the need to know exactly what is being treated becomes more important. Knowing the disease includes knowing its prognosis when treated and untreated, its risk of relapse and recurrence, its permanent disabilities, and its ultimate outcomes. This knowledge defines the boundaries of the potential options (cure, relieve, palliate, etc.) of therapy. Once the options are identified, patient preference and utilities influence the final selection from among them.

Just as the correct assessment of the *illness* was the key to generating appropriate diagnostic hypotheses in the previous section of this book, such an assessment is often the key to setting treatment objectives as well. Since most patients want treatment to relieve their symptoms, an accurate assessment of their illness is central to any treatment objectives that address symptomatic relief.

Finally, we need to assess the patient's *predicament* in order to identify the limits of our treatment options. Although poverty and bad housing require social and political intervention rather than medical therapy, such predicaments sharply limit our medical treatments, and must be considered before we tell a penniless diabetic septuagenarian to follow an expensive diet, to test her blood or urine frequently with costly dipsticks, and to buy disposable insulin syringes.

A synthesis of the disease, the illness, the predicament, and the options for treatment objectives will identify those objectives that are worth pursuing in the individual case. Usually they will be some combination of objectives taken from the first three options (cure, prevent a recurrence, limit structural or functional deterioration) plus the next three (prevent later complications, relieve current symptoms, deliver reassurance); occasionally, however, the last objective (allow to die with comfort and dignity) takes precedence over all others.

Once the objectives of therapy are set we are ready to proceed to the next step of selecting the precise treatment to achieve them. As you will see, the results of this next step may cause us to come back and reassess our original objectives of therapy.

Selecting the Specific Treatment

Modern manufacturers have introduced exotic machines that can select, punch, drill, bend, fit, and weld raw materials into finished goods all by themselves; they sharpen their own tools when they become dull, replace bits of themselves when they wear out, and even sense and correct their own mistakes. One problem they have not been able to overcome, however, is the almost irresistible temptation they present to their human attendants to adjust, reset, and otherwise tinker with them, even when they are functioning just fine. The results are often disastrous. In desperation, some plant managers have installed prominent notices along their automated assembly lines: IF IT AIN'T BROKE, DON'T FIX IT!

We think that the analogy fits, and that the first element of selecting the specific treatment has to be to decide whether *any* treatment is required. There are two sorts of circumstances in which patients "ain't broke" and we ought not attempt to "fix" them. The first is due to false-positive diagnostic errors that label patients as diseased when, in fact, they are not, and we hinted at these in the previous section of this chapter. Nicely summarized by Dr. Clifton Meador [52], these "nondiseases" can be subclassified as *mimicking syndromes* (round-faced fat women with hairy upper lips but normal steroids have non-Cushing's disease), *upper-lower-limit syndromes* (borderline laboratory values), *normal variation syndromes* (short children of short parents have nondwarfism), *laboratory error syndromes, roentgenologic-overinterpretation syndromes, congenitally absent-organ syndromes* ("nonfunctioning" kidneys and gall bladders that are not there) and *overinterpretation-of-physical-findings syndromes*.

The upper-lower-limit syndrome is quite common, especially where laboratories are automated and report 6, 12, 20, or 80 different blood constituents when any single one is ordered. The result is a very high rate of unexpected, unexplained (in terms of the patient's history and physical examination) abnormal lab test results.*

Most of these "abnormal" results are bogus. For example, when Dr. Bradwell's team carefully followed up 100 patients with unexpected, unexplained abnormal lab test results (an additional 74 were unexpected but later explained), 71% of them had normal results when the tests were repeated some time later [7]. Although these patients were not treated in the interim, any therapy instituted between such initial and repeat tests would appear efficacious!

The second circumstance in which patients "ain't broke" and don't need "fixing" is when either the treatment is worse than the disease or when their illness is trivial, self-limited, or well within the recuperative and reparative powers of the patient's body and mind. This second circumstance must be identified when it occurs, for it calls for *no* treatment.

We have started a list of patients "who ain't broke, so don't fix them" in Table 7-1. When we operate on and medicate such patients we only reinforce their "sick role" behaviors, spend money and other resources that would better have been directed elsewhere, and increase their risk of iatrogenic disease.

Having decided that the patient's sickness *does* warrant treatment and having selected the goal of this treatment, you must now select the specific drug, operation, splint, exercise, or conversation that will best achieve this goal. How (on earth) do you decide which one to prescribe? It seems to us that there are three ways to pick a therapy:

1. On the basis of retrospective analyses of your own uncontrolled clinical experience, that of others, or the extension of current concepts of mechanisms of disease you can logically arrive at the therapy that *seems to work* or *ought to work*; we shall call this the method of *induction*.
2. On the basis of prospective analyses of formal randomized clinical trials designed to expose worthless or dangerous treatments, you can select the therapies that *successfully withstand formal attempts to demonstrate their worthlessness*; we shall call this the method of *deduction*.
3. On the basis of recommendations from your teachers, consultants, colleagues, advertisements, or pharmaceutical representatives you can simply accept a treatment *on faith*; we shall call this the method of *abdication* (or, to fit the rhyme and cadence of the other two, the method of *seduction*).

It will, by this point in the book, come as no surprise to learn that we prefer the *deductive* (or, more correctly, the *hypothetico-deductive*) method for selecting specific treatments. The best information on whether a given treatment does

*For a more complete discussion of why this inevitably results when clinical laboratories use inappropriate definitions of the normal range, see p. 59.

Table 7-1. Conditions among patients who "ain't broke, so don't fix them"

1. Adie's pupil
2. Café au lait spots
3. Campbell de Morgan spots
4. "Letter-reversals" in 4-year-olds
5. Non-Cushing's disease
6. Nondwarfism
7. Pityriasis rosea (save antipruritics)
8. Pregnancy
9. Ptosis of the kidney (in a normotensive)
10. Small degrees of stable scoliosis
11. Silent gallstones
12. Symptomless colonic diverticulae
13. Symptomless hiatus hernia
14. Symptomless hypokalemia in thiazide-treated hypertensives who are not taking digitalis
15. Symptomless hypotension
16. Symptomless hyperuricemia
17. Umbilical hernia in infancy

more good than harm to patients with a given disorder is the results of a randomized clinical trial in which patients with the given disorder were randomly allocated to receive either the given treatment or a placebo (or conventional therapy) and then followed up for clinically relevant outcomes of their disease and its treatment. Fortunately, randomized clinical trials are becoming very much more common and have dramatically demonstrated the efficacy of many treatments and the uselessness or even harmfulness of several others. However, the proper evaluation of therapy requires more than just randomization, and this chapter will provide five other guides for sorting out therapeutic claims. We have listed all six guides in Table 7-2, and will discuss them shortly. Before doing so, however, we have a few more things to say about the methods of induction and seduction.

Why are we so hard on the method of induction? After all, this method constitutes the major strategy for nominating the treatment ideas that get tested in randomized clinical trials, and many of these treatment ideas prove to be powerfully efficacious. The fatal flaw in the method of induction is that it is often incapable of exposing erroneous conclusions about efficacy, even when the observations upon which it operates are totally accurate [53].

Consider an example. Clinicians frequently judge the efficacy of a modern treatment by comparing their current clinical experience (outcomes of patients receiving the new treatment) with their former clinical experience (outcomes of patients treated in other ways, before the new treatment was available). If the outcomes in today's patients are better than those of yesterday's, the new therapy is judged both efficacious and superior to the old. The use of "historical com-

Table 7-2. Six guides to distinguish useful from useless or even harmful therapy

1. Was the assignment of patients to treatments really randomized?
2. Were all clinically relevant outcomes reported?
3. Were the study patients recognizably similar to your own?
4. Were both clinical and statistical significance considered?
5. Is the therapeutic maneuver feasible in your practice?
6. Were all the patients who entered the study accounted for at its conclusion?

parisons" in this fashion is risky, as shown in the rise and fall of the "gastric freeze" [56]. Recognizing that gastric cooling to 5 to 10°C sharply reduced acid secretion, a former president of the American College of Surgeons lowered the temperature of the coolant entering gastric balloons placed in peptic ulcer patients to −10°C. The first few patients so treated experienced sharp reductions in their ulcer symptoms and exhibited x-ray healing of their ulcers. These results, when contrasted with prior experience, so impressed the innovators that they paid the ultimate tribute to the use of historic controls; in their landmark report of their initial success, they stated, "Since April 1961, no patients with duodenal ulcer referred for elective operation have been operated upon on the senior author's surgical service. This circumstance in itself bespeaks the confidence in the method by patients as well as surgeons" [72].

The next few years saw the sale of 2500 gastric freezing machines and a growing controversy over the efficacy of the procedure. Finally, a proper randomized trial was carried out [61]. In this trial, subsequent surgery for ulcer disease, gastrointestinal hemorrhage, or hospitalization for intractable pain occurred in 30 (44%) of the 68 patients randomized to the sham treatment and in 35 (51%) of the 69 patients randomized to the gastric freeze. These results, published several years after the initial, promising report, sounded the death knell for the gastric freeze and it rapidly was abandoned. In the meanwhile, tens of thousands of ulcer patients had their stomachs frozen on the basis of those historical controls, paying the price for our reliance on induction as a method for selecting the best treatment.

The comparison of current therapeutic results with those of historical controls does not make sense even in so final a disease as cancer [16]. Louis Diehl and David Perry compared survivals and disease-free survivals between two groups of control patients who did not receive the latest therapy: historical controls who could not receive it, and later controls from current randomized trials who were allocated not to receive it. Over 20% of the later controls exhibited more than 20% better survival than the historical controls, even without the latest therapy! There have been too many other improvements in general nutrition, health care, and the management of advanced disease to base important treatment decisions on comparisons of the results of current and historical therapy.

A second inductive approach avoids the problem of "historical comparisons" by comparing contemporaneous patients who happen to have received or not received a particular treatment. Although the patients being compared here are not randomly allocated to receive or not receive the treatment, they usually look comparable, and it is possible to statistically "adjust" them for any differences in risk factors that are recognized. This approach can lead us astray as well, as you will recall from Chapter 5, Early Diagnosis; any treatment initiated early in the course of a disease will look good even when it is useless. Another pitfall in this second inductive approach is discovered when we attempt to determine the efficacy of a treatment by comparing patients who took all their medicine with those who took little or none of it. At first glance, this looks like quite a good approach, for the two groups of patients must have the same disease and be pretty homogeneous, otherwise they would not have been prescribed the same medication. The striking results of such an approach are shown in Table 7-3.

In this particular study, men who had survived a myocardial infarction and had been started on the same medication were carefully followed up for recurrent infarcts or death [10]. In addition, measurements were made to see whether and how well they were taking their medicine. As seen in Table 7-3, 26% of the 882 men who took less than 80% of their medicine died, compared with only 16% of the 1813 men who took at least 80% of their medicine. Clearly those who were highly exposed to this medication did very much better than those who were not. Even after statistical adjustment for 40 risk factors and other baseline characteristics, those who took their medicine were 38% less likely to die than those who did not take their medicine and this difference in mortality was extraordinarily statistically significant. This looks like very convincing evidence that this medication is highly efficacious.

Until we learn that it was a placebo! These results come from the placebo group of a trial of various lipid-lowering drugs, and this same striking relation between mortality and compliance was found both in patients on active therapy and those on placebo. Similarly better outcomes among faithful placebo takers have now been reported from a number of other randomized trials [2, 22, 37, 60]. Patients who faithfully follow instructions appear destined for rosier outcomes, regardless of whether their treatment works. As a result, comparisons between compliant and noncompliant patients constitute another fallacious approach to determining whether a treatment does more good than harm.

The defect in all these inductive approaches is that they fail to limit error. They seek confirmatory evidence that the treatment may be good, but fail to carry out the crucial experiments that will show whether the treatment is bad. The crucial advantage of the hypothetico-deductive approach is that it provides, in the randomized control trial, the scientifically rigorous opportunity to demonstrate that therapeutic claims are rubbish. It has been such randomized trials that exposed the uselessness of treating peptic ulcers with gastric freezing (about 15,000 patients were chilled before this treatment was abandoned), symptomless nonfamilial hypercholesterolemia with clofibrate (5500 untimely deaths have been attributed to this regimen in the United States alone), and angina pectoris with internal mammary ligation. We laugh at the naiveté of our predecessors who endorsed and prescribed these treatments, but is there any reason to believe that we are more intelligent than they? Few readers would claim to be more

Table 7-3. Mortality in men with coronary heart disease who did and did not take their medicine

		Number of men	% Mortality*
Compliance with medication	Took <80%	882	26%
	Took ≥80%	1813	16%

$$\text{Risk reduction for death} = \frac{0.26 - 0.16}{0.26} = 38\%$$

$$P = 0.0000000073$$

*Adjusted for 40 risk factors and other baseline characteristics.
Adapted from Coronary Drug Project Research Group. Influence of adherence to treatment and response of cholesterol on mortality in the Coronary Drug Project. *N. Engl. J. Med.* 303:1038, 1980.

astute clinicians than William Osler, yet he advocated the use of opium for the treatment of diabetes (.5–2 grains tid) [34]. If we are as gullible as our predecessors, we owe it to our patients to minimize our application of useless and harmful therapy by basing our treatments, wherever possible, on the results of proper randomized control trials.*

Do we have anything good to say about the final way to pick a treatment: the method of *abdication* (to some authority who tells you what to do but not why) or *seduction* (by the slick ad or slicker detail man)? Not much. Of course, if the sickness you are treating is one you very rarely encounter and are unlikely to see again, abdicating in favor of some expert who has published how he or she treats this entity certainly saves time and probably limits harm. But to base your treatment of commonly encountered problems on the advice of some "expert" who publishes treatment recommendations but no supporting evidence puts you on a par with the barefoot doctor. After all, it was these same experts who advocated turpentine stupes and leeches. Experts worth their salt will cite proper evidence from randomized clinical trials to back up their claims, and you can track these trials down and apply the guides from Table 7-2 to them.

The same holds for pharmaceutical representatives. The useful ones play down testimonials and show biz, and will give or send you reprints on randomized trials of their products, published in refereed journals. The others will snow you with pharmacokinetics, stress how many of your colleagues are already on the bandwagon, and offer claims that would make a used-car salesman blush.

And although pharmaceutical representatives constitute a major source of information about new drugs, why should you want to be the first clinician on the block to use them? Even if their efficacy is well supported by randomized control trials, such trials are too small to detect rare but devastating side effects and,

*A "midway" method for determining efficacy in a single patient is the "N-of-1" randomized trial, described in detail in a later section of this chapter.

unless no effective alternative treatment exists, it is a good idea to wait until the new drug has been used for awhile.*

And now to the readers' guides (shown in Table 7-2) for use in sorting out therapeutic claims. Once again, they constitute "applied common sense" and are designed to increase the efficiency as well as accuracy of your reading. Guides 1 and 6 deal mostly with *validity* (are the article's conclusions true?); guides 2, 3, and 5 deal mostly with *applicability* (are the article's conclusions relevant to your own patients?); and guide 4 deals with both validity (statistical significance) and applicability (clinical significance).

WAS THE ASSIGNMENT OF PATIENTS TO TREATMENTS REALLY RANDOMIZED?

Every patient who entered the study should have had the same, *known* probability (typically 50%) of receiving one or the other of the treatments being compared; assignment to one treatment or another should have been carried out by a system analogous to flipping a coin. It is usually easy to decide whether this was done, for key terms such as *randomized trial* or *random allocation* should appear in the abstract, the methods section, or even the title of such articles.†

As a result, the busy clinical reader has the option of applying this guide rigorously: if you are reading a subscribed journal in the "surveillance" mode to "keep up with the clinical literature" (rather than searching the clinical literature to decide how to treat the problem presented by a specific patient), we've recommended that you discard at once all articles on therapy that are not randomized trials.

Although the randomized trial can sometimes produce an incorrect conclusion about efficacy (especially, as we shall find out shortly, when it is a small trial), it is by far the best tool currently available for identifying the clinical maneuvers that do more good than harm. Can we *ever* be confident that a treatment is efficacious in the absence of a randomized trial? Only when traditional therapy is invariably followed by death. For example, prior to 1946 the outcome of tuberculous meningitis was invariably fatal. Then, when small amounts of streptomycin became available for use in humans, a few U.S. victims treated with this new drug survived [36]; this remarkable survival following streptomycin was repeated shortly thereafter in the United Kingdom [54]. Thus, the ability to show, with replication, that patients with previously universally fatal disease can

*If, for example, a drug causes a serious adverse reaction in 1/1000 (.1% or .001) of those who take it, the "rule of three" tells us that in order to be 95% confident of finding at least one adverse reaction we need to follow 1000 × 3 or 3000 patients. That is much larger than virtually any clinical trial just to find *one* serious adverse reaction. Thus, although randomized trials are the only sure way to determine the efficacy of a drug, postmarketing surveillance is required to determine its safety [63]. We'll talk about this in detail in Chapter 9.

†Beware of "look-alikes" to randomization. For example, some reports describe how patients were asssigned "at random" to one therapy or another; often these are *not* randomized trials, and the authors of such reports might as well have said that the patients were assigned "at the investigator's convenience," "without conscious bias," or even "hapazardly."

survive following a new treatment constitutes sufficient evidence, all by itself, for efficacy.

Insisting on evidence from randomized clinical trials can increase the efficiency with which one reads a subscribed journal, for it will lead to the early rejection of most articles concerned with therapy.* The rule requires some modification, however, when reading around a particular patient. In this latter instance it will often occur that no proper randomized control trials have ever been published. What should the clinical reader do then?

Two sorts of actions are appropriate when reading up on a specific patient. First, the initial literature search should seek out any randomized trials that do exist. Second, in the absence of any published randomized clinical trials, clinical readers will have to use the results of subexperimental investigations. Before accepting the conclusions of such studies, clinicians should satisfy themselves that the improved patient outcomes following therapy are simply so great that they cannot be explained by one or more biases in the assembly of the study patients or in the assessment or interpretation of their responses to therapy This second rule is obviously a judgment call and should be tempered by the recollection that this same sort of subexperimental evidence supported the earlier use of clofibrate, internal mammary ligation, and the gastric freeze. Thus, the situation is a familiar one for clinicians: the need to act in the face of incomplete information. As in other, similar circumstances it is perhaps best accomplished by harking back to Table 7-1 and considering both the certainty of causation and the consequences of the alternative courses of action that are open: Does the patient require *any* intervention? If so, have any of the available interventions been shown to do more good than harm in a randomized trial? If none, which among them is likely to produce the most favorable trade-off between benefit and risk? The following guides may help form this latter judgment, as well as assist in the critical assessment of proper randomized trials.

WERE ALL CLINICALLY RELEVANT OUTCOMES REPORTED?

Table 7-4 summarizes the results of an important randomized trial of clofibrate among men with elevated serum cholesterol [57]. Some of the outcomes of therapy appear highly favorable. For example, serum cholesterol—a key coronary risk factor—fell by almost 10%, providing some biologic evidence for benefit. However, some readers will recognize a claim of therapeutic benefit based upon this cholesterol change as an example of the "substitution game" in which a risk factor is substituted for its associated clinical outcome [75], and will want to look further to see whether there were real changes in the occurrence of acute coronary events.

Such evidence is also available in Table 7-4 where we note reductions in both nonfatal myocardial infarctions (row 2 in the table) and in all infarctions, both

*The clinical journals show signs of agreeing with this point of view. In what may have been a "first," all of the *Original Articles* in the May 3, 1990 issue of the New England Journal of Medicine were randomized trials!

Table 7-4. Clinically relevant outcomes in a randomized trial of clofibrate in the prevention of coronary heart disease

	Placebo	Clofibrate
Average change in serum cholesterol (%)	+1	−9
Nonfatal myocardial infarctions per 1000 subjects	7.2	5.8
Fatal and nonfatal myocardial infarctions per 1000 subjects	8.9	7.4
Total deaths per 1000 subjects	5.2	6.2

fatal and nonfatal (row 3 in the table). The efficacy of clofibrate, therefore, would appear to be supported in this study. However, when we consider all clinically relevant outcomes, especially from the point of view of the patient [63], we must consider the effects of clofibrate on quality of life and total mortality, and the latter is shown with disturbing effect in row 4 of the table: total mortality rose with clofibrate therapy, a result that has profoundly affected both the use and availability of this drug. Because one's judgment about the usefulness of clofibrate or other agents can depend, in a crucial way, on the clinical outcomes chosen for comparison, readers must be sure that all clinically relevant outcomes are reported.

Furthermore, because clinical disagreement is ubiquitous in medicine, readers should also recognize the necessity for explicit, objective criteria for the clinical outcomes of interest and their application by observers who are "blind" to whether the patient under scrutiny was in the active treatment or control group.

WERE THE STUDY PATIENTS RECOGNIZABLY SIMILAR TO YOUR OWN?

This guide has two elements. First, the study patients must be *recognizable,* that is, their clinical and sociodemographic status must be described in sufficient detail for you to be able to recognize the similarity between them and your own patients. Second, the study patients should be at least roughly *similar* to patients in your practice. This guide can be overdone, as when one of our clinical clerks refused to extrapolate the results of a positive randomized trial among 40–65-year-olds to a 68-year-old patient on our service. Increasingly, therefore, we state this guide, "Are the patients in this study *so different* from my patients that I could *not* apply the study results in my practice?"

WERE BOTH CLINICAL AND STATISTICAL SIGNIFICANCE CONSIDERED?

Clinical significance here refers to the *importance* of a difference in clinical outcomes between treated and control patients, and is usually described in terms of the *magnitude* of a result. Suppose that the active treatment group in a randomized trial of aspirin in threatened stroke had 50% fewer strokes and deaths than the corresponding control group. This 50% reduction becomes clinically significant when its publication leads to changes in clinical behavior;* thus, it is confirmed as being clinically significant when clinicians prescribe aspirin to patients with threatened stroke. By contrast, *statistical significance* tells us whether the conclusions the authors have drawn are likely to be *true* (regardless of whether or not they are clinically important).

Suppose you read an article that reports on a randomized double-blind clinical trial comparing a new drug (call it Drug A) with an identical appearing placebo (call it Drug B) for the control of an important clinical disorder. Based on their results (and excluding for the moment the possibility that Drug A makes patients worse), the authors of the article will have drawn one of two conclusions: either Drug A is *better* than Drug B, or Drug A is *no better* than Drug B. They will report this conclusion in their article and will try to convince us that it is correct.

Of course we all recognize that there is a *true* answer to the question posed by this trial, and that either Drug A *really is better* that Drug B, or Drug A *really is no better* than Drug B. The clinical trial in the article is one attempt to get at the truth, and when we compare the author's conclusions with the true state of affairs as in Table 7-5, some very confusing statistical concepts become clear.

If the team conducting the trial concludes that Drug A is better than Drug B, and in truth it really *is* better, as in cell *w* of Table 7-5, then they have drawn a correct "true-positive" conclusion and all is well. Similarly, they can draw a correct true-negative conclusion that Drug A is no better than Drug B when in truth it is not, as in cell *z*. Trouble arises when they draw the erroneous conclusions of cells *x* and *y*. In cell *x* they have drawn an erroneous false-positive conclusion that Drug A is better than Drug B when, in truth, it is no better. Conversely, in cell *y* they have drawn an erroneous false-negative conclusion that Drug A is no better than Drug B when, in truth, it is better.

These relationships between the conclusions drawn from a trial, on the one hand, and the true state of affairs, on the other, can usefully be thought of as an attempt to "diagnose" the truth. The clinical trial is the diagnostic test, and we can interpret it as positive (Drug A is better than Drug B) or negative (Drug A is no better than Drug B). We hope that our conclusions are "true-positives" and "true-negatives" (cells *w* and *z*, respectively) and hope to avoid the erroneous conclusions that lead to "false-positive" (cell *x*) and "false-negative" (cell *y*) interpretations.

As you can see from Table 7-5, two sorts of erroneous conclusions can be made. As it happens, these errors have names and one of them is attached to an old friend. This is shown in Table 7-6.

With a flair for exciting names, statisticians have decided to call the false-positive error of concluding that Drug A is better than Drug B when, in truth, it is not the "Type I error." What *is* exciting, however, is that in reporting the results of a trial the authors almost always tell us the size of the risk that they

*Although we have defined clinical significance from the perspective of the clinician it could, of course, also be defined from the patient's perspective in terms of "important differences in the quality of life."

Table 7-5. Comparing the conclusions drawn from a clinical trial with the true state of affairs

		The true state of affairs	
		Drug A is *better* than drug B	Drug A is *no better* than drug B
Conclusion drawn from a clinical trial	Drug A is *better* than drug B	TP Correct w	FP Error x
	Drug A is *no better* than drug B	FN Error y	TN Correct z

TP = true-positive; FP = false-positive; FN = false-negative; TN = true-negative.

Table 7-6. Naming the erroneous conclusions from a clinical trial

		The true state of affairs	
		Drug A is *better* than drug B	Drug A is *no better* than drug B
Conclusion drawn from a clinical trial	Drug A is *better* than drug B	TP Correct ($1 - \beta$ = power) w	FP Type I error (risk of making this error = α = the P value!) x
	Drug A is *no better* than drug B	FN Type II error (risk of making this error = β) y	TN Correct z

have made this false-positive error, for this is what the P value means! The P value (or α as it is called before the study begins) is the probability of a false-positive conclusion that Drug A is better than Drug B is when, in truth, it isn't. Thus, the smaller the P value, the more comfortable we are about a conclusion that the experimental therapy really is better than the control or placebo therapy.

As you can see from Table 7-6, the erroneous false negative conclusion has an exciting name, too, and it is the "Type II error." The size of the risk of drawing this erroneous conclusion also can be calculated, and it is called β. What is really interesting about this column of the table is cell *w,* which is equal to $(1 - \beta)$. It tells us the probability that the authors would conclude that Drug A is not statistically significantly better than B when, in truth, it really is better. This probability of drawing a true-positive conclusion when you ought to is called the "power" of the study and, by harking back to Chapter 4 on diagnostic tests, you can see that the *power* of a scientific study is analogous to the *sensitivity* of a diagnostic test. It may be helpful to think of it in this way as we proceed.

It should come as no surprise that these relationships are used in both planning and interpreting randomized trials. In planning such a trial, investigators can decide beforehand just how great a risk they are willing to run of drawing erroneous conclusions of both sorts (that is, of committing false-positive Type I and false-negative Type II errors). In doing so they often decide to run a 5% risk of concluding that experimental and conventional therapy *do* produce different clinical outcomes when, in truth, they do *not* (a false-positive Type I or α error of .05), and to run a 20% risk of concluding that experimental and conventional therapy do *not* produce different clinical outcomes when, in fact, they *do* (a false-negative Type II or β error of .20). If β is .20, then the power of the study is 1 − .20 or 80%; that is, if in truth experimental therapy and conventional therapy really do produce different results, the study will have an 80% chance of finding it and labeling it statistically significant. Or, by analogy, the sensitivity of the study for finding a real difference, if it truly exists, is 80%.

Most authors decide to set the false-positive α risk at .05 and the false-negative β risk at .20, so that these values for α and β are sometimes referred to as "conventional levels of statistical significance." In other clinical situations, especially in the growing number of cases in which clinicians want to find out whether a new treatment is not better than, but *as good as,* a standard treatment of higher toxicity or cost, the false-negative risk may be set lower. We'll come to an alternative way of looking at this issue of "equivalence" shortly.

To these decisions about risks are then added judgments about the expected rate of outcome events in patients assigned to conventional therapy and the degree of difference in outcomes between these conventionally treated patients and those assigned to experimental therapy that would be considered clinically significant (as we have noted earlier, this typically takes the form of a halving of the event rate). Then, because these five elements (α, β, the clinically significant difference, the rate of events in patients on conventional therapy, and the number of patients in each treatment group) are interrelated, it follows that if you know or set any four, you can calculate the fifth. So if investigators set α, β, and the clinically significant difference, and if they know the rate of events that occurs on conventional therapy, the number of patients required to maintain this relationship can be calculated; in fact, this is how clinical researchers routinely decide how many patients they need in a randomized trial. There are, of course, several additional twists and turns to the preceding discussion, but they are of interest to the doers of research and this book is for the users of research. Thus, we are content if we have convinced you that it *is* possible, before starting a therapeutic trial, to define how many subjects are required to demonstrate clinically significant differences at conventional levels of statistical significance.

So ends the statistics lesson. From it, we can derive two very useful yardsticks for interpreting an article on a clinical trial.

First, *if the difference is statistically significant, is it clinically significant as well?* Second, *if the difference is not statistically significant, was the trial big enough to show a clinically important difference if it had occurred?* We'll address the first yardstick here, with some of its recent expansions and extensions, and then go on to the second yardstick.

Suppose that the authors conclude that Drug A is better for patients than Drug B, and have calculated the P value at .02. This means that their risk of having erroneously concluded that Drug A is better, when in truth it is not, is only 2 in 100. That looks pretty good, and you can assume that the difference in results on Drug A and Drug B is real. The question then becomes, "Is it clinically important as well?"

"Clinical significance" goes beyond arithmetic and is determined by clinical judgment. It is another of those formerly mysterious elements of the "art" of medicine that we can better understand through the application of epidemiology and biostatistics to clinical decisions. In this case, these applications can help you sort out whether Drug A's benefits are big enough for you to want to put the patient and yourself through the risks and trouble of treatment with it. We think that this topic is important enough to warrant a major discussion here.

We'll describe two ways for thinking about clinical significance in matters of treatment (which is where the topic most dramatically arises, although we commented earlier on its parallel application to making diagnostic and prognostic decisions). The first is quick, easy, and applicable to individual patients. The second takes a bit longer, but is applicable not only to individual patients but also to different patients with different treatments for different illnesses. To illustrate their use and usefulness, we'll introduce both of them with the results (statistically significant) of one of the landmark U.S. Veterans Administration trials of whether treating hypertension would prevent fatal and nonfatal target organ damage [70]. In this trial, patients with and without prior target organ damage (to the heart, brain, eye, kidney, or major vessels) at entry were randomized to receive either active antihypertensive drugs or identical appearing placebos, and the clinical course over the next 3 years for the subset of men who entered before the age of 50 with diastolic blood pressures between 90 and 114 is shown in Table 7-7.

As you can see from Table 7-7, the treatment target here was the prevention of death, stroke, or other major complication of these men's hypertension. As we've already said, the treatment produced statistically significant improvements in these outcomes. Among men with target organ damage at the start of the trial, more than one-fifth (.22) of those randomized to inert placebos went on to additional major complications, compared to less than one-tenth (.08) of those given active antihypertensive drugs. Men free of target organ damage at the start of the trial, although at lower risk of complications, also benefited from active treatment; one-tenth (.10) of those on placebo, but less than one-twentieth (.04) of those on active drugs, suffered complications of their disease during the 3 years the trial lasted.

How might these benefits be expressed in terms of clinical significance? The first method simply calculates the percent reduction in the risk of target complications achieved through active treatment by comparing (by arithmetic division) the difference in the complication rates between placebo and active patients

Table 7-7. Occurrence of death, stroke, or other major complications

	Adverse event rates	
	Placebo	Active Rx
Patient status at entry	P	A
Prior target organ damage	.22	.08
No prior organ damage	.10	.04

Table 7-8. Occurrence of death, stroke, or other major complications

	Adverse event rates		Relative risk reduction RRR
Patient status at entry	Placebo P	Active A	$\frac{(P - A)}{P} = \text{RRR}$
Prior target organ damage	.22	.08	$\frac{.22 - .08}{.22} = 64\%$
No prior organ damage	.10	.04	$\frac{.10 - .04}{.10} = 60\%$

with what would have occurred with no treatment (the complication rate among placebo patients). This calculation, which is usually called the *relative risk reduction* (and labeled RRR in subsequent tables) is carried out for you in Table 7-8.

These relative risk reductions mean that the risk of death, stroke, or other major complications of hypertension was reduced by almost two-thirds through active treatment, and we'll bet that you will judge this benefit to be "clinically significant." The great majority of your colleagues have done so, as shown in the tremendous increase in the proportion of hypertensive patients placed on antihypertensive drugs since the publication and dissemination of the results of trials such as this one.

When this yardstick is applied, relative risk reductions of $\geqslant$ 50% almost always, and of $\geqslant$ 25% often, are considered to be clinically significant. For example, coronary artery bypass surgery produced a relative risk reduction in death within 5 years of 56% among men with stable angina pectoris and left main stem coronary artery stenosis in one of its trials [17]. More recently, the combination of streptokinase and aspirin produced a relative risk reduction of 40% in death over the next 5 weeks among patients suspected of undergoing acute myocardial infarctions [39]. Finally, a randomized trial of propranolol found that it reduced the risk of dying in the subsequent 2 years by 26% among early, stable survivors of myocardial infarctions [6]. Table 7-13 summarizes the relative risk reductions (plus other properties we'll explain later) for several treatments validated in randomized trials.

The relative risk reduction, then, is a quick and useful measure of clinical significance. It usually appears right in the abstract of the article reporting a randomized trial of therapy and, if not, usually can be calculated from the "Results" section of the paper, as long as there is a placebo or "no treatment" group, and as long as specific treatment targets (such as death, stroke, or some given level of disability) are being counted (rather than some "continuous" measure like blood pressure or antibody level).

The second measure of clinical significance, which we've enjoyed studying with clinical epidemiologist Andreas Laupacis and biostatistician Robin Roberts [45], is in rare but increasing use and, although it looks complex at the start, is both conceptually simpler and clinically more useful than the relative risk reduction. A reexamination of Table 7-8 will show you why: the relative risk reduction discards the measure of the risk of no treatment ("absolute risk"). Patients with and without prior target organ damage benefit equally, in terms of relative risk reduction, from antihypertensive drug therapy, although the former are much more likely to go on to death, stroke, or other major complications, with or without treatment. Indeed, the effect of treating a patient with target organ damage is to reduce his absolute risk to that of the untreated patient with no target organ damage! The higher priority for detecting and treating the hypertensive patient who already has target organ damage is not captured in the relative risk reduction, and this measure therefore lacks an important element of clinical significance.

We can capture this missing element by sticking to the absolute risks of bad outcomes in the absence and presence of treatment, and this is shown in Table 7-9.

These absolute differences in the risks of death, stroke, or other major complications of .14 for patients with, but only .06 for patients without, target organ damage at the outset now show the greater absolute gains from treating the former group and captures the clinical significance of this difference. Already, however, you probably have identified a major shortcoming in the clinical usefulness

Table 7-9. Occurrence of death, stroke, or other major complications

	Adverse events			Absolute risk reduction ARR
Patient status at entry	Placebo P	Active A	RRR	P − A = ARR
Prior target organ damage	.22	.08	64%	.22 − .08 = .14
No prior organ damage	.10	.04	60%	.10 − .04 = .06

Table 7-10. Occurrence of death, stroke, or other major complications

	Adverse events				Number needed to treat NNT
Patient status at entry	Placebo P	Active A	RRR	ARR	$\frac{1}{ARR}$ = NNT
Prior target organ damage	.22	.08	64%	.14	$\frac{1}{.14} = 7$
No prior organ damage	.10	.04	60%	.06	$\frac{1}{.06} = 17$

of this "absolute risk reduction." Its decimal form is foreign to most clinicians, neither fitting cozily in the mind nor rolling smoothly off the tongue in bedside discussion. It may contain more information than the relative risk reduction, but it is in a form that most of us cannot use.

But see what happens when we divide the absolute risk reduction into 1 (that is, "take its reciprocal"). The very useful result is shown in Table 7-10.

The reciprocal of the absolute risk reduction turns out to be the number of patients we need to treat in order to prevent one complication of their disease! Thus, we need to treat only 7 hypertensives with preexisting target organ damage for 3 years in order to prevent one of them from going on to death, stroke, or other major complication, whereas we need to treat 17 hypertensives initially free of target organ damage for this same length of time to prevent one of them from suffering such a complication.

This measure of clinical significance, which we have called the "number needed to treat" or "NNT," has three additional properties that add to its clinical usefulness; and we'll discuss two of them here. First, the NNT nicely emphasizes the effort you and your patients will have to expend in order to accomplish a very tangible treatment target. In doing so, it helps to quantify and, thereby, demystify the "art" of the decision to treat some, but not other, patients, even when they have the same disorder.* Second, the "number" in the NNT gives you a base from which to express the costs of treatment, both in terms of the

*Andreas Laupacis and D. L. S. received a huge shove in this direction when they were making rounds in our CCU at the same time that they were working up the NNT. A senior cardiologist lamented to them that he could not get the house staff to forego long-term secondary prophylaxis for low-risk patients following myocardial infarction. We showed him how, if we assume that secondary prophylaxis with beta blockers achieves a relative risk reduction in one-year mortality of 30% among both high-risk (1-year case fatality of .20) and low-risk (1-year case fatality of .02) infarction patients, we'd have to treat only 17 of the former (1/[.20 − .14]) but 170 of the latter (1/[.02 − . 014]), in order to prevent one death. Our colleague was delighted by the way the NNT approach could help him express his "art" to his residents, and we were encouraged to forge ahead.

dollar costs of the regimen and its monitoring and, of special interest to the patient, in terms of the side effects and toxicity of the treatment. For example, the British Medical Research Council hypertension trial reported the frequency of specific side effects on the randomized treatments [55]. This sort of information permits us to reckon that, among the 17 hypertensives (initially free of target organ damage) we need to treat for 3 years in order to prevent one death, stroke, or other major complication, the choice of a thiazide as the first line drug would be followed by impotence in one, symptomatic gout in a second, and diabetes in a third, all leading to the discontinuation of treatment. Several more could be expected to experience these side effects but remain on therapy.

A more recent example is the U.S. Physicians' Health Study [65] in which over 22,000 male physician volunteers were randomized to either aspirin (325 mg every other day) or placebo for an average of 5 years. The relative risk reduction for myocardial infarction was an impressive 44%, but the absolute risk was so low at the outset (.26% per year) that the corresponding NNT with aspirin for 5 years in order to prevent one myocardial infarction came to 108 (we'll show you how these calculations were made in a moment). Interestingly, the accompanying editorial echoed our suggestion that the relative risk reduction is an insufficient measure of clinical significance: "There are clear problems in reporting (relative) risk reduction as a percentage when the absolute prevalence (sic) of events is low." [23]. Moreover, because the study kept careful track of potential side effects of aspirin, it also was determined that, for example, 3.3% of aspirin takers but only 2.2% of placebo takers experienced melena during the trial. So, with respect to these clinical outcomes, if we treat 108 men with low-dose aspirin for 5 years in order to prevent myocardial infarction in one of them, we can expect to produce one additional bout of melena along the way. Moreover, even though hemorrhagic strokes were only one-tenth as frequent as myocardial infarction, they were twice as frequent among aspirin-takers (the P value for this difference was .06), so we'd expect one extra hemorrhagic stroke per 1000 patients treated with aspirin for 5 years. Although the trial observed no favorable trend in total cardiovascular mortality, many clinicians judge these and the other side effects to be worth risking, even in low-risk patients, in order to prevent myocardial infarction. Other clinicians point out that, if the relative risk reduction and risks of side effects are the same for patients at high and low risk for myocardial infarction, why not restrict aspirin to the former, in whom the NNT is lower? This point of view encourages readers to search the article in question for tables showing whether clinically sensible subgroups of patients have greater risks of the treatment target you are trying to prevent, but are still nicely responsive to treatment, so that risky therapy can be confined to those patients in whom the NNT, and therefore the risk of side effects, is low. To help you grasp what this can mean in practical clinical terms, Table 7-11 displays the NNTs for different baseline risks and relative risk reductions.

Two quick conclusions follow a perusal of Table 7-11. First, when the absolute baseline risk of the bad clinical outcome is high, even modest relative risk reductions generate gratifyingly small NNTs; thus a treatment that produces only

Table 7-11. The effect of different baseline risks and relative risk reductions on the number needed to treat

Baseline risk (with no treatment)	Relative risk reduction on treatment						
	50%	40%	30%	25%	20%	15%	10%
.9	2	3	4	4	6	7	11
.6	3	4	6	7	8	11	17
.3	7	8	11	13	17	22	33
.2	10	13	17	20	25	33	50
.1	20	25	33	40	50	67	100
.05	40	50	67	80	100	133	200
.01	200	250	333	400	500	667	1000
.005	400	500	667	800	1000	1333	2000
.001	2000	2500	3333	4000	5000	6667	10000

a 10% relative risk reduction in a baseline risk of .9 is as clinically significant as one that produces a 30% relative risk reduction in a baseline risk of .3 (did you discover that the NNT is 11 for both of these?). Second, rather small changes in the absolute baseline risk of a rare clinical event lead to big changes in the numbers of patients we need to treat in order to prevent one. So a powerful but risky treatment that produces a relative risk reduction of 50% for a bad outcome, but also produces an equally serious side effect in 1% of those who receive it, isn't worth giving to patients with a .01 risk of the bad outcome, is it? The NNT here is 200, and you'd produce two bad side effects for every bad outcome you prevented. If, however, you could identify a subgroup of patients whose risk of the bad outcome was .05, the NNT is now reduced to 40 and the scales have tipped in favor of treatment.

One final comment on generating and understanding NNTs arises from the happy but confusing circumstance in which there is more than one positive trial of the same treatment for the same disorder, but the "raw" data yield conflicting measures of the number needed to treat. Consider the hypothetical situation shown in Table 7-12 (in both cases, the differences in complication rates between active and placebo patients were statistically significant).

Although the relative risk reductions in trials #1 and #2 in Table 7-12 are identical, the absolute risks without treatment and absolute risk reductions differ. Consequently, the numbers of patients that need to be treated to prevent one complication were twice as many in trial #2 as in trial #1. Which one should we use in determining the clinical significance of the benefits of this treatment?

In fact, the two trials are quite consistent, and their reconciliation resides in their durations: trial #1 (a relatively small trial) required an average follow-up of 4 years to achieve a statistically significant result, whereas trial #2 (a relatively large trial) required an average follow-up of only 2 years. Trial #2 indi-

Table 7-12. Two trials of drug A: Occurrence of complications of the underlying disease

	Adverse events				Number needed to treat NNT
	Placebo P	Active A	RRR	ARR	$\frac{1}{ARR} = NNT$
trial #1 Duration—4 years	.40	.30	25%	.10	$\frac{1}{.10} = 10$
trial #2 Duration—2 years	.20	.15	25%	.05	$\frac{1}{.05} = 20$

cates that we can accomplish the same end as trial #1, the prevention of one event, by treating twice as many patients for half as long, and serves as an example for the general formula

$$NNT{:}E = NNT{:}A \times A/E$$

where E is the duration of therapy for which you want to estimate the NNT and A is the actual average duration of therapy (in the same units of time) in the trial you are reading about. In the example in Table 7-12, if we want to extrapolate from trial #1 to trial #2, A = 4, E = 2, and NNT:2 = 10 × 4/2 = 20.

Of course, these calculations assume that the treatment's efficacy (as measured, say, by the relative risk reduction) is constant over time, and that it doesn't increase or decrease as the duration of therapy increases. Deviations from constant efficacy can wax or, more often we think, wane. An example of waxing measures of efficacy are seen with cholestyramine in the prevention of coronary events, where a sizable relative risk reduction didn't appear until the fourth year of the trial [48]. We think that the more common situation is exemplified by the use of propranolol following myocardial infarction. Its relative risk reduction for mortality fell in the second year of treatment [6].* Considerations of disease mechanisms and pharmacodynamics may help you decide whether time trends in efficacy ought to be up, down, or steady.

On the other hand, efficacy usually waxes when an efficacious surgical procedure is compared with a less efficacious nonsurgical one. Perioperative com-

*When an initially high relative risk reduction later falls to or near zero, this doesn't constitute grounds for stopping treatment at that point; such waning trends can't, by themselves, distinguish early and temporary vulnerability of patients to the complications of their disease (in which case they don't need treatment any longer) from continuing susceptibility to these complications (in which case they need continuing therapy).

plications often make surgery look worse in the short run, and the surgical benefit cannot be revealed until medical failures begin to accumulate.

You should remember these examples and cautions if an NNT extrapolated from a short trial disagrees sharply from that actually observed in a long trial. If efficacy waxes, the short trial will overestimate the true NNT; if efficacy wanes, the estimate of NNT will be overoptimistically low.

The third of the three additional advantages of the NNT approach is its usefulness as a generic yardstick for comparing different treatments for different disorders. Although this goes beyond the present discussion of an approach to determining the clinical significance of a single treatment for a single condition, and is more suited to deciding how you want to ration your time and other resources in your overall practice, we've summarized the NNTs (and other properties) of a few treatments in Table 7-13. The results of our first attempt to see how Canadian internists set their own treatment priorities suggests that they may find the NNT a bit more useful than the relative risk reduction; we shall continue to pursue this lead [46].

The foregoing NNT strategy should help you make up your own mind about the clinical significance of a report describing a positive and statistically significant response to treatment. Its elements are three: the first gives you that key comparison of the risks of doing nothing with the benefits of doing something; second, the associated harm resulting from the side effects and toxicity of the treatment; and third, the identification of high-risk/high-response subgroups of patients who have the most to gain, and the least to lose, from the treatment in question.*

The NNT is a fine approach to assessing the clinical significance of a positive trial reporting those events that do or do not happen—a patient dies or does not die, has a stroke or does not have a stroke. However, other aspects of our patients' health, such as their function and well-being, are as or more important and either difficult or impossible to summarize as NNTs. The term "health-related quality of life" has been coined to denote physical and emotional (as opposed to biochemical and physiological) function, as well as the social or personal value (or "utility") with which patients regard this function.

Quality-of-life measures are found in three different sorts of articles: those about the distribution of dysfunction in a population of patients or other people; those about the relation between quality of life and prognosis; and, of greatest

*How much information do we require in forming such judgments? Andrew Oxman has suggested to us, and we agree, that it depends on our initial estimates of the risks of doing nothing versus something and the energy and money involved. If initial, small amounts of information suggest that the patient risks a great deal if we do nothing, but benefits substantially (with little risk of side effects) if we do a specific something, and if the treatment involves little cost, we proceed at once to treat. If, on the other hand, this initial smattering suggests minimal risk if we do nothing, little benefit and considerable risk if we do a specific something, and the latter entails considerable effort and money, we quickly close the door. To the extent that our initial information deviates from these extremes, we tend to look further, think longer, procrastinate, or refer the patient for another opinion.

Table 7-13. Measures of efficacy for six different conditions

Therapy	Events	Follow-up (years)	Risk of doing nothing	RRR	NNT[a]	NNT:5[b]
Stepped care for diastolic blood pressure of 115–129 mm Hg[c]	Death, stroke, myocardial infarction	1.5	.13	89%	9	3
Left main coronary artery bypass surgery[d]	Death	5	.32	56%	6	6
Aspirin for transient ischemic attacks[e]	Death, stroke	2.2	.23	31%	14	6
Cholestyramine for hypercholesterolemia[f]	Death, myocardial infarction	7.4	.12	14%	60	89
Isoniazid for inactive tuberculosis[g]	Active tuberculosis	5	.01	75%	96	96
Stepped care for diastolic blood pressure of 90–109 mm Hg[h]	Death, stroke, myocardial infarction	5.5	.05	14%	128	141

[a]Calculated for the actual mean duration of follow-up in each trial.
[b]Adjusted to the NNT for five years, assuming constant benefit over time (see test for calculation).
[c]Veterans Administration Cooperative Study Group on Antihypertensive Agents. Effects of treatment on morbidity in hypertension: Results in patients with diastolic blood pressures averaging 115 through 129 mm Hg. *J.A.M.A.* 202: 1028–34, 1967.
[d]European Coronary Study Group. Long-term results of prospective randomised study of coronary artery bypass surgery in stable angina pectoris. *Lancet* 2: 1173–80, 1982.
[e]The Canadian Cooperative Study Group. A randomized trial of aspirin and sulfinpyrazone in threatened stroke. *N. Engl. J. Med.* 299: 53–59, 1978.
[f]Lipid Research Clinics Program. The Lipid Research Clinics Coronary Primary Prevention Trial results. I. Reduction in incidence of coronary heart disease. *J.A.M.A.* 251: 351–64, 1984.
[g]International Union Against Tuberculosis Committee on Prophylaxis. Efficacy of various durations of isoniazid preventive therapy for tuberculosis: five years of follow-up in the IUAT trial. *Bull. W.H.O.* 60: 555–64, 1982.
[h]Medical Research Council Working Party. MRC trial of treatment of mild hypertension: principal results. *Br. Med. J.* 291: 97–104, 1985.

importance to us in this discussion, those about the impact of a disease or condition, or treatments for it, on patients' physical, emotional, and social functions. Thus, these measurements can be used to *discriminate* one sort of patient from another, to *predict* the prognosis or other future state of a patient, and to *evaluate* the effects of interventions upon those who receive them [42]. Because more and more clinical articles about therapy use quality-of-life measurements to make their case, we will offer you a primer on them here; some of you may want to read further [18, 26, 59].

The "evaluative" quality-of-life measures you will encounter in articles assessing the efficacy of therapy must have one crucial attribute that is not necessary for discriminative or evaluative instruments. This attribute is responsiveness (or as it is sometimes called, sensitivity to change)—the ability to detect any clinically important differences produced by the treatment in question, even if the magnitude of those differences is small. Therefore, when reading the Methods section of a clinical article in which quality-of-life measures were used to evaluate a therapy, you should look to see whether the authors used a measure that had been shown to be responsive as well as reproducible.

You are likely to encounter three different sorts of evaluative quality-of-life measures when you read such articles. The first sort are generic measures that address the complete spectrum of function, disability, and distress along the entire range of patients from healthy to very ill. For this reason, you will encounter them in reports on a wide variety of different treatments for different disorders. For example, the Sickness Impact Profile (SIP) [5] has been used in studies of cardiac rehabilitation [58], total hip joint arthroplasty [47], and treatment of back pain [15]. In the latter study, 203 walk-in patients with mechanical back pain were randomized to receive recommendations of 2 or 7 days bed rest. When the Sickness Impact Profile was completed by patients three weeks after their presentation, as you can see in Table 7-14, the scores (the lower the score, the smaller the deleterious impact) were comparable in the two groups.

However, patients receiving the 7-day recommendation spent more time away from work (5.6 days versus 3.1 days, P = .01), and there was actually a trend in physical function in favor of the 2-day recommendation group. Reassured by the Sickness Impact Profile results that the earlier mobilization of back patients has no deleterious effect on health-related quality of life, both we and our patients can be more comfortable with the recommendation for shorter bed rest.

The second sort of measure you will encounter describes not the individual symptoms or disabilities comprising a patient's state of health, but the overall social value (utility) that patient places on this health state [32]. Measured in clever ways with delightful names (the von Neumann and Morgenstern standard gamble, and the time-trade-off method [69]), the result is expressed as a single number along a continuum from death (.0) to full health (1.0). This "quality" number can then be multiplied by the number of years a patient is in the health state produced by a particular treatment, resulting in "quality-adjusted life years" or "QALYs."

For example, Weinstein and Stason [73] judged that a year with angina pectoris had a quality of .7 compared to a year without angina (with a quality of

Table 7-14. The Sickness Impact Profile in a trial of low back pain*

	Outcome measure	2 days of rest group	7 days of rest group
Sickness	Physical domain score	11.6	12.4
Impact	Psychosocial score	16.8	16.8
Profile	Overall score	15.7	15.9
	Days absent from work	3.1	5.6

*The lower the score, the smaller the deleterious impact

1.0), and that a year of partial relief from angina had a quality of .85. They then went to the randomized trials of coronary artery bypass surgery, determined the changes in life expectancy from surgery, and applied these quality estimates to them. The results suggested that bypass surgery resulted in a gain of about 6 QALYs in patients with left main stem coronary artery stenosis and about 3 QALYs in those with triple vessel disease.

A major advantage of such utility measures is that they can be plugged into economic analyses.* For example, in cost-utility analysis the cost of an intervention can be related to the number of quality-adjusted life years (QALYs) gained by applying, versus not applying, a treatment. The resulting "cost per QALY gained" permits readers to compare different treatments for the same patients, or the same treatment for different patients. Thus, in the case of coronary artery bypass surgery, it was estimated (in "1981 U.S. dollars"†) that it cost $3800 per QALY gained among patients with left main-stem disease and $7200 per QALY gained among patients with triple vessel disease. For comparison, the cost (in "1983 U.S. dollars") per QALY gained from hospital hemodialysis is $54,000, and the cost per QALY gained from neonatal intensive care ranges from $4500 for babies weighing 1000 to 1500 grams to $31,800 for babies weighing 500–999 grams [69]. You can then compare this cost per QALY gained with that for other programs. As you can imagine, health planners, administrators, program evaluators, and health-policy decision-makers are carrying out these same comparisons!

*As we'll explain in Chapter 13, economic analyses are about choices (what allocation of drugs, clinicians, hospitals, and other resources would produce the greatest benefit to patients and the public?). Dollars are *not* the central focus, but are simply used as a convenient measure. Thus, the *real* cost of doing one thing (e.g., bone-marrow transplants) is the *inability* to have enough resources left to do something else (e.g., alcohol rehabilitation); this is what is meant by the term "opportunity cost."

†Since currency changes in value from year to year, good articles pick a single year and relate all costs to the value of the currency during that year.

Because it is tough to make these overall utility measurements, because they vary depending on how patients are questioned about them, because they are a bit of a "black box" in which we can't tell what aspect of the patient's life are the deciding ones, and because they may not be responsive to small but clinically important changes in the quality of life, you are likely to encounter a third, more focused sort of quality-of-life measure that concentrates on limited areas of health status that are specific to the condition under study (the frail elderly, or those with chronic lung disease, or sexual dysfunction) [27]. Indeed, some of these quality-of-life measures even focus on problems specific to the individual patient [28]. For example, in a randomized trial of digoxin versus placebo among heart failure patients in sinus rhythm, digoxin proved superior in improving their shortness of breath in day-to-day activities as well as in the more general outcomes of the distance patients could walk in 6 minutes and in their physicians' assessment of their heart failure [31]. Similarly, patients in a controlled trial of bronchodilators for their chronic lung disease demonstrated clinically important improvements in dyspnea, fatigue, and emotional function as well as the less focused improvements in airway function [29]. We think you'll agree that such specific measures are more in line with your concerns as a clinician, and when reading an article that uses such measures, you can apply this yardstick of clinical credibility to the measures employed.

Regardless of what quality-of-life or utility measure you encounter in an article about therapy, we hope that the foregoing primer will help you decide whether they have led to valid and clinically useful conclusions about efficacy. To summarize:

1. Decide whether the measures are looking at clinically important features of the illness that you would hope to improve in your own patients.
2. Look to see whether the differences between groups are statistically significant; if so, consider whether they are clinically important.
3. If the results are not statistically significant, look to see whether the measures have previously been shown to be responsive (able to detect those clinically significant changes which, if they did occur with treatment, would make you want to prescribe it).
4. If the utility measures were incorporated into an economic analysis (the term "cost-utility" will tip you off to these), decide whether this economic analysis is clinically valid; we will show you how to do that in Chapter 13.

Finally, as we stressed earlier, when considering other outcomes in a trial, the need for careful, blinded measurement of function and quality of life is important.

So far, we've discussed how to interpret an article in which the difference in outcomes *is* statistically significant. What about those in which it is *not*?

The second yardstick applies to the results of a "negative" trial: *If the difference is not statistically significant, was the trial big enough to show a clinically important difference if it had occurred?* This goes back to our statistics lesson where we pointed out that it is possible for authors to determine ahead of time how big their study should be.

Unfortunately, the authors of most trials that reach negative conclusions either could not or would not put enough patients in their trials to detect clinically significant differences. That is, the β errors of such trials are very large and their power (or sensitivity) is very low. Indeed, when Jennifer Freiman and her colleagues reviewed a long list of trials that had reached "negative" conclusions they found that most of them had too few patients to show risk reductions of 25% or even 50% [21].

How can you apply this second yardstick? The approach that we'd suggest is based on posttrial results, rather than pretrial speculations, and suggests that "how many patients they needed depends on what they found!" [52]. This approach takes the actual study results and plugs them into Tables 7-15 and 7-16.

The rows of Tables 7-15 and 7-16 represent the rates of events among patients on the control or placebo treatment and the columns show the rates of events among patients on the experimental treatment. You can simply take these rates from the published report and identify the cell where they intersect. The entry in that cell gives the minimum number of patients required in each of the treatment groups for a study with these results to be reasonably sure (with a 1-sided α of .05) that a relative risk reduction of 25% (Table 7-15) or 50% (Table 7-16) would not have been missed if it had occurred.* By a *relative* risk reduction of 50% we mean a *halving* of an event rate. Thus, a reduction from .40 to .20 is a 50% relative risk reduction and a reduction from .40 to .30 is a 25% relative risk reduction. Accordingly, if the size of the treatment groups in the published report exceeds those in Tables 7-15 and 7-16 you can be pretty sure that the trial was, indeed, big enough to detect clinically important differences if they had occurred.

Let's try an example. When Hill and his colleagues performed their randomized trial of home-versus-hospital care for patients with suspected myocardial infarction (in the days before thrombolytic therapy) [35], they observed a 6-week case-fatality rate of 20% among the 132 patients who were randomized to be treated at home. This rate was not statistically significantly different from the 6-week case-fatality rate of 18% they documented among the other 132 patients who were randomized to treatment in hospital. Can we conclude that it was safe in those days to treat such coronary patients at home? Was this trial big enough to show a clinically significant difference (say, a 25% or 50% better outcome among hospitalized coronaries) if it did occur? If we track these results (both

*If you want to understand why we talk about "alpha" in Tables 7-15 and 7-16, this footnote is for you. Tables 7-15 and 7-16 address the "negative" trial by converting a "beta" problem into an "alpha" problem. Rather than go through the cumbersome calculations of a beta analysis, we have simply set up tables that contrast the trial results actually observed with the theoretical results that would have occurred if the experimental group enjoyed relative risk reductions of 25% (Table 7-15) or 50% (Table 7-16) from the rates observed among the control patients. As long as the studies had numbers of patients in each group that were equal to or greater than those listed in the tables, these studies' results are *incompatible* with relative risk reductions of 25% or 50%, and they *were* big enough to show clinically significant differences if they had occurred.

Table 7-15. Was the trial big enough to show a relative risk reduction of ≥25% if it had occurred?*

Observed rate of events in the control group		Observed rate of events in the experimental group																		
		.95	.90	.85	.80	.75	.70	.65	.60	.55	.50	.45	.40	.35	.30	.25	.20	.15	.10	.05
	.95		14	27	68	391														
	.90		11	18	38	110	1057													
	.85			14	25	54	185	4889												
	.80			11	18	33	78	326												
	.75				13	22	44	112	635											
	.70				11	16	28	57	165	1524										
	.65					13	20	35	75	250	6349									
	.60					10	15	24	43	99	402									
	.55						12	17	28	53	132	722								
	.50							13	20	33	65	180	1607							
	.45							10	15	22	38	79	254							
	.40								11	16	25	44	98	381						
	.35									12	18	28	50	121	634					
	.30										13	19	30	57	1296					
	.25										10	13	20	33	64	196	4537			
	.20											10	14	20	34	71	261			
	.15												10	14	20	35	78	371		
	.10													10	13	20	34	80	589	
	.05															12	17	30	74	1245

Trials up here have risk reductions of 25% or more

Trials down here needed fewer than 10 patients per group

*This table displays how many patients would be needed per group, to be confident ($\alpha = .05$, 1-tailed) that you have not missed a 25% relative risk reduction in the experimental group. (A reduction from .40–.30 is a 25% relative risk reduction, as is a reduction from .20 to 0.15.)

Table 7-16. Was the trial big enough to show a relative risk reduction of ≥50% if it had occurred?*

Observed rate of events in the control group		Observed rate of events in the experimental group																
		.70	.65	.60	.55	.50	.45	.40	.35	.30	.25	.20	.15	.10	.08	.06	.04	.02
	.98	14	24	50	165	5803												
	.95	12	19	37	102	921												
	.90		14	26	58	236												
	.85		12	19	38	108	995											
	.80		10	15	27	63	256											
	.75			12	21	41	116	1059										
	.70				16	29	66	268										
	.65				13	22	43	120	1082									
	.60				11	17	30	68	270									
	.55					13	22	42	119	1059								
	.50					11	17	30	66	260								
	.45						13	22	42	113	987							
	.40						11	16	28	62	239							
	.35							13	20	38	102	867						
	.30							10	15	26	55	205						
	.25								12	18	33	86	699					
	.20									13	22	45	160					
	.15									10	15	26	64	482				
	.10										11	17	32	102	254	2017		
	.08											14	25	66	131	453		
	.06											12	20	44	76	179	1313	
	.04											10	16	31	47	87	274	
	.02												12	22	30	47	97	561

Trials up here have risk reductions of 50% or more

Trials down here needed fewer than 10 patients per group

*This table displays how many patients would be needed per group, to be confident (α = .05, 1-tailed) that you have not missed a 50%-relative risk reduction in the experimental group. (A reduction from .40–.20 is a 50% relative risk reduction, as is a reduction from .20 to .10.)

about 20%) into Table 7-15, we see that the trial needed 261 patients per group to be confident that it had not missed a risk reduction of 25% in the 6-week case-fatality rate of coronary patients treated in hospital; in Table 7-16, we see that the trial needed 45 patients per group to be confident that it had not missed a 50% risk reduction in the 6-week case-fatality rate of hospitalized coronaries. Thus, the trial was too small to reject a 25% improvement, but large enough to reject a 50% improvement, in the 6-week case-fatality rates of coronary patients treated in hospital. As a result, the important question addressed by this study was only partially answered by it, and the controversy continued, as it should have, right up to the time that thrombolytic therapy for chest pain changed the question.

There is a second way to decide whether a negative trial was big enough to show a clinically important difference if it had occurred. It involves looking in the article for something called a "confidence interval" or "confidence limits" on the risk reduction, NNT, or other measure of efficacy. This confidence expression often is preceded by a percentage and may be abbreviated "95% CI" or "95% CL," respectively.

A useful way to understand confidence intervals goes back to P values. The P value, as you'll recall, tells you the risk of the false-positive conclusion that a treatment is efficacious when, in truth, it is not. In other words, the P value tells you how often these results would have occurred by chance if the experimental treatment were really no different from the control. Thus, when experimental therapy produces a relative risk reduction of 40% and the P value is .06, this means that, if there were really no difference between treatment and control therapy and you repeated the trial 100 times, results as or more extreme than those observed (that is, a relative risk reduction of 40% or more) would have happened 6 times in 100 by chance alone. If, however, the P value is .04, a relative risk reduction of 40% or more would have happened, by chance alone, only 4 times in these one hundred replications.

Although the difference between 4 times in 100 and 6 times in 100 is trivial, if we invoke the generally agreed-upon ("conventional") levels of statistical significance, this difference is crucial. This convention, which sets "statistical significance" at .05, thereby declares that a trial generating a relative risk reduction of 40% and a P value of .04 is positive and has established that the experimental and control treatments really are different, whereas the trial that generates this same 40% risk reduction and a P value of .06 is negative and has not established that experimental and control therapy are different from one another.*

For this reason, many authorities have debated whether the $P < .05$ represents an inappropriate way of branding studies as simply "positive" or "negative," and whether study results should be expressed as confidence limits (12, 20, 24, 44).

*Note once again that the absence of proof is not the proof of absence, and that even the conventional view generates a "Scotch verdict" that efficacy is "not proven" rather than "not present."

This alternative and, especially for negative trials, possibly more informative way for articles to report this sort of statistical analysis is to present the likely, rather than the unlikely, implications of the trial. That is, instead of telling you that some degree of relative risk reduction is likely to occur, by chance, only a little (say, less than 5% or 1%) of the time, authors can tell you where the true risk reduction is likely to lie most (say, 90% or 95%) of the time. Indeed, what they can do is give you a range of relative risk reductions, within which the true relative risk reduction will lie most of the time (and they can specify what they mean by "most").

This is the confidence interval approach. Specifically, the 95% confidence interval (the one which you'll usually see) of a relative risk reduction indicates the range within which, 19 times out of 20, its true value will lie. This is pretty close to what we'd call an intuitive definition of the confidence interval: you can be 95% certain that the truth is somewhere inside a 95% confidence interval.

How can the confidence interval help you interpret a negative study? Let's look at the one that we have summarized in Table 7-17.

The initial entries in Table 7-17 come from the Swedish Co-operative Stroke Study, carried out to determine whether patients with cerebral infarcts might have fewer subsequent strokes if they took aspirin [8]. Placebos were given to 252 control patients (n_C), and 18 of these ($p_C = 18/252 = .07$) had a subsequent

Table 7-17. Confidence interval in a "negative" randomized trial

	Control (placebo)	Experimental (aspirin)
Patients	$n_C = 252$	$n_E = 253$
Recurrent strokes	$p_C = .07$	$p_E = .09$

Absolute risk reduction $= p_C - p_E = .07 - .09 = -.02$
Relative risk reduction $= (p_C - p_E)/p_C = -.02/.07 = -29\%$
95% confidence interval for a relative risk reduction:

$$\frac{(p_C - p_E) +/- 1.96\sqrt{\dfrac{p_C(1 - p_C)}{n_C} + \dfrac{p_E(1 - p_E)}{n_E}}}{p_C} =$$

$$\frac{(.07 - .09) +/- 1.96\sqrt{\dfrac{.07 \times .93}{252} + \dfrac{.09 \times .91}{253}}}{.07} =$$

$$\frac{-.02 +/- .05}{.07} =$$

from $\dfrac{+.03}{.07} = +43\%$ to $\dfrac{-.07}{.07} = -100\%$

nonfatal stroke. Aspirin was given to 253 experimental patients (n_E), of whom 23 (p_E = 23/253 = .09) had a recurrent nonfatal stroke. As you can see, the results certainly did not favor aspirin. There was an absolute increase of .02 between the two groups, generating a relative risk increase (rather than reduction) of 29%.

This result, in a trial containing over 500 patients, appears quite definitive in terms of excluding any possible benefit from aspirin. Definitive, that is, until we examine its confidence interval in the lower portion of Table 7-17.* One boundary of the 95% confidence interval on that absolute difference of − .02 is (− .02 − .05 =) − .07, generating a relative risk *increase* of recurrent stroke from aspirin of (− .07/.07 =) − 100%, supporting our prior suspicion that aspirin cannot be beneficial in this situation. However, the other boundary of that absolute difference is (− .02 + .05 =) + .03, generating a relative risk *reduction* of recurrent stroke from aspirin of (.03/.07 =) + 43%, and telling us that we shouldn't consider the matter closed.† If we believe that a risk reduction of 30% or more would be clinically significant, we cannot regard the Swedish study as definitively excluding a benefit of aspirin. As it turns out, an overview of all trials of antiplatelet agents in patients with transient ischemic attack or stroke indicates a relative risk reduction from aspirin of over 20% (with quite narrow confidence limits), great enough for most clinicians to want to treat such patients with aspirin.

Some clinicians overinterpret the extremes of the confidence interval and, when faced with the foregoing information would misinterpret it to mean that a relative risk increase of 100% is *just as likely* as the observed relative risk increase of 29%. Not so. If we chart the probabilities that each result in a confidence interval is the correct one, the result is a bell curve such as that shown in Figure 7-1.

Thus, the value most likely to be the correct one is the result they got, and progressively distant values are progressively less likely to be correct. The extreme values are calculated and provided to readers because they *could* be true, but as we progress toward the limits they are progressively less likely to be true. So, the confidence interval can help you decide how to interpret the results of

*Actually, we do it by the shortcut of determining the confidence limits around the absolute risk reduction and dividing them by p_C. You could argue that this latter p_C should have its confidence limits taken into consideration as well, but the resulting calculations are much more complex and their answers do not importantly differ from the easier method we employ [13].

†In terms of our earlier discussion of the "number needed to treat," this confidence interval translates, at the one extreme, to 1/− .07, or causing one recurrent stroke for every 14 patients you treat and, at the other, to 1/+ .03, or preventing one stroke for every 33 patients you treat. If you are starting from scratch, the 95% confidence interval on the number needed to treat is simply the reciprocal of the numerator of that 95% confidence limit on a relative risk reduction, and looks like this:

$$\frac{1}{(p_C - p_E) +/- 1.96\sqrt{\dfrac{p_C(1 - p_C)}{n_C} + \dfrac{p_E(1 - p_E)}{n_E}}}$$

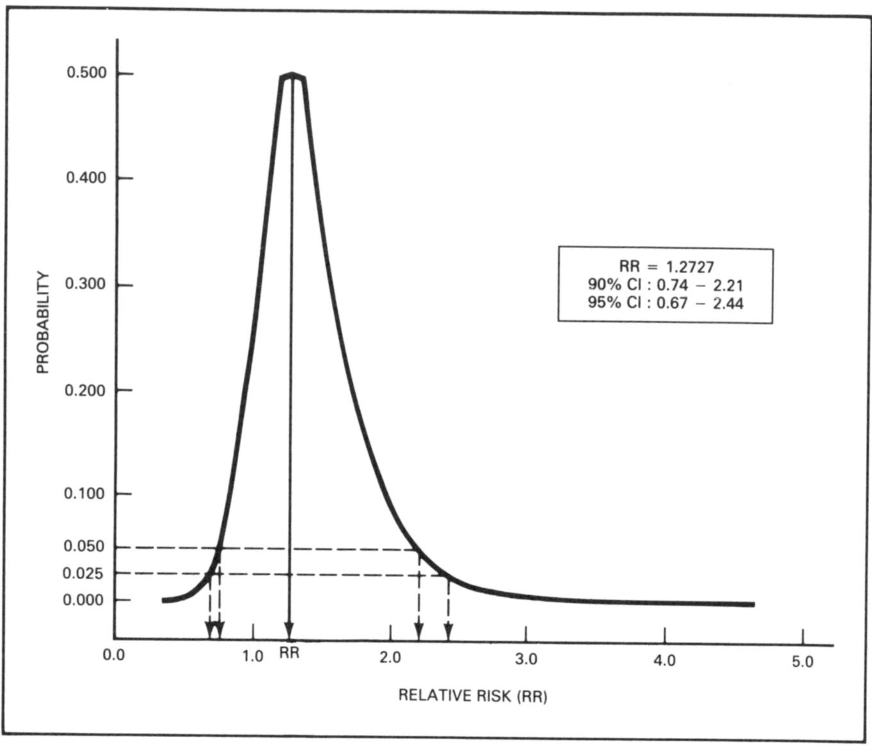

Figure 7-1. The probabilities of different confidence limits.

just about any clinical article.* When an article draws a negative conclusion about a treatment (because $P \geq .05$), you can focus on the upper end of the confidence interval for the relative risk reduction, for this places the treatment in the most favorable light. If this upper boundary lies below what you'd consider to be the smallest clinically significant risk reduction, you are reading about a definitively negative trial. If, on the other hand, this upper end of the confidence interval includes clinically important relative risk reductions, the trial hasn't ruled them out and cannot be regarded as definitively negative.

In the latter case, you may want to look further, especially for an "overview" that combines the results of several, similar trials. For reasons that are either intuitively obvious or can be divined from looking at the denominator of that formula in Table 7-17, the more patients in a study, the smaller its confidence interval. Thus, an overview that combines the results of several trials will report a very narrow confidence interval and often can forge a definitive overall conclusion from a series of indeterminate reports. We will show you how to read

*Since this book is about using the results of studies done by others, rather than doing the studies yourself, we won't go into the details of how to calculate the confidence intervals for other measures like sensitivity, specificity, likelihood ratio, relative odds, and the like. If you want to learn how to calculate these, you'd better consult a statistics text, perhaps beginning with one entirely devoted to confidence limits by Martin Gardner and Douglas Altman [25].

overviews (some of which, because they generate quantitative answers, are also called "meta-analyses") in Chapter 13.

IS THE THERAPEUTIC MANEUVER FEASIBLE IN YOUR PRACTICE?

The requirements here are four. First, the therapeutic maneuver has to be described in sufficient detail for readers to replicate it with precision. Who did what to whom, with what formulation and dose, administered under what circumstances, with what dose adjustments and titrations, with which searches for and responses to side effects and toxicity, for how long and with what clinical criteria for deciding that therapy should be increased, tapered, or terminated?

Second, the therapeutic maneuver must be clinically and biologically sensible. For example, the dose, route, and duration of drug therapy should be consistent with existing knowledge about pharmacokinetics and pharmacodynamics. Similarly, combinations of different treatment modalities should make clinical sense.

Third, the therapeutic maneuver has to be available. Readers must be capable of administering it properly and their patients must find it accessible, acceptable, and affordable.

Fourth, when reading the description of the maneuver in the published report, readers should note whether the authors avoided two specific biases in its application: *contamination* (in which control patients accidentally receive the experimental treatment; the result is a spurious reduction in the difference in clinical outcomes between the experimental and control groups) and *cointervention* (the performance of additional diagnostic or therapeutic acts on experimental but not control patients; the result is a spurious increase in the difference in clinical outcomes observed between experimental and control groups). Once again, it should be apparent that cointervention is prevented by "blinding" both study patients and their clinicians as to who is receiving which treatment [62].

WERE ALL PATIENTS WHO ENTERED THE STUDY ACCOUNTED FOR AT ITS CONCLUSION?

The canny reader will note how many patients entered the study (usually the numbers of experimental and control patients will be almost identical) and will tally them again at its conclusion to make certain that they correspond. For example, Panel A of Table 7-18 describes clinical outcomes in 151 patients in a randomized trial of surgical versus medical therapy for bilateral carotid stenosis [19].

Among 79 surgical and 72 medical patients "available for follow-up," a risk reduction for continued transient ischemic attack, stroke, or death of 27% (P = .02) was reported, a difference that is both clinically and statistically significant. However, closer reading of the report reveals that 167, not 151, patients entered this study and that 16 of them were "not available for follow-up" because they had suffered a stroke or died during their initial hospitalization, and thus were excluded from the foregoing analysis. Furthermore, 15 of these 16 patients originally had been allocated to surgery; 5 of them had died and 10 had suffered strokes during or shortly after surgery. Only 1 patient randomized to medical therapy suffered such a fate. The reintroduction of these 16 patients into the

Table 7-18. Surgical versus medical therapy in bilateral carotid stenosis

Panel A: Outcome among patients "available for follow-up"

	Rate of subsequent TIA, stroke, or death
Medical therapy	53/72 = 74%
Surgical therapy	43/79 = 54%

$$\text{Risk reduction} = \frac{74\% - 54\%}{74\%} = 27\% \quad P = 0.02$$

Panel B: Outcome among all patients randomized

	Rate of subsequent TIA, stroke, or death
Medical therapy	54/73 = 74%
Surgical therapy	58/94 = 62%

$$\text{Risk reduction} = \frac{74\% - 62\%}{74\%} = 16\% \quad P = 0.09$$

analysis results in panel A of Table 7-18; the risk reduction from surgery is now only 16% and it is no longer statistically significant (P = .09).

The authors of the preceding report were careful to include outcome information on all patients who entered their trial, making the construction and interpretation of both panels of Table 7-9 possible. However, what can the reader do when outcomes are not reported for missing subjects? One approach (admittedly conservative and therefore liable to lead to the false-negative conclusion that treatment doesn't work when it does) is to arbitrarily assign a bad outcome to all missing members of the group which fared better, and good outcomes to all missing members of the group that fared worse. If this maneuver fails to cancel the statistical or clinical significance of the results, the reader can accept the study's conclusions.

These, then, are guides that will help you apply the deductive approach to selecting specific treatments.

How do we convert all the foregoing into a set of practical tactics for the busy clinician? We would suggest the following:

1. Based on your goal of treatment, identify potential regimens that might accomplish the goal (pharmacologic, surgical, psychotherapeutic, nutritional, physical, etc).
2. Start with the one that strikes you as "best" (for whatever reason), seek out articles that report randomized control trials of its efficacy. Some of the tactics for tracking down these and other articles are discussed in Chapter 11, Tracking Down the Evidence to Solve Clinical Problems. Others include checking

your own library, asking colleagues and consultants,* and seeking help from hospital or reference librarians (for example, the College of Family Physicians of Canada operates a central library that provides its members with literature searches and reprints).

3. If you find a randomized control trial with the preceding tactics, you can then assess the evidence in the article, applying the guides listed in Table 7-2. If the trial demonstrated that the treatment did more good than harm, you are home free and can proceed to selecting a treatment target (so that you will know when to stop, change your dose, shift to another treatment), and get on with it. If, on the other hand, the trial found the treatment useless or harmful, you have done your patient (and yourself) an enormous service, although it means that you will have to start over with the next "best" treatment.
4. If you cannot find any randomized control trials of the "best" treatment (and this will often be the case) you face four alternatives: (a) you can consider, in sequence, the next "best" treatments and repeat steps 2 and 3; (b) you can try to determine the efficacy of the "best" treatment in your own, individual patient. The method for doing this lies midway between induction and deduction and occurred to us as an extrapolation of one of the algorithms for deciding whether a patient has had an adverse drug reaction that we'll describe in Chapter 9, and is called the "N-of-1" trial; we'll show you how to carry out N-of-1 trials in the next section of this chapter; (c) you can reassess the ultimate objective of treatment you established earlier. If, for example, you sought a cure and now find that the "curative" treatments in vogue are useless or harmful, you may wish to refocus your objective on limiting structural or functional deterioration and on relieving current symptoms; and (d) you can practice induction, abdication, or seduction and hope that the treatment you select helps, or at least does no harm.

Having gone through these steps the first time for a given treatment, you will have established a "baseline" of understanding about it. If you do keep your own small library, you can file your articles and notes away for future reference. This process will also alert you to look for newer, more definitive evidence as you scan your subscription journals and browse through others. In fact, you can plan and run your own continuing education program by executing this process for each of the treatments you most commonly prescribe.

N-of-1 Trials: Selecting the Optimal Treatment with a Randomized Trial in an Individual Patient

As we all know, you will not always be able to find a randomized trial to guide your selection of the treatment most likely to help a specific patient. The relevant trial may never have been done, or your patient may be unlike the patients in the

*Consultants worth their salt will know whether treatments used in their field have been tested in randomized control trials and ought to be able to cite the relevant articles; they often can help interpret the articles as well (as long as you can keep them to the sorts of questions posed in Table 7-2).

trials that have been done. Even if a relevant trial has been done on patients similar to yours, not all of them will have responded in the same way. In a positive trial, not all patients will have benefited from therapy; in a negative trial, there may have been a subgroup (similar to your patient but too small to be reliably detected) who actually benefited.

Under these circumstances, and often after thinking through the alternative strategies we described in the previous section, clinicians typically conduct the time-honored "trial of therapy." The patient is started on a treatment and followed, the subsequent clinical course being monitored to determine whether the patient improves (and the treatment usually is judged effective) or doesn't (and the treatment often is judged useless). Many natural phenomena can mislead us when we conduct such conventional therapeutic trials. First of all, lots of illnesses are self-limited and get better on their own. Similarly, back in Chapter 2 we learned that extreme laboratory values (and the same applies to many symptoms), if untreated and remeasured a bit later, often return to or toward the normal range. In either case, however, any treatment applied in the interim, even if quite useless, will appear efficacious.

Second, the "placebo effect," that extraordinarily powerful response that follows the giving and receiving of treatment [4] can lead to substantial relief of symptoms in the absence of any inherent efficacy of the specific treatment. Third, both our own and our patient's expectations (both optimistic and pessimistic) about the effects of the treatment (including the risk of side effects) can bias both of our later conclusions about whether the treatment worked. Finally, when the patient is grateful for our time and effort in trying to help, this gratitude (plus simple good manners) often is reflected in an exaggeration of the benefits of our latest prescription when we ask, "Did that medicine help you?"

Of course, it is to avoid these pitfalls that large-scale randomized trials of therapy are conducted with safeguards that permit the natural, untreated course of the disorder to be observed, that keep both patients and their clinicians "blind" to when active treatment is being administered, that apply objective, explicit criteria for clinical outcomes, and that employ formal statistical analysis to avoid drawing false-positive and false-negative conclusions about efficacy.

"Laterally thinking" from algorithms about adverse drug reactions (that pay considerable attention to the responses to de-challenge and re-challenge), and educated by earlier work in the behavioral sciences [43], a group of us led by Gordon Guyatt have applied these same strategies to randomized trials of therapy in individual patients [27, 33]. Initiated at the time that the first edition of this book was going to press, this approach has been sufficiently successful for us to want to show you how to do it [30].

This section gets a bit more "technical" than many other sections of the book, and even talks about how to *do* (what some would call) research yourself, rather than appraise research done by others. Nonetheless, given the power of the N-of-1 strategy to help you make individual treatment decisions we've decided to include it here.

There are many ways of conducting randomized clinical trials in individual

patients (or, as we and other clinicians have come to call them, "N-of-1 RCTs"); the method we have found most widely applicable can be summarized as follows:

1. A clinician and patient agree to test a therapy (hereafter called the "experimental therapy") for its ability to improve or control the symptoms, signs, or other manifestations (hereafter called the "treatment targets") of the patient's illness. Although in most of the discussion we will focus on comparison of experimental therapy to placebo, it can also be compared to alternative medication.
2. The patient then undergoes *pairs* of treatment *periods* organized so that one period of each pair applies the experimental therapy and the other period applies either an alternative treatment, or placebo (Figure 7-3). The order of these two periods within each pair is randomized by a coin toss or other method that ensures that each period has an equal chance of applying the experimental or alternative therapy. There are other ways of designing N-of-1 RCTs in which one does not use the paired design. These approaches have been used successfully by a clinical epidemiologist in Seattle, Eric Larson. In this discussion, however, we will focus almost exclusively on the paired design with which we have the most experience.
3. Whenever possible, both the clinician and the patient are "blind" to the treatment being given during any period.
4. The treatment *targets* are monitored (often through the use of a patient diary) to document the effect of the treatment currently being applied.
5. Pairs of treatment periods are replicated until the clinician and patient are convinced that the two treatments are clearly different or clearly no different.

The N-of-1 RCT can best executed by asking yourself a series of questions (listed as guidelines in Table 7-19), each of which must be answered before proceeding to the next.

IS AN N-OF-1 RANDOMIZED TRIAL INDICATED FOR THIS PATIENT?

Because N-of-1 RCTs are unnecessary for some ailments (such as self-limited illnesses) and unsuited for some treatments (such as definitive operations), it is important to determine, at the outset, whether an N-of-1 RCT is really indicated for the patient and treatment in question. We believe an N-of-1 RCT is appropriate if the answer to each of the following questions is "yes."

Is the Effectiveness of the Treatment Really in Doubt?

Not if one or several randomized clinical trials already have shown that the treatment is highly effective in virtually all patients (if you are unsure whether such trials have been undertaken, apply the strategies for searching the medical literature described in Chapter 11). However, if a substantial proportion of patients in positive trials were unresponsive to the treatment, an N-of-1 RCT may be appropriate.

Similarly, your patient already may have exhibited such a dramatic response

Table 7-19. Guidelines for N-of-1 randomized trials

1. Is an N-of-1 randomized trial indicated for this patient?

a. Is the effectiveness of the treatment really in doubt?
b. Will the treatment, if effective, be continued long-term?
c. Is the patient eager to collaborate in designing and carrying out an N-of-1 RCT?

2. Is an N-of-1 Randomized Trial Feasible in This Patient?

a. Does the treatment have a rapid onset?
b. Does the treatment cease to act soon after it is discontinued?
c. Is an optimal treatment duration feasible?
d. Can clinically relevant targets be measured?
e. Can sensible criteria for stopping the trial be established?
f. Should an unblinded run-in period be conducted?

3. Is an N-of-1 Trial Feasible in my Practice Setting?

a. Is there a pharmacist who can help me?
b. Are strategies for the interpretation of the trial data in place?

4. Is the study Ethical?

---

to the treatment that both of you are convinced that it works. N-of-1 trials really aren't necessary in such cases. They are best reserved for situations in which: (a) neither you nor your patient is confident that a current treatment is really beneficial; (b) you or your patient are uncertain whether a proposed treatment is likely to work in a particular patient; (c) your patient insists, despite your best efforts, on taking a treatment that you consider useless or potentially harmful; (d) your patient is experiencing symptoms which both of you suspect represent side effects from a current (and otherwise beneficial) treatment, but neither of you is certain; or (e) neither you nor your patient is confident of the optimal dose of a medication or replacement therapy.

If one of these situations applies, it would be appropriate to proceed to the next question.

Will the Treatment, If Effective, Be Continued Long Term?

If the underlying condition is self-limited or if treatment will only be continued over the short term, the associated N-of-1 RCT will be of limited usefulness.* We'd suggest you stick to chronic conditions in which maintenance therapy is likely to be continued over long periods of time. If the latter applies, carry on.

Is the Patient* Eager *to Collaborate in Designing and Carrying Out an N-of-1 RCT?

The N-of-1 RCT is, by its very nature, a cooperative venture requiring substantial effort from both clinician and patient. Accordingly, it is only indicated when

*Remember that an N-of-1 RCT only tells you the best treatment for this particular patient, not the best therapy for all such patients.

your patient can fully understand the nature of the experiment and is enthusiastic about participating.

IS AN N-OF-1 RANDOMIZED TRIAL FEASIBLE IN THIS PATIENT?

Even with affirmative answers to all the foregoing questions, the nature of the illness or treatment may not lend themselves to the N-of-1 trial. As before, we shall approach the issue of feasibility with a series of questions; as previously, the answer to each must be "yes."

Does the Treatment Effect Have a Rapid Onset?

N-of-1 RCTs are much easier to perform when the treatment, if effective, displays its effectiveness within hours. Although it is possible to do N-of-1 RCTs of drugs with longer latency (such as gold or penicillamine in rheumatoid arthritis, or tricyclic antidepressants for depression) the corresponding requirement for very long treatment periods may make the trial prohibitively long.

Does the Treatment Cease to Act Soon After It Is Discontinued?

Treatments whose effects abruptly cease when they are withdrawn are the most suitable for N-of-1 RCTs. When treatments continue to act long after they are stopped, you have to wait for a long time (that is, you need a prolonged "washout period") before you can start the next treatment. If this washout period is more than a few days, the feasibility of your trial is compromised.

Similarly, treatments which have the potential to "cure" the underlying condition, or at least lead to a permanent change in the treatment target, are not suitable for N-of-1 RCTs. This is true, for example, for most behavioral, occupational, and physiotherapy.

Is an Optimal Treatment Duration Feasible?

If active therapy takes a few days to reach full effect, and a few days to cease acting once stopped, treatment periods of sufficient duration to avoid distortion from these delayed peak effects and washout periods are required. For example, our N-of-1 RCTs of theophylline in asthma use treatment periods of at least 10 days—3 days to allow the drug to equilibrate or wash out, and 7 days thereafter to monitor the patient's response to treatment. So although short treatment periods make N-of-1 RCTs more feasible, they may have to be long to be valid.

Second, when an N-of-1 RCT is testing a treatment's ability to prevent or blunt attacks or exacerbations of disease (such as migraines or seizures), each treatment period must be long enough to include an attack or exacerbation, if one is going to occur. We've extrapolated a rough rule of thumb, called the "inverse rule of 3" [64], to this situation: if an event occurs, on average, once every x days, we need to observe $3x$ days to be 95% confident of observing at least one event. Applying this rule in a patient with familial Mediterranean fever with attacks, on average, once every 2 weeks, called for treatment periods 6 weeks long. You and your patient will need to decide whether their attacks or exacerbations are sufficiently frequent to make their N-of-1 RCT feasible.

Finally, you may not want your patient to take responsibility for crossing over from one treatment period to the next without your supervision, or you may need to examine your patient at the end of each period. Both your own and your patient's schedules also will dictate the length of each treatment period.

Can Clinically Relevant Treatment Target(s) Be Measured?

You and your patient need to define exactly what you will use as clinical outcomes (treatment targets) to determine the efficacy of the treatment you are studying in your N-of-1 RCT. These treatment targets usually go beyond a physical sign (the rigidity and tremor of parkinsonism, the jugular venous distension, S3, and the crackles of congestive heart failure), a laboratory test (blood sugar, uric acid, erythrocyte sedimentation rate, serum creatinine), or a measure of performance (of peak flow, or on a 6-minute walk test), because each of these is only an indirect measure of your patient's quality of life and how that patient is feeling.

In most situations both of you will prefer to measure symptoms, feelings of well-being, or quality of life directly. Fortunately, the principles of quality-of-life measurement that we described in the previous section (p. 209) can be applied to N-of-1 RCTs without too much trouble. They begin with asking your patient to identify the most troubling symptoms or problems being experienced from this illness, and then deciding which of these symptoms or problems are likely to be responsive to the experimental treatment. A minimum of three, and maximum of seven, symptoms are likely to be most efficient and helpful. Second, you convert this responsive subset of symptoms or problems into a self-administered questionnaire or diary for the patient. For example, one of our patients with chronic airflow limitation said his worst symptoms were the shortness of breath he experienced while walking up stairs, bending, or vacuuming, and these became the treatment targets for his N-of-1 RCT (accompanied by pulmonary function tests, to see whether they reflected changes in the target symptoms). Another patient with fibrositis (to whom we shall return later) identified fatigue, aches and pains, morning stiffness, and trouble sleeping as the treatment targets for her N-of-1 RCT.

The resulting symptom questionnaire can take a number of formats. A daily diary is best for some patients and symptoms; for others a weekly summary may be better. We think that the best way to construct symptom questionnaires is to use graded descriptions, from none to severe, for each symptom. This is illustrated in Figure 7-2, a patient questionnaire for an N-of-1 RCT of diphenylhydantoin which had appeared, in an open trial, to be ameliorating the patient's symptoms of Meniere's disease (this N-of-1 RCT, by the way, revealed that active drug administration bore no relation to symptoms, and convinced both the patient and the clinician, Dr. John Premi, that the drug was not effective). Constructing simple symptom questionnaires like this is not difficult, and allows you and your patient to collaborate in identifying and quantifying those symptoms upon which your conclusions from your N-of-1 RCT often will depend.

Whatever formats you choose for measuring treatment targets, our experience suggests that you should ask your patient to rate each of them at least twice during each treatment period. Record-keeping can be made easier by combining identifying information, dates, treatments, and ratings onto a one-page form,

Figure 7-2. A Data Collection Form for an N-of-1 RCT

Pair 1, Period 2

PHYSICIAN: John Premi

PATIENT: ______________________________

DIAGNOSIS: MENIERE'S

TRIAL MEDICATION: Dilantin Dose: 100 mg tid

DURATION OF STUDY PERIODS: Three weeks

OUTCOMES: Symptom rating of last ten days of each study period:

1. How many episodes or attacks have you had in the last 10 days? ______

2. How long has each attack lasted (1) ______ (2) ______
(3) ______ (4) ______ (5) ______ (6) ______
(7) ______ (8) ______

3. Overall, on average, how severe have the attacks been during the last 10 days? Please indicate how severe the attacks have been by circling one of the following numbers. (Don't answer if there have been no attacks at all.)

a. As severe as they have ever been
b. Very severe, but not as bad as at their worst
c. Severe
d. Moderate intensity
e. Mild to moderate
f. Mild
g. Barely noticeable

4. How limited have you been in your day-to-day life, and in your activities, by the attacks during the last 10 days? Please indicate how limited you have been by circling one of the following numbers.

a. Extremely limited, prevented from doing many or most activities
b. Very limited, prevented from doing many activities
c. Quite limited, prevented from doing some activities
d. Moderately limited
e. Somewhat limited in activities, but no activity completely stopped
f. Mildly limited
g. Not at all limited

and more detailed guides for constructing questionnaires for N-of-1 RCTs are available [66, 74].

A final point: Side effects should also receive attention, and items like nausea, gastrointestinal disturbances, dizziness, or other common side effects can appear along with the treatment targets on the questionnaire. The measurement of side effects becomes particularly important when they can lead to unblinding. Finally, in N-of-1 RCTs designed to determine if medication side effects are responsible for a patient's symptoms (for example, whether a patient's fatigue is caused by an antihypertensive agent he is taking), the side effects become the primary treatment targets.

Can Sensible Criteria for Stopping the Trial Be Established?

The advantage of not specifying the required number of pairs of treatment periods in advance is that you and your patient can stop anytime you both are convinced that the treatment periods within each pair are exhibiting important differences in the symptoms, and the like, that comprise the treatment targets. It is then time to stop, break the code, and decide whether the experimental treatment ought to be stopped or continued indefinitely. Thus, if there is an overwhelming difference in the treatment target between the two periods of the first pair, both you and your patient may want to stop immediately. On the other hand, if there are less dramatic differences between the two periods of each pair, you and your patient may need three, four, or even five or more pairs before confidently concluding that real differences exist.

If, on the other hand, you wish to conduct a formal statistical analysis of data from your N-of-1 RCT, this analysis will be considerably strengthened if you specify the number of pairs in advance (we will discuss this a bit later in the chapter). Whether or not you specify the number of treatment periods in advance, it is advisable to conduct at least two pairs of treatment periods before breaking the code. This is because too many conclusions drawn after a single pair will be either false-positive judgments (that the treatment is effective when it isn't) or false-negative judgments (that the treatment is not effective when it is). On our N-of-1 RCT Service, we urge clinicians and patients to resist temptation and refrain from breaking the code until they are quite certain they are ready to terminate the study.

Should an Unblinded Run-in Period Be Conducted?

A preliminary run-in period on active therapy, during which both you and your patient know that active therapy is being received, could save you both a lot of time. After all, if there is no hint of response during such an open trial, or if intolerable side effects occur, an N-of-1 RCT would have been fruitless or impossible. For example, we once prepared a full-blown, double-blind N-of-1 RCT of methylphenidate for a child with hyperactivity, only to witness a dramatic increase in agitation over the first 2 days of the first study period (during which the child was receiving the active drug), forcing an abrupt termination of the study and the forfeit of our planning and preparation. A final use of an open run-in period is to determine the optimal dose of the active medication. To give you an idea of how these criteria may be applied, Table 7-20 provides a list of con-

Table 7-20. Conditions and treatments in which N-of-1 RCTs are, and are not, useful

Condition	Target	Treatment
	N-of-1 RCT likely to be useful	
Asthma	Many symptoms	Beta agonists Theophylline
Arthritis	Pain	Anti-inflammatory agents
Movement disorders (e.g., parkinsonism)	Stiffness Mobility	Central dopaminergic drugs
Angina pectoris	Chest pain Mobility	Beta blockers, calcium antagonists, nitrates
	N-of-1 RCT not likely to be useful	
Angina pectoris	Myocardial infarction, death	Beta blockers, calcium antagonists, nitrates
Surgical conditions (unless simple and repetitive)	Symptoms	Operation
Depression	Mood	Amitriptyline, ECT
Inflammatory bowel disease	Exacerbations	Steroids or other anti-inflammatory agents

ditions and treatments which are suitable, and another list which are unlikely to be suitable, for N-of-1 RCTs.

IS AN N-OF-1 RANDOMIZED TRIAL FEASIBLE IN MY PRACTICE SETTING?

Clinicians may answer "yes" to all the preceding questions and still be unsure about whether or how to proceed. The following questions will address the mechanisms and safeguards that will ensure the feasibility of an N-of-1 RCT in your practice.

Is There a Pharmacist Who Can Help Me?

Conducting an N-of-1 RCT that incorporates all the aforementioned safeguards against bias and misinterpretation requires collaboration between you and your pharmacist or pharmacy service. To promote blindness, the preparation of placebos that are as close as possible (or feasible) to the active medication in appearance, taste, and texture is the goal. Rarely, pharmaceutical firms can supply such placebos. More often, however, you will want to call on your local pharmacist's ingenuity to repackage the active medication and placebo in identical forms. For example, many medications can be repackaged (after crushing if necessary) in opaque capsules. Identical opaque placebo capsules can be filled with lactose. This takes time, but usually is not technically difficult (our average pharmacy cost, over and above buying the active drug, for preparing medications for our N-of-1 studies in 1989 has been $125). Perhaps at a future date N-of-1 RCTs will become part of conventional clinical practice, and these additional costs will be picked up by drug-benefit plans.

Our pharmacy colleagues have also accepted responsibility for preparing the randomization schedule (which requires nothing more than a coin toss for each pair of treatment periods). Medication containers for each period of each pair are labeled and filled with the appropriate active medication or placebo and given to us, and the pharmacist keeps the code in case it needs to be broken in an emergency. This collaboration allows both clinicians and patients to remain blind.

Are Strategies for the Interpretation of the Trial Data in Place?

Once you and your patient have carefully gathered data on the treatment targets in your N-of-1 RCT, how should you analyze and interpret them? Let's examine the options in an actual N-of-1 RCT of ipratropium bromide (4 puffs of 20 mcg of the active drug or an identically presented placebo qid) we conducted in collaboration with a patient with chronic airflow limitation.

Our patient wanted relief from shortness of breath, both overall and when he walked upstairs, played his vibraphone, and dried the dishes. With help from our N-of-1 RCT Service, a diary was constructed in which he could record, on a daily basis, the severity of his breathlessness during these activities of daily living, using a 7-point scale in which a higher number meant better function (i.e., 1 = "extremely short of breath" and 7 = "not at all short of breath"). He successfully completed four successive pairs of treatment periods (as usual, the order of ipratropium and placebo puffers was randomized within each pair), recording his symptoms during the last 5 days of each 7-day treatment period. The unblinded mean scores from his diary are shown in Figure 7-3 and Table 7-21. How should we analyze them to decide whether his active puffer is helping him and ought, therefore, to be continued?

One approach is to simply "eyeball" the results shown in Figure 7-3, a method that has a long and distinguished record in the psychology literature on single subject designs and is strongly advocated by some experts in this field [3, 41, 43]. What do you notice when you eyeball Figure 7-3? When we eyeball it, we notice three things: first, responses to a given treatment are pretty stable within each treatment period (the lines are pretty flat for each treatment period); second, with the exception of the active treatment period in the third pair, our patient was virtually always doing better (recording improved symptoms) on active than placebo puffers; third, in every pair but the third one, active puffers were accompanied by about the same degree of symptomatic improvement (the gap between active and placebo puffers is pretty constant). It's important to note here that this patient (and the other patients who have used this 7-point scale

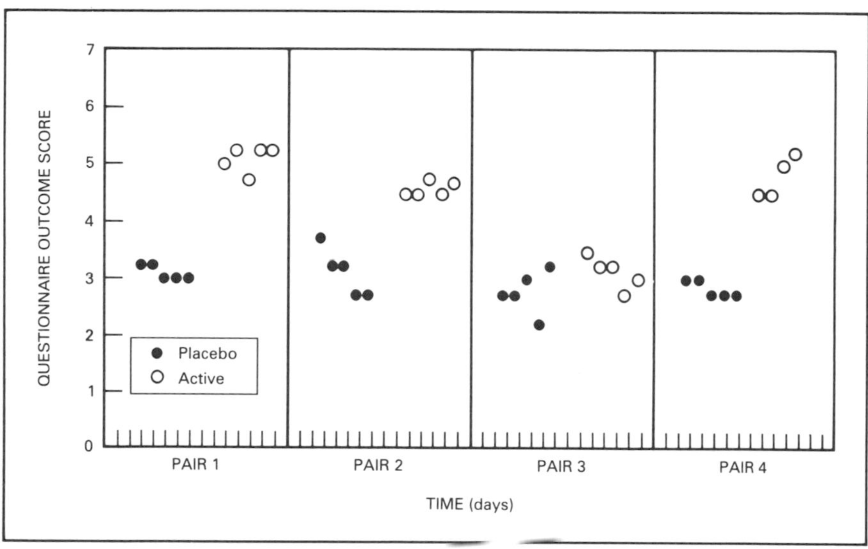

Figure 7-3. Results of an N-of-1 RCT of ipratropium bromide in a man with chronic airways limitation.

method to record their symptoms) have concluded that average symptomatic differences of one-half point or more are "symptomatically significant" and should generate long-term treatment plans.

Although eyeballing is simple and appealing, even experts in "visual analysis" often disagree about the consistency and interpretation of such displays [11]. Moreover, eyeballing doesn't tell us how likely we would be to observe differences of this sort by chance alone. For this reason, we usually carry out some sort of statistical analysis of our N-of-1 RCTs, both to avoid the false-positive conclusion that the active and placebo treatments are producing different degrees of symptomotology when, in fact, they aren't, and also to avoid the false-negative conclusion that they are having similar effects when, in fact, one of them is superior. The simplest statistical test assumes that the apparently superior treatment is not efficacious and calculates the probability that our patient would have done better on it during each treatment pair by chance alone. This is exactly similar to calculating the probability that "heads" would repeatedly appear when tossing a coin. Thus, the probability of our patient doing better on his active puffer during all four pairs of treatments by chance alone is $1/2 \times 1/2 \times 1/2 \times 1/2 = 1/16 = .0625$, which is remarkably close to the "conventional" level of statistical significance of .05 and, we think, pretty convincing evidence that our patient benefits from active puffers. This test of statistical significance (which goes by the name "sign test" [9]), is easy to carry out and doesn't require consultation with a statistician. Accordingly, if it shows us that our results are unlikely to be due to chance, we can stop testing here.

But what if the sign test produces a less striking result? Although easy to

Table 7-21. Results of an N-of-1 RCT of ipratropium bromide in a man with chronic airways limitation

Pair	Treatment	Daily mean scores					Treatment mean scores
		Day 3	Day 4	Day 5	Day 6	Day 7	
1	Active	5.00	5.25	4.75	5.25	5.25	5.10
	Placebo	3.25	3.25	3.00	3.00	3.00	3.10
						Difference (d_i)	+2.00
2	Active	4.50	4.50	4.75	4.50	4.70	4.59
	Placebo	3.75	3.25	3.25	2.75	2.75	3.15
						Difference (d_i)	+1.44
3	Active	2.50	3.25	3.25	2.75	3.00	3.15
	Placebo	2.75	2.75	3.00	2.25	3.25	2.80
						Difference (d_i)	+0.35
4	Active	4.50	4.50	5.00	5.25	–	4.81
	Placebo	3.00	3.00	2.75	2.75	2.75	2.85
						Difference (d_i)	+1.96
All pairs	Mean active						4.413
	Mean placebo						2.975
						Mean difference (d)	+1.438

Critical values of t (above which P < 0.05)		
Treatment pairs	df	Critical t-value
2	1	6.31
3	2	2.92
4	3	2.35
5	4	2.13

$$t_{(\text{pair}-1\ \text{df})} = \sqrt{\frac{\Sigma(d_i - d)^2}{\text{pairs} - 1}}$$

$$= \sqrt{\frac{(2.00 - 1.438)^2 + (1.44 - 1.438)^2 + (0.35 - 1.438)^2 + (1.96 - 1.438)^2}{3}}$$

$= 3.74$ and $P < 0.05$ (more precisely, $P = 0.01$)

execute, it has very low power, and reliance on it as the only test will lead you to draw many false-negative conclusions that no treatment differences exist when, in fact, they do. In less clear-cut N-of-1 RCTs you ought to consider using (or asking a friendly statistician to use) a second, more powerful statistical strategy that makes use of all the degrees of symptom severity you built into your questionnaire. This statistical test, the Student's paired* t-test, considers not only the direction, but also the strength of the treatment effect in each pair of treatment periods. At the bottom of Table 7-21 we have carried out a paired t-test on our patient's diary. As you can see, this calculation begins by calculating the difference (d_i) between the average symptom scores on active and placebo treatment during each pair of treatment periods. Then the d_is are averaged to generate an overall mean difference (d-bar). Next, we add together the squared differences between the overall mean difference (d-bar), divide this sum by the number of pairs of treatment periods − 1, and take the square root of the dividend. We then determine whether the resulting t statistic is greater than the "critical t-value" for the relevant "degrees of freedom" (df, which corresponds to the number of pairs of treatment periods − 1). To make this task a bit easier for you, we have included critical values of t at the bottom of Table 7-21. In our example, we had four pairs of treatment periods, or three degrees of freedom, and our calculated t-value of 3.74 is considerably greater than the corresponding critical value of 2.92. Accordingly, we can conclude that the risk of drawing the false-negative conclusion that our patient fared no better on active puffers than on placebo puffers is considerably less than .05 (indeed, when we calculated it out further, P was .01). In analyzing your own trials, you can sweat this calculation out longhand, use one of the increasingly available packages for hand calculators and personal computers, or seek help from someone with more statistical expertise.

Finally, if you have access to a statistician who prefers "Bayesian" approaches over the t-test,† you can build in your and your patient's preconceived notions of the likelihood that active treatment is better and, if it is, reach a definitive answer much sooner than you would using the "sign test" approach.

*It's called a "paired" t-test because the treatment and control observations come from the same patient(s). If we were comparing treatment observations from one group of patients with control observations from a second group of patients, we would do an "unpaired" t-test and employ a different formula for the calculations.

†A disadvantage of the t-test in the eyes of many statisticians is that it makes additional assumptions about the data which may not be valid. The assumption of greatest concern is that observations are independent of one another; that is, a patient is equally likely to feel good or bad on a particular day irrespective of whether he or she felt good or bad the day before. The term used to describe data that are not independent is autocorrelation, and although some autocorrelation is likely to exist in many N-of-1 RCTs, its impact can be reduced if you use the average of all measurements in a given period (rather than the individual measurements) in the statistical analysis. Furthermore, the paired design of the N-of-1 RCT which we use further reduces the impact of any autocorrelation which exists. We have empirically examined the results of 17 of our N-of-1 RCTs and found no evidence of clinically important autocorrelation, so we are satisfied that the paired t-test approach is unbiased when applied in this way.

IS THE STUDY ETHICAL?

That ethical issues are involved is, to us, clear. Whether anyone beyond you and your patient should discuss their ethics is less clear, and depends on whether the conduct of an N-of-1 RCT is seen as a clinical act, designed to improve the quality of your care for an individual patient, or a research undertaking with wider implications.* If it is the former, your patient provides informed consent by participating in its design and, in collaboration with you, deciding when to start and end it. We believe that the N-of-1 RCT can and should be part of routine clinical practice. But, like any medical innovations, it deserves close scrutiny and study before being accepted by clinicians, and this scrutiny should consider ethical as well as other issues.

If the answers to all the foregoing questions are "yes," you and your patient are ready to proceed on the venture. You may still be wondering how useful the adventure will be, and how likely it will be that, having spent the time and effort, your patient will be better off.

Initial Experiences With N-of-1 RCTs

To give you some idea of what you might expect if you start to do N-of-1 RCTs yourself, let us tell you about the first 73 we considered carrying out [33]; they are summarized in Table 7-22. Three of them never got off the drawing board (one patient died, another got cold feet, and a third developed a concurrent illness that negated the purpose for the trial). Of the 70 we launched, 13 were never completed (usually because of noncompliance or intercurrent comorbidity). The remaining 57 either went on to complete three pairs of treatment periods or were stopped early when either the patient, the clinician, or both became convinced that one of the treatments was superior to the other. Fifty of these 57 produced definite clinical or statistical answers, and when management decisions both before and after the N-of-1 RCTs were recorded, they changed in 39% (in 29% the pretrial drug was stopped altogether; in 8% the pretrial drug, which otherwise would have been stopped, was continued indefinitely; in 2% it was decided to do another N-of-1 RCT!). The agreement between statistical analyses and clinical certainty about the efficacy of therapy was good, at 95%, and usually confirmed that the treatment was beneficial.

We have not kept systematic track of initial inquiries that never resulted in actual N-of-1 RCTs. On several occasions, an open trial resulted in such dramatic benefits or side effects that the idea of a formal trial was abandoned. On others, patients with multiple, unstable medical problems made the reliable ascertainment of the effect of a single medication impossible. Finally, an occasional patient appeared unable to keep a valid symptom diary.

*The first time our own Research Ethics Committee (which, we're delighted to report, doesn't confuse ethics with law) reviewed our proposal for performing N-of-1 RCTs, they decided that our design sought to improve the quality of care provided individual patients and that the Clinical Ethics Committee, not the Research Ethics Committee, should pass judgment on our plans. It was only when we set up a pilot N-of-1 RCT Service that our Research Ethics Committee began its periodic review of our progress.

Table 7-22. Experience with 73 N-of-1 RCTs

Planned N-of-1 RCTs—73 3 N-of-1 RCTs never started (1 death, 1 concurrent illness, 1 consent withdrawn)
N-of-1 RCTs Begun—70 13 N-of-1 RCTs not completed (7 patient's noncompliance, 5 concurrent illness, 1 physician noncompliance)
Completed N-of-1 RCTs—57 9 N-of-1 RCTs with 3 pairs completed that did not provide a definite clinical answer; 2 of them provided a definite statistical answer
Definite N-of-1 RCTs—50 Clinically definite—48 Statistically definite—19

These results indicate that you are likely to find N-of-1 RCTs appropriate and feasible in many of your patients, and that you will find that your management changes as a result of the trial in an appreciable proportion. N-of-1 RCTs certainly require additional time and energy from both us and our patients, and present operational and intellectual challenges to both of us. They can be both frustrating and enormous fun. Perhaps most important is the fact that over a quarter of the time they result in major changes in long-term therapy, of real benefit to the quality of the lives of our patients, that simply never would have been achieved had they not been conducted.

Decision Analysis Revisited

Finally, some clinical decisions are too complex to permit simple treatment decisions or even N-of-1 trials. They occur when the choice between two management alternatives looks like a toss-up or, especially, when treatments pose substantial risks as well as benefits. It has been suggested that such decisions can be made much more rational and therefore more helpful to patients by formalizing them through a systematic approach called *decision analysis*.

In this strategy, which can be used to make both diagnostic decisions (as we showed you back in Chapter 4) and treatment decisions, all relevant courses of action and their consequences are mapped out and evaluated in order to identify (if it exists) the single course of action that best serves the patient [73]. Once again, we stress that we don't consider ourselves experts at this, and provide the following simply as an example of what we find ourselves doing about once in every 80 admissions to our busy in-patient medical service.

One of us employed decision analysis when consulted by a family practice team about a patient who they were considering for revision of an artificial hip. The facts were these:

1. A 63-year-old housewife with 6 grown children and a 10-year history of stable angina pectoris had undergone total hip replacement 8 years ago for primary osteoarthritis. Although she had a post-op pulmonary embolus, the orthopedic result was excellent and she was pain-free and fully mobile until one year ago.
2. During the last 12 months she had experienced increasing pain in her hip on weight bearing, and at the time of consultation she was largely confined to a wheelchair, although she could walk with a cane or crutches for short distances and around her house.
3. Eight months ago she suffered an uncomplicated subendocardial anterior myocardial infarction. Although her recovery was uncomplicated, her long-standing stable angina pectoris persisted and frequently limited her ability to get about on crutches.
4. Her orthopedic surgeon reviewed her case, concluded that she probably had an aseptic loosening of her femoral component, and spelled out the risks and benefits of reoperation as follows:
   a. If only the acetabular component required replacement (and the chances of this were estimated to be only 25%), the probability of a good result (permitting full ambulation again) was 80%; however, that left a probability of a poor result (confined to her wheelchair) of 20%. Moreover, the foregoing good and poor results applied only to survivors of the surgery, and this patient's cardiovascular disease suggested a risk of dying in the perioperative period of up to 5%.
   b. If, as was more likely (its chances were judged to be 65%), the femoral component required replacement, the probability of a good result was judged to be lower, at 60%, with a 40% chance of a poor result. Once again, the foregoing applied only to survivors, and the increased duration and extent of this more difficult procedure was judged to double her risk of perioperative death to 10%.
   c. If both components required replacement (the probability that this would be required was 10%), the chances of a good result fell slightly below half to 45%, and the probability that the patient would wind up in a wheelchair was 55%, even if she survived surgery. Her risk of perioperative death was judged to be very high for this combined procedure, at 15%.
   d. Finally, if no surgery were performed, she either would remain the same as she was now (the chances of this were judged to be 20%) or would become worse and be permanently confined to her wheelchair (the chances of this outcome were judged to be 80%).

A hot debate ensued within the primary care team, with some members advocating surgery and others, concerned about the risks of perioperative death, urging against it. And although they wanted to involve the patient in this decision, they feared that they would sway the patient's conclusion by the fashion in which they presented the facts of the situation to her.

That this debate was occurring despite agreement within the team about the risks and benefits of surgery suggested to us that a formal decision analysis might yield two useful results. First, it might provide an objective resolution to the debate. Second, it would permit the team to involve the patient in the discussion without unfairly swaying her opinion. The team agreed with our proposal and we proceeded.

This or any other formal decision analysis begins by identifying all the alternative actions, treatments, clinical changes, and outcomes that could occur for the patient in question. On the basis of this, a decision tree that displays these elements in their proper time sequence is constructed. This is shown for our patient in Figure 7-4.

Points where the tree branches ("nodes") are square ("choice nodes") when they are under the control of the clinician, and round ("chance nodes") when they are not. We can now attach the probabilities for the various operative risks and benefits to this decision tree, and the result is shown in Figure 7-5.

Note that the probabilities of good and poor results are multiplied by the probabilities of surviving surgery at chance nodes A_2, A_3, and A_4, and that the sum of all probabilities at any chance node always equals 1.0 (at chance node A_2, for example, $[.8 \times .95] + [.2 \times .95] + [.05] = .76 + .19 + .05 = 1.0$).

The next step in decision analysis forces us to assign numbers to the quality of life represented by each of the outcomes in the tree. As we emphasized in Chapter 4, clinicians and patients make these judgments all the time, and they

Figure 7-4. Decision tree for a specific patient with a loose arthroplasty and coronary heart disease.

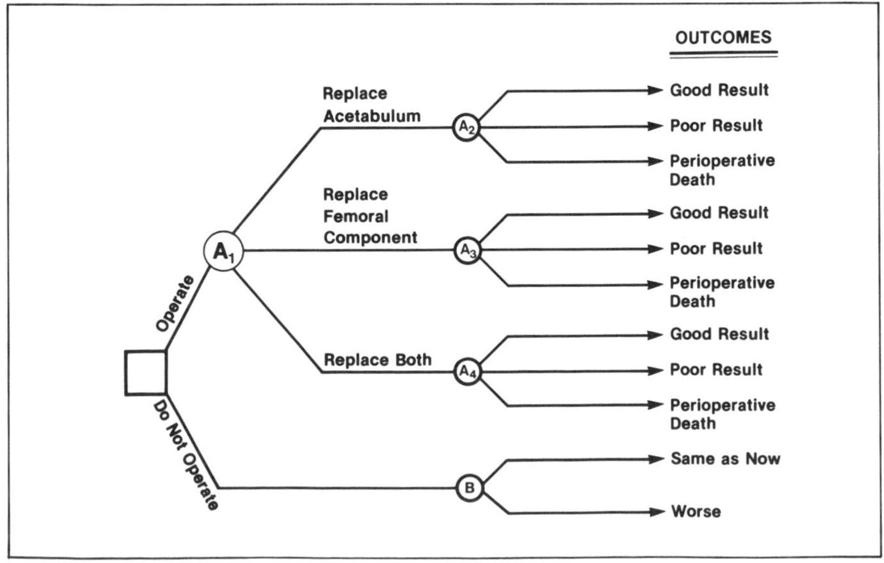

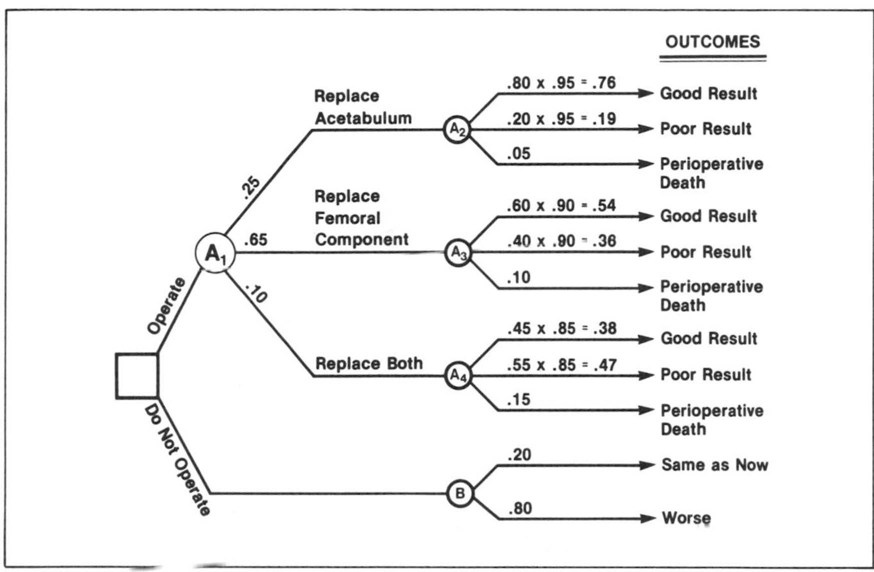

Figure 7-5. The decision tree with probabilities in place.

affect most of our clinical decisions, often in a crucial way. All that decision analysis does is force us to assign numbers (called "utilities") to these judgments.

In this case, this assignment of utilities was carried out both by the patient and by the members of the team. Although there are some complex methods for determining these utility values, we used the very simple one of drawing a thermometer for the patient, and asking her, "If the top of the thermometer represents having a successful operation and walking on your own again, and if the bottom of the thermometer represents being dead, where would you mark your present situation, being restricted to crutches, and being confined to a wheelchair?" We then assigned a "quality of life" of 1.0 to the top of the thermometer for successful surgery that would permit her to walk on her own again ("good result") and 0.0 to being dead, and simply measured the distances to the marks she had placed to correspond with the other outcomes: "same as now," restricted to crutches ("poor result"), and confined to a wheelchair ("worse"). The results, although they varied somewhat (the next day, she moved all the outcomes upwards), always maintained the same ranking of: Good Result, Same as Now, Worse, Poor Result, and Death. So did the utilities assigned by the other members of the primary care team looking after her. We have inserted typical ones into the tree, and they are shown in Figure 7-6.

We then worked our way back through the decision tree by "folding it back" from right to left. By multiplying the utilities by the probabilities of their occurrence, and summing them for each chance node, we could assign utilities to the chance nodes A_2, A_3, A_1, and B. For example, the utility for chance node A_2 was the utility of living with a good result (1.00) times the probability of both

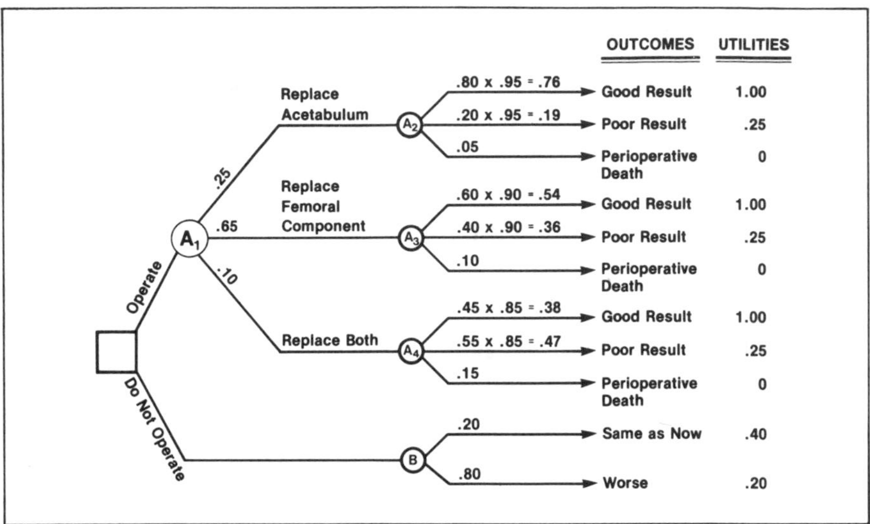

Figure 7-6. The decision tree completed.

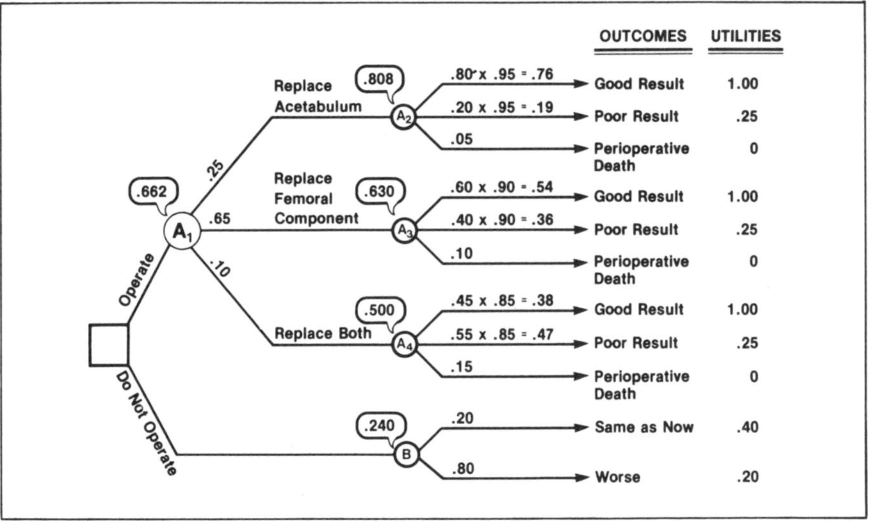

Figure 7-7. Folding back a decision tree.

surviving acetabular replacement and having a good result (.76), plus the utility of living with a poor result (.25) times the probability of both surviving and having a poor result (.19), plus the utility of dying at or shortly after surgery (0) times the probability of dying from surgery (.05). This sum was .808 and we inserted this utility in the balloon over chance node A_2 in Figure 7-7.

In similar fashion, we calculated the utility for the following: Chance node A_3

$$(1 \times .54) + (.25 \times .36) + (0 \times .1) = .54 + .09 + 0 = .630$$

Chance node A_4

$$(1 \times .38) + (.25 \times .47) + (0 \times .15) = .38 + .12 + 0 = .500$$

Chance node B

$$(.40 \times .2) + (.20 \times .8) = .080 + .160 = .240$$

It was apparent that any operation, regardless of whether it was an easy or difficult procedure, was preferable to no operation, because the utilities for nodes A_2 (.808), A_3 (.630), and A_4 (.500) all exceeded the utility for node B (.240). We confirmed this by folding the operative branch back once more by summing the products of the utilities of nodes A_2, A_3, and A_4 times their respective probabilities:

$$(.808 \times .25) + (.630 \times .65) + (.500 \times .10) = .202 + .410 + .050 = .662$$

The result (.662) was the utility or quality of life our patient would, on average, achieve by going to surgery, and it was substantially greater than the quality of life she would, on average, achieve by refusing surgery (.240). Accordingly, unless our patient was extremely "risk averse" to the low but real risk of early death from surgery [50, 51], the preferred course of action was to operate.

As the primary care team worked through this decision analysis, some of them objected to some of the utilities and probabilities that were being used. Moreover, after the patient had pondered the alternatives and discussed them with her family, she revised her utilities upwards for both her current and possible future status. Because the method allows us to insert clinically sensible changes in any of these entries, we recalculated the "folding back" step with the alternative utilities and probabilities they proposed. None of the alternative proposals reversed the original preference for surgery, and most made the decision to operate even stronger, not weaker, since they included claims that the surgical mortality estimates were too high, that the probability of an "easy" acetabular replacement was .5 rather than .25, and that we ought to revise chance node B to include the risk (albeit low) of dying without surgery. As a result, the debate ceased and the team became unanimous (with the patient!) that an operation should be undertaken. Thus, the strategy of decision analysis was able to simplify a complex treatment decision and set the stage for the final decision about therapy.*

Now that you have selected the specific treatment that will be initiated to achieve one or more specific objectives of therapy, all that remains is the identification of treatment targets.

*Surgery went well. Only the acetabulum needed replacement and the result was excellent.

Identifying Treatment Targets

When writing about the importance of precise educational objectives, Robert Mager introduced a seahorse (whom we'll meet in Chapter 14) and stated, "If you are not sure where you are going, you're liable to end up someplace else" [49]. So, too, with treatment regimens. Unless you state your treatment target at the outset, you will not know when to stop, change your dose, add a second treatment, and so forth.

The identification of treatment targets is central to the performance of N-of-1 trials, as we showed you earlier. It's also central to any other therapeutic endeavor, as we hope to convince you here.

Some treatment targets are easy to set and monitor, such as blood pressure, sTSH levels, and the disappearance of specific symptoms. Others may be much more difficult, such as the size and spread of deep tumors, the function of families, and the occurrence of "soft" neurologic signs. The key is to link them to both the goals of treatment and to the specific therapy, and then to make them as easily observable as possible.

For example, in treating symptomless essential hypertension the treatment goals are to limit structural and functional deterioration and to prevent later symptoms. Although we could define targets such as "preventing left ventricular hypertrophy by voltage criteria," or "maintaining the creatinine clearance above 90 ml per minute," these targets are too expensive and cumbersome to monitor at every visit. Rather, we take advantage of the link (established in the randomized control trials that demonstrated the efficacy of antihypertensive drugs) between blood-pressure lowering and the limitation of structural and functional deterioration and the prevention of later complications. As a result of this additional bonus from the randomized trials, we can "substitute" blood pressure reduction for the more complex measures. Thus, we can use simple measurements of blood pressure for the week-to-week monitoring and adjustment of treatments, and order cardiograms and clearances at much longer intervals.

In addition to their obvious value when clinical responsibility is shared, precisely specified treatment targets can help us avoid undermedication, a common problem when the goal of treatment is to allow the terminally ill to die with comfort and dignity [1]. Reminded by a prominent entry in the patient's chart that our treatment target is the relief of pain (from, say, metastatic cancer), we are more likely to acknowledge the rarity of opiate-induced respiratory depression, the irrelevance of concerns about long-term addiction, the absurdity of routine blood tests and vital signs (as opposed to the vital role of hugging the patient), and the thoughtlessness of making the patient ask the nurse (rather than the reverse) whether more pain killers should be given.

Finally, involving the patient in setting and monitoring progress toward the treatment objective can have a very favorable effect on compliance with the treatment regimen. Of course, if patients will not take their medicine, all of your efforts in diagnosis, prognosis, setting objectives of treatment, selecting the specific therapy, and identifying treatment targets go down the tube. The next chapter is designed to help you avoid this common failure.

References

1. Angel, M. The quality of mercy. *N. Engl. J. Med.* 306: 55, 1982.
2. Asher, W. L., and Harper, H. W. Effect of human chorionic gonadotropin on weight loss, hunger, and feeling of well-being. *Am. J. Clin. Nutr.* 26: 211, 1973.
3. Barlow, D. H., and Hersen, M. *Single Case Experimental Designs: Strategies for Studying Behavioral Change* (2nd ed.). New York: Pergamon, 1984.
4. Benson, H., and McCallie, D. P.: Angina pectoris and the placebo effect. *N. Engl. J. Med.* 300: 1424–29, 1979.
5. Bergner, M., Bobbitt, R. A., Carter, W. B., and Gilson, B. S. The Sickness Impact Profile: Development and Final Revision of a Health Status Measure. *Medical Care* 19: 787–805, 1981.
6. Beta Blocker Heart Attack Trial Research Group. A randomized trial of propranolol in patients with acute myocardial infarction: I. Mortality results. *J. Am. Med. Assn.* 247: 1707, 1982.
7. Bradwell, A. R., Carmalt, M. H., and Whitehead, T. P. Explaining the unexpected abnormal results of profile investigations. *Lancet* 2: 1071, 1974.
8. Britton, M., Helmers, C., and Samuelsson, K. High-dose salicylic acid after cerebral infarction: A Swedish co-operative study. *Stroke* 18: 325, 1987.
9. Conover, W. J. *Practical Nonparametric Statistics*. New York: Wiley, 1971, P. 121.
10. Coronary Drug Project Research Group. Influence of adherence to treatment and response of cholesterol on mortality in the Coronary Drug Project. *N. Engl. J. Med.* 303: 1038, 1980.
11. DeProspero, A., and Cohen, S. Inconsistent visual analysis of intrasubject data. *J. Appl. Behav. Anal.* 12: 573, 1979.
12. DeRouen, T. A. Four comments received on statistical testing and confidence intervals. *Am. J. Pub. Health* 77: 237, 1987.
13. Detsky, A. S., and Sackett, D. L. When was a "negative" clinical trial big enough? How many patients you needed depends on what you found. *Arch. Intern. Med.* 145: 709, 1985.
14. Detsky, A. S. Decision analysis: What's the prognosis? *Ann. Intern. Med.* 106: 321, 1987.
15. Deyo, R. A., Diehl, A. K., and Rosenthal, M. How Many Days of Bed Rest for Acute Low Back Pain? A Randomized Clinical Trial. *N. Engl. J. Med.* 315: 1064–70, 1986.
16. Diehl, L. F., and Perry, D. J. A comparison of randomized concurrent control groups with matched historical control groups: Are historical controls valid? *J. Clin. Oncol.* 4: 1114, 1986.
17. European Coronary Study Group. Long-term results of prospective randomised study of coronary artery bypass surgery in stable angina pectoris. *Lancet* 2: 1173, 1982.
18. Feinstein, A. R., Josephy, B. R, and Wells, C. K. Scientific and clinical problems in indexes of functional disability. *Ann. Intern. Med.* 105: 413–20, 1986.
19. Fields, W. S., Maslenikov, V., Meyer, J. S., et al. Joint study of extracranial arterial occlusion: V. Progress report of prognosis following surgical or nonsurgical tests for transient ischemic attacks and cervical carotid artery lesions. *J.A.M.A.* 211: 1993, 1970.
20. Fleiss, J. L. Confidence intervals vs significance tests: Quantitative interpretation. *Am. J. Pub. Health.* 76: 587, 1987
21. Frieman, J. A., Chalmers, T. C., Smith, H., Jr., et al. The importance of beta, the type II error, and sample size in the design and interpretation of the randomized control trial. Survey of 71 negative trials. *N. Engl. J. Med.* 299: 690, 1978.
22. Fuller, R., Roth, H., and Long, S. Compliance with disulfram treatment of alcoholism. *J. Chron. Dis.* 36: 161, 1983.
23. Fuster, V., Cohen, M., and Halperin, J. Aspirin in the prevention of coronary disease. *N. Engl. J. Med.* 321: 183, 1989.

24. Gardner, M. J., and Altman, D. G. Confidence intervals rather than P values: Estimation rather than hypothesis testing. *Br. Med. J.* 292: 746, 1986.
25. Gardner, M. J., and Altman, D. G. Statistics with Confidence—Confidence Intervals and Statistical Guidelines. London: *Br. Med. J.*, 1989.
26. Guyatt, G. H., Bombardier, C., and Tugwell, P. X. Measuring Disease-Specific Quality of Life in Clinical Trials. *Can. Med. Ass. J.* 1986; 134: 889–95.
27. Guyatt, G. H., Sackett, D., Taylor, D. W., et al. Determining optimal therapy—Randomized trials in individual patients. *N. Engl. J. Med.* 314: 889, 1986.
28. Guyatt, G. H., Berman, L. B, Townsend, M., et al. A Measure of Quality of Life for Clinical Trials in Chronic Lung Disease. *Thorax* 42: 773–78, 1987.
29. Guyatt, G. H., Townsend, M., Pugsley, S. O, et al. Bronchodilators in Chronic Airflow Limitation, Effects on Airway Function, Exercise Capacity and Quality of Life. *Am. Rev. Respir. Dis.* 135: 1069–74, 1987.
30. Guyatt, G., Sackett, D., Adachi, J., et al. A clinician's guide for conducting randomized trials in individual patients. *C.M.A.J.* 139: 497, 1988.
31. Guyatt, G. H., Sullivan, M. J. J., Fallen, E., et al. A controlled trial of digoxin in congestive heart failure. *Am. J. Cardiol.* 61: 371–75, 1988.
32. Guyatt, G. H., Veldhuyzen Van Zanten, S. J. O., Feeny, D. H., and Patrick, D. L. Measuring quality of life in clinical trials: A taxonomy and review. *Can. Med. Ass. J.* 140: 1441–47, 1989.
33. Guyatt, G. H., Keller, J. L., Jaeschke, R., et al. Clinical usefulness of N of 1 randomized control trials: Three year experience. *Ann. Int. Med.* 112: 293–99, 1990.
34. Harvey, A. M., and McKusick, V. A. *Osler's Textbook Revisited.* New York: Appleton-Century-Crofts, 1967. P. 194.
35. Hill, J. D., Hampton, J. R., and Mitchell, J. R. A randomized trial of home versus hospital management for patients with suspected myocardial infarction. *Lancet* 1: 837, 1978.
36. Hinshaw, H. C., Feldman, W. H., and Pfuetze, K. H. Treatment of tuberculosis with streptomycin: Summary of observations on 100 cases. *J.A.M.A.* 132: 778, 1946.
37. Hogarty, G. E., and Goldberg, S. C. Drug and sociotherapy in the aftercare of schizophrenic patients. *Arch. Gen. Psychiatry* 28: 54, 1973.
38. International Union Against Tuberculosis Committee on Prophylaxis. Efficacy of various durations of isoniazid preventive therapy for tuberculosis: Five years of follow-up in the IUAT trial. *Bull. W.H.O.* 60: 555–64, 1982.
39. ISIS-2 (Second International Study of Infarct Survival) Collaborative Group: Randomized trial of intravenous streptokinase, oral aspirin, both, or neither among 17,187 cases of suspected acute myocardial infarction: ISIS-2. *Lancet* 2: 349–60, 1988.
40. Kassirer, J. P., Moskowitz, A. J., Lau, J., and Pauker, S. G. Decision analysis: A progress report. *Ann. Intern. Med.* 106: 275, 1987.
41. Kazdin, A. E. Single-Case Research Designs: Methods for Clinical and Applied Settings. New York: Oxford, 1982.
42. Kirshner, B., and Guyatt, G. H. A methodologic framework for assessing health indices. *J. Chron. Dis.* 38: 27, 1985.
43. Kratchwill, T. R. (ed.). Single Subject Research: Strategies for Evaluating Change. Orlando, Fl.: Academic, 1978. P. 316.
44. Lachenbruch, P. A., Clark, V. A., Cumberland, W. G., et al. Letters to the Editor. *Am. J. Pub. Health* 77: 237, 1987.
45. Laupacis, A., Sackett, D. L., and Roberts, R. S. An assessment of clinically useful measures of the consequences of treatment. *N. Engl. J. Med.* 318: 1728, 1988.
46. Laupacis, A., Sackett, D. L., and Roberts, R. S. Therapeutic priorities of Canadian internists. *Can. Med. Assoc. J.* 142: 329, 1990.
47. Liang, M. H., Larson, M. G., Cullen, K. E., and Schwartz, J. A. Comparative Measurement Efficiency and Sensitivity of Five Health Status Instruments for Arthritis Research. *Arthritis Rheum.* 28: 542–47, 1985.

48. Lipid Research Clinics Program. The Lipid Research Clinics Coronary Primary Prevention Trial results: I. Reduction in incidence of coronary heart disease. *J.A.M.A.* 251: 351, 1984.
49. Mager, R. F. *Preparing Instructional Objectives* (2nd ed.). Belmont: Fearon, 1975.
50. McNeil, B. J., and Pauker, S. G. The patient's role in assessing the value of diagnostic tests. *Radiology* 132: 605, 1979.
51. McNeil, B. J., Pauker, S. G., Sox, H. C., Jr., et al. On the elicitation of preferences for alternative therapies. *N. Engl. J. Med.* 306: 1259, 1982.
52. Meador, C. K. The art and science of nondisease. *N. Engl. J. Med.* 272: 92, 1965.
53. Medawar, P. B. *Induction and Intuition in Scientific Thought.* Philadelphia: American Philosophical Society, 1969.
54. Medical Research Council. Streptomycin treatment of tuberculosis meningitis. *Lancet* 1: 582, 1948.
55. Medical Research Council Working Party. MRC trial of treatment of mild hypertension: Principal results. *Br. Med. J.* 291: 97, 1985.
56. Miao, L. L. Gastric Freezing: An Example of the Evaluation and Medicine Therapy by Randomized Clinical Trials. In J. P. Bunker, B. A. Barnes, and F. Mosteller (eds.), *Costs, Risks & Benefits of Surgery.* New York: Oxford, 1977. Pp. 198–211.
57. Oliver, M. F., Heady, J. A., Morris, J. N., and Cooper, J. W.H.O.cooperative trial on primary prevention of ischaemic heart disease using clofibrate to lower serum cholesterol: Mortality follow-up. *Lancet* 2: 379, 1980.
58. Ott, C. R., Sivarajan, E. S., Newton, K. M., et al. A controlled randomized study of early cardiac rehabilitation: The Sickness Impact Profile as an assessment tool. *Heart and Lung* 12: 162–70, 1983.
59. Patrick, D. L., and Deyo, R. A. Generic and disease-specific measures in assessing health status and quality of life. *Medical Care* 27: F217–32, 1989.
60. Pizzo, P. A., Robichaud, K. J., Edwards, B. K., et al. Oral antibiotic prophylaxis in patients with cancer: A double-blind randomized placebo-controlled trial. *J. Pediatr.* 102: 125, 1983.
61. Ruffin, J. M., Grizzle, J. E., Hightower, N. C., et al. A cooperative double-blind evaluation of gastric "freezing" in the treatment of duodenal ulcer. *N. Engl. J. Med.* 281: 16, 1969.
62. Sackett, D. L. Design, Measurement and Analysis in Clinical Trials. In J. Hirsh, J. F. Cade, A. S. Gallus, E. Schonbaum (eds.). *Platelets, Drugs and Thrombosis.* Basel: Karger, 1975. Pp. 306–13.
63. Sackett, D. L., and Gent, M. Controversy in counting and attributing events in clinical trials. *N. Engl. J. Med.* 301: 1410, 1979.
64. Sackett, D. L., Haynes, R. B., Gent, M., and Taylor, D. W. Compliance. In W. H. W. Inman (ed.), *Monitoring for Drug Safety.* Lancaster: MTP, 1980.
65. Steering Committee of the Physicians' Health Study Research Group. Final report of the aspirin component of the ongoing Physicians' Health Study. *N. Engl. J. Med.* 321: 129, 1989.
66. Sudman, S., and Bradburn, N. M. Asking Questions: A Practical Guide to Questionnaire Design. San Francisco: Jossey-Bass, 1982.
67. Taylor, D. C. The components of sickness: Diseases, illnesses and predicaments. *Lancet* 2: 1008, 1979.
68. The Canadian Cooperative Study Group. A randomized trial of aspirin and sulfinpyrazone in threatened stroke. *N. Engl. J. Med.* 299: 53–59, 1978.
69. Torrance, G. W. Measurement of Health State Utilities for Economic Appraisal. *J. Health Economics* 5: 1–30, 1986.
70. Veterans Administration Cooperative Study Group on Antihypertensive Agents. Effects of treatment on morbidity in hypertension: III. Influence of age, diastolic pressure, and prior cardiovascular disease; further analysis of side effects. *Circulation* 45: 991, 1972.
71. Veterans Administration Cooperative Study Group on Antihypertensive Agents. Ef-

fects of treatment on morbidity in hypertension: Results in patients with diastolic blood pressures averaging 115 through 129 mm Hg. *J.A.M.A.* 202: 1028–34, 1967.

72. Wagensteen, O. H., Peter, E. T., Nicoloff, D. M., et al. Achieving "physiological gastrectomy" by gastric freezing: A preliminary report of an experimental and clinical study. *J.A.M.A.* 180: 439, 1962.
73. Weinstein, M., and Fineberg, H. *Clinical Decision Analysis*. Philadelphia: Saunders, 1980.
74. Woodward, C. A., and Chambers, L. W. Guide to Questionnaire Construction and Question Writing. Ottawa: Canadian Public Health Association, 1983.
75. Yerushalmy, J. On Inferring Causality from Observed Associations. In F. J. Ingelfinger, A. S. Relman, M. Finland (eds.), *Controversy in Internal Medicine*. Philadelphia: Saunders, 1966. P. 659.

8

Helping Patients Follow the Treatments You Prescribe

By applying the "basic science for clinical medicine" described in Chapters 1 through 7, you will find yourself increasingly able to gather accurate and reliable clinical information, to select and interpret useful diagnostic tests, to estimate realistic prognoses, and to identify treatments that will do more good than harm. Now comes the crunch.

All these efforts, no matter how carefully planned or how painstakingly executed, will be for naught if you do not prescribe the best treatment at the appropriate time and if your patients will not or cannot adhere to the regimens that you prescribe for them. Reviewing your own performance in administering the best treatment and keeping up to date are important and complex topics that occupy the next section of this book. In this chapter we consider how often patients follow the treatments we prescribe and how we can help our patients to adhere closely to these treatments in order to maximize their benefits.

We also will use this chapter to illustrate and extend many of the basic principles we presented earlier by using them to review the literature on patient compliance. (You can take on the mantle of the critic now and judge for yourself if we can practice what we have been preaching!)

Ivory Tower Versus Real World Research

Patient compliance is "The extent to which the patient's behavior, in terms of taking medications, following diets, or executing life style changes, coincides with the clinical prescription" [25]. Compliance plays a central role in making or breaking almost every clinical encounter and a "therapeutic alliance" between patient and doctor is needed for success. Here is a graphic example. When Materson and his colleagues studied the antihypertensive efficacy of chlorthalidone, they found a convincing and highly statistically significant correlation coefficient of .63 between the dose prescribed and the lowering of blood pressure (calculated from data in [41]). When we studied the relation between the dose prescribed and blood pressure response in a different setting [61], the correlation was a measly .11, not statistically significant. What happened?

In Materson's investigation, patients were carefully selected volunteers who agreed *in advance* to follow their treatments closely, keep frequent clinic appointments, and undergo repeated blood pressure checks. By contrast, the patients in our investigation were found to be hypertensive on screening at a large steel mill. We managed to include over 95% of the workers in our screening (What would you rather do: spend an hour in a coke oven or come to get your blood pressure checked on company time?). We referred those who were hypertensive to their family physician for further assessment and treatment. Six months later, we found that, despite persisting hypertension, 49% were not treated or referred on by their family doctor, a story which we will pick up again in the next section of the book. Of those who were treated, 100 were prescribed chlorthalidone (the study took place in the days before combination diuretics had taken over the market). It was among these individuals that we found the very low correlation between the prescribed dose of chlorthalidone and blood pressure.

The reason for this poor showing became evident when we examined what the patients had been prescribed and how much of it they actually took. Often physicians had prescribed too little of the drug to be efficacious (for example, chlorthalidone 25 mg on Monday, Wednesday, and Friday), or too much of the drug to be useful (for example, 200 mg per day, a dose that increases side effects without producing appreciable improvements in blood pressure control in comparison with lower doses). On the other hand (perhaps in self-defense?), less than half the patients were complying with their prescriptions. When we compared the amount of medication *consumed* with the blood pressure, the correlation almost tripled from .11 to .29 and became statistically significant. Although it was not possible to quantitate, much of the rest of the difference between Materson's .63 and our .29 appeared to be due to the prescription of doses that were too high or too low.

The key difference between Materson's study and ours is that the former was set up as an "explanatory" trial while the latter was a "management" study [60]. Other terms might do as well: for example, ivory tower versus real world. Both types of studies play an important role in the march of medical science. Explanatory trials attempt to determine whether a treatment *can work* under relatively ideal circumstances of careful prescription and high patient compliance. These studies are efficient in screening treatments for their potential: If they don't work under optimal conditions, they certainly won't work in the trenches. Management trials, on the other hand, try to determine whether treatments *do work* under usual clinical circumstances (relatively speaking, again—it is very difficult to get all patients to agree to enter a trial, impossible to measure what is happening to patients completely unobtrusively, and tricky to interpret the results of a study if the intervention is not standardized).

It is worthwhile keeping this "explanatory versus management" spectrum in mind in reviewing reports of studies and attempting to answer the question "Is the therapeutic maneuver feasible in your practice?" If the effect of a treatment is marginal in an explanatory trial, it probably won't have much effect for most of your patients unless you can afford to provide the amount of supervision and encouragement that patients received in the trial. The reason, as we will demonstrate, is that supervision and encouragement are among the most potent stimuli to patient compliance.

The Magnitude of Low Compliance

Try to answer the following questions about your own patients:

1. What percent of appointments that they make for themselves do they keep? _______%

2. What percent of appointments that I make for them do they keep? ________%

3. If I prescribe a short-term regimen to cure an intercurrent illness (say, oral antibiotics for strep throat), what proportion of patients will complete a 10-day course of therapy? ________%

4. What proportion of my patients will comply with a long term medication regimen (such as antacids for peptic ulcer)? ________%

5. What proportion of my patients wear their seatbelts? ________%

The results of studies of patient compliance are quite sobering [62]. Patients keep about 75% of the appointments they make for themselves, but only about 50% of the appointments that we make for them for needed follow-up. When invited to appointments for screening—for example, pap smears [55]—attendance drops off to less than 35% (still better than twice as good as what happens if doctors and patients are left without any reminders [55]!).

For short-term medications for cure, compliance runs about 75% for the first few days, but less than 25% of outpatients will complete a 10-day course of antibiotic therapy for a strep throat or otitis media.

Medication compliance can be surprisingly low even among inpatients, especially when they are on self-administration programs. When hospitalized ulcer patients were provided with bedside antacids and kept under unobtrusive surveillance, it was documented that they consumed less than 45% of their prescribed dose [57]. Furthermore, despite the direct administration of oral medication by hospital staff to hospitalized schizophrenics, only 76% of their urines contained the prescribed drugs or their metabolites [50].

Compliance with long-term medications usually runs at about 50%, regardless of whether the intent is to prevent or alleviate symptoms. Compliance with lifestyle recommendations is worse yet; only about 30% of patients will comply with even modest dietary advice, and fewer than 10% of cigarette smokers who have no major target organ damage will stop smoking on the advice of their physician [78]. Finally, except in jurisdictions where laws requiring seat-belt use are vigorously enforced, only about 20% of drivers regularly buckle up.

How do these published results agree with estimates based on your own experience? If your estimates are much more optimistic, you should pay particular attention to the section that follows on how to detect low compliance.

Please stop here for a moment and write down the following:

1. The methods of measuring compliance that you currently use or have used in your clinical practice. (On what proportion of your patients do you assess compliance?)
2. Any other methods that you think could be used.
3. For each of the diagnostic methods you have listed, give your estimate of the sensitivity with which they detect low-compliance problems and the specificity with which they identify high compliance.

As you can see from the assignment we have just given you, the principles of interpreting diagnostic tests can be applied to the strategies we use to detect low compliance. We will review the operating characteristics of eight methods that have been employed in an effort to diagnose low compliance: clinical judgment, monitoring attendance at scheduled appointments, monitoring achievement of the treatment goal, searching for telltale side effects, pill counts, medication monitors, drug levels, and patient interviews.

CLINICAL JUDGMENT

The most common method that we use for assessing the compliance of our patients is our clinical judgment, based on "knowing the patient." This method is attractive for we are quite willing to generate compliance estimates for our patients, often with apparent ease and considerable confidence. However, Harold Roth's group has reported a low correlation between physicians' estimates of compliance with ulcer regimens and objective measures [58]. Moreover, these physicians had been told in advance that their patients' measured compliance was low, yet they still overestimated their patients' compliance by 71%! The physicians' predictions did not improve for patients they had followed longer [56]. Other studies of the value of clinicians' estimates [4, 7, 8, 36-38] of whether or not their patients are compliant have shown them to be no more accurate than flipping a coin.

When informed of the results of these studies, two family practitioners in our town did not believe they applied to family physicians. They judged they could do better, given that they had ongoing relationships with their patients. To prove their point, they invited colleagues whom they regarded as "good family docs" to identify up to 10 patients in each of their practices for whom they had prescribed digoxin and for whom they felt they could provide an accurate clinical judgment on compliance [22]. (Although this study was in family medicine, it looks like an "explanatory" study to us!) Once these patients were identified and their physicians' estimates of compliance given, nurses went to the patients' homes and questioned them about their medication taking, counted their pills, and took blood samples (at least 6 hours after the last putative dose) for digoxin levels. The results of this study are shown in Table 8-1.

Here is a chance to use your diagnostic test skills: Calculate below the usual measures of performance for Table 8-1.

Prevalence (or pretest probability)
of low compliance:

Sensitivity of clinical judgment:

Specificity of clinical judgment:

Probability of low compliance
when doctor predicted it:

Table 8-1. Comparison of family physicians' estimates of compliance and actual compliance among patients on digoxin

		Actual compliance by pill count		
		Low (< 80%)	High (≥ 80%)	
Physicians' estimates of compliance	Low (< 80%)	2 a	7 b	9
	High (≥ 80%)	19 c	43 d	62
		21	50	71

Adapted from J. R. Gilbert, C. E. Evans, R. B. Haynes, and P. Tugwell. Predicting compliance with a regimen of digoxin therapy in family practice. *Can. Med. Assoc. J.* 123:119, 1980.

Probability of high compliance when doctor predicted it:

Overall accuracy:

Likelihood ratio for clinical judgment of low compliance:

Likelihood ratio for clinical judgment of high compliance:

(Our calculations are at the end of the chapter if you get stuck or want to check yours.)

The likelihood ratios generated from Table 8-1 provide a succinct summary of the power of clinical judgment in diagnosing compliance. At .68 for the judgment of low compliance and 1.05 for a judgment of high compliance, these family physicians' "clinical judgments" were not only useless for this task, they were going in the wrong direction! We shall temporarily draw the curtain of charity over further discussion of our ability to predict compliance based on clinical judgment.

MONITORING ATTENDANCE AT SCHEDULED APPOINTMENTS

Because dropping out of care constitutes one of the most common and most severe forms of noncompliance, monitoring attendance is the single most important tactic for determining compliance among ambulatory patients. Moreover, for that small number of disorders for which the treatment is administered at the visit (e.g., immunizations, depot phenothiazines for psychosis), monitoring attendance is the only compliance measure required. For self-administered regimens, on the other hand, attendance is a necessary *but not sufficient* prerequisite for compliance. Thus, Roth has reported a low correlation between attendance and compliance with an ulcer regimen [59].

Monitoring attendance is administratively straightforward if your practice is set up for it. You must have a daily appointment book and a rule whereby patients who require follow-up visits are always given a booking for their next appointment.

Many clinics and offices, however, fail to give patients specific appointment times for their next visits. For conditions such as hypertension, patients simply may be told to call in 2 or 3 months for a follow-up appointment. Unfortunately, when a patient fails to call for an appointment, his or her absence will not be noted in most practices, and noncompliance may be detected too late, when she or he suffers a preventable complication of the disorder.

MONITORING ACHIEVEMENT OF THE TREATMENT TARGET

In the previous chapter, we called for setting explicit treatment targets for each patient. If you can specify a measurable target, and your therapy is efficacious, then failure to achieve the target can alert you to the possibility of noncompliance. (And if you cannot specify a measurable treatment target, then you need to be more concerned with that than with compliance!)

We must be careful how we interpret the patient's response to therapy. Only in situations in which perfect compliance guarantees clinical success will therapeutic responsiveness be perfectly correlated with compliance. Unfortunately, most treatments are only partially successful, and to accuse the patient of low compliance whenever a treatment fails is neither fair nor rational. Finally, many disorders exhibit spontaneous remissions and exacerbations that are independent of treatment and, thus, compliance. Table 8-2 depicts these possibilities.

From the compliance perspective, we want to move patients from cell *a* (not at goal because of low compliance) to cell *d* (at goal, with high compliance) by a maneuver that increases their adherence to treatment. On the other hand, improving the compliance of patients in the other cells (in which the problem is inadequate treatment or underprescribing coupled with high compliance [cell *b*] or incorrect diagnosis or overprescribing, regardless of compliance [cell *c*]) would not only be inappropriate, but could lead to adverse or toxic effects with no corresponding increase in benefits.

If the three methods we have described so far for detecting low compliance have been followed in sequence, all you will know at this point is whether or not your patient has achieved the treatment target. That is, you will know which horizontal row of Table 8-2 your patient belongs in, but not whether he or she belongs in the right or left columns. For example, Tom Inui and his colleagues found that 57% of those who were at the treatment goal were compliant, and 43% were not [29]. Why might this be so?

If you have established a firm diagnosis before beginning treatment, and the patient has reached the treatment goal, then the patient's compliance is not of great concern. However, there are three exceptions to this generalization. First,

Table 8-2. Correlation of compliance with achievement of the treatment target

		Compliance by pill count	
		Low	High
Achievement of the treatment target	No (not at target)	The group you want to identify a	Inadequate Rx or underprescribing b
	Yes (at target)	c Wrong diagnosis or overprescribing	d Ideal

if your initial diagnosis was wrong, you are rewarding yourself with bouquets for your therapeutic success when you should be tossing brickbats at yourself for treating the patient needlessly for a disorder he does not have. In this case the noncompliant patient is serving himself quite well, but the compliant patient needs to be let off the hook. Second, even chronic diseases can go into remission at times, and this happens to noncompliant as well as compliant patients. (Which of these first two explanations is operative will not be clear at this point. A way to find out is to discontinue the treatment and follow the patient closely. When we did this for well-controlled hypertensives in our community, a third of them were still normotensive a year later [44].) Third, if a patient's condition is already well-controlled when he takes only half the medication you prescribe, a sudden rise in compliance to 100% (such as might occur if the patient were hospitalized for an unrelated disorder) could lead to catastrophic overdosing and toxicity.

Nonetheless, the need for exact compliance measurements among "successful patients" is hardly as compelling as among patients who have failed to reach the treatment target. So this third method simply helps us *narrow the search* for the noncompliant patient, and it may be both expedient and efficient to reserve the more accurate assessments for patients who have not reached treatment targets despite usually adequate treatment prescriptions.

A practical illustration of this relation between compliance and achievement of the treatment target among hypertensive patients is shown in Table 8-3. As you can calculate from this table, the association between compliance and blood pressure control is far from perfect. Did you calculate the sensitivity and specificity of achievement of the treatment goal as a diagnostic test for low compliance? When we did so, the sensitivity was 64% (38/59) and the specificity was 57% (43/75). What about the likelihood ratios? We calculated the failure to achieve the treatment goal would be only about 1.5 times as likely to be observed in a noncompliant patient as in a compliant one, and that the likelihood ratio for the achievement of the treatment goal was about .6, also rather unimpressive. As a result, the probability of low compliance in this example is 21/64 = .33 if the blood pressure is controlled and 38/70 = .54 if it is not. We would have to apply additional compliance measures to avoid the false-positive mislabeling of

Table 8-3. Relation between compliance and diastolic blood pressure (DBP) control among hypertensive patients

		Compliance by pill count		
		Low (< 80%)	High (≥ 80%)	
Achievement of the treatment target	No (DBP ≥90)	38 (a)	32 (b)	70
	Yes (DBP <90)	21 (c)	43 (d)	64
		59	75	134

Adapted from R. B. Haynes. Influence on Compliance. In K. C. Mezey (ed.), *Fixed Drug Combinations: Rationale & Limitations*. London: Royal Society of Medicine/Academic Press, 1980.

almost half of the 70 patients who, despite taking their medications, are not at goal blood pressure. Nonetheless, applying some additional measures, which we will describe later, to those who have not reached the treatment goal will both identify a substantial group of noncompliers and also focus on those noncompliers at highest risk of the complications of the disorder.

SEARCHING FOR TELLTALE SIDE EFFECTS

Some regimens produce clear-cut pharmacologic effects or side effects, the absence of which suggests low compliance: urinary frequency with diuretics, dry mouth with anticholinergics, dark stool with oral iron, slow heart rate with beta blockers, suppression of thyroid stimulating hormone with thyroid hormone replacement [12]. However, the link between these effects and the treatment goal may be tenuous (postural hypotension from antihypertensive drugs can occur without reaching goal blood pressure, and vice versa). When we assessed the ability of changes in potassium and uric acid to detect compliance in patients on diuretics, their sensitivities were 82% and 80% respectively, but their specificities only 48% [26].

As seen in cell *b* of Table 8-2, high compliance with an inadequate dose, or with an oral medication that is poorly absorbed, will result in neither side effects nor achievement of the treatment goal. And, as documented in Chapter 5, many side effects appear to result from the act of being medicated rather than from the medication itself. Accordingly, this approach has the same limitations as the previous one, plus the additional disadvantage that it is not coterminous with the treatment goal.

PILL COUNTS

Asking patients to bring their pills to each visit is a good idea to ensure that the patient has the medications you intended. Sometimes this can help with measuring compliance, as well. However, to be accurate, this method requires keeping track of how many pills were dispensed with each prescription, the dates each prescription or refill was begun, whether the patient has left caches of medication in other places, whether pills are shared with a relative, and so on.

Also, patients who do not want you to know their true compliance rate can forget to bring their pills or "deep six" some of them or just simply skip the appointment. Nevertheless, pill counts that are much higher than they ought to be (as long as your calculations are correct!) are proof of low compliance, and the exercise is often worthwhile, particularly during home visits to patients who have missed appointments. As long as you are clear about what is required to get an accurate measurement (see preceding text and the section Asking the Patient later in this chapter for further details), you or a visiting health worker can do the accounting that is needed to relate the number of pills the patient has on hand to the number they should have if they have been following the prescription as intended [26].

MEDICATION MONITORS

The number and variety of pill containers that provide an automatic record of pill usage (or at least, cap removal) reminds one of the age-old passion of would-be inventors to build a better mouse trap. One of the earlier versions of the "better pill container" included a radioactive source that burnt an image in a photographic film strip, attached to the back of a unit-dose drug container [47]. The size of any spot was inversely related to the rate at which pills were removed from its ingenious, spring-loaded container.* More recently, microelectronics have led to new products, some of which have been very useful in elucidating patterns of medication consumption. For example, Stefan Norell found a large number of different patterns of compliance with pilocarpine, as determined by an eye drop container with a computer chip in its lid, which recorded each time that the lid was removed [53]. One company now makes a pill container with a similar device in its top and a recent study has shown that seizure activity among epileptics relates more closely to the information provided by this device than serum drug levels or pill counts [10]. Unfortunately, at least for now, the software for "debriefing" the computer chip in the pill container cap is proprietary and caps must be sent into the manufacturer, so their use is largely limited to research projects.

Even if monitors were to function accurately and conveniently, none (to date) can determine whether the patient has actually consumed the medication when the pill lid is removed.

DRUG LEVEL MEASUREMENTS

Modern analytic methods are permitting an ever-wider array of medications to be both qualitatively and quantitatively measured in urine, blood, saliva, breath, and other effluvia [45]. As we shall learn a bit later, when the results of these measurements are fed back to patients as part of a negotiating process, they can

*We had hoped to examine one of these devices in Hamilton, Ontario, where we work, but cautious Canadian customs officials denied permission for its American inventor to bring it across the border!

result in sharp rises in compliance. Drug levels are particularly useful for drugs with relatively long serum half-lives, such as diphenylhydantoin, lithium, and digoxin, for which regular consumption results in steady-state plasma levels.

But direct measurements of drugs in body fluids often are expensive, cumbersome to obtain, with limited availability in many practice settings, and reported only long after the patient has left the office. Furthermore, for drugs with short half-lives, these measurements reflect compliance for only the immediately preceding dose. For example, in a study in which serum drug levels were monitored and pill taking was also recorded with a special pill container, drug levels were in the therapeutic range when most patients with seizure activity visited the clinic but the pill container showed lapses around the time of the seizure [10]. Although we shall welcome the era of the "dip stick" compliance measurement, it will not solve all our compliance measurement problems.

ASKING THE PATIENT

Hippocrates didn't think much of this approach. One of his less well-known admonitions states, "The physician should keep aware of the fact that patients often lie when they state that they have taken certain medicines" [29]. Is this admonition true, and do we waste time asking patients about their compliance? Consider the compliance of hypertensive patients with their prescribed medications in the sixth month of therapy [26]. The "gold standard" for determining their true compliance was a pill count, conducted at a surprise home visit, which compared the amounts of medication patients had on hand with the amount they should have had if they had taken their medicine as prescribed. At this same home visit each patient was told, "People often have difficulty taking their pills for one reason or another and we are interested in finding out any problems that occur so we can understand them better." They were then asked, "Have you ever missed any of your blood pressure pills?" If they said "yes" they were asked to estimate the average number of tablets missed per day, week, and month during the previous month. Table 8-4 compares the results of asking patients about their compliance (diagnostic test) with the results of their pill counts (gold standard). See whether you can generate some useful indexes of the accuracy of asking patients about their compliance.

When we followed our own advice and calculated the sensitivity, specificity and predictive value of "asking the patient," using the same 80% cutoff for both the pill count (gold standard) and the self-report (diagnostic test), we were pleasantly surprised. Although the sensitivity of self-reporting is low (37%), its specificity is very high (95%). As a result, when almost half of a group of patients are taking less than 80% of their pills, asking the patient can be very useful: 95% of those who admit taking less than 80% of their medicine are telling the truth. (Tom Inui and his colleagues got similar results [sensitivity 55% and specificity 88%] with a slightly different question, "Many patients find it difficult to take their medicines or stick to their diets as their doctors say they should. Over the past two months since you were last in the clinic, do you think you have taken your medicine as you should, on schedule and regularly?" Patients were

Table 8-4. Self-reported compliance versus pill count compliance for 127 hypertensive patients

		Compliance by pill count (as a gold standard)	
		Noncompliant (< 80%)	Compliant (≥ 80%)
Self-reported compliance (as a diagnostic test)	0–29%	14	0
	30–79%	7	1
	80–99%	12	7
	100%	24	62
		57	70

Adapted from D. L. Sackett, R. B. Haynes, E. S. Gibson, et al. Randomized clinical trial of strategies for improving medication compliance in primary hypertension. *Lancet* 1:1205, 1975.

Table 8-5. Likelihood ratios for self-reported compliance

		Compliance by pill count (as a gold standard)		
		< 80% (noncompliant)	≥ 80% (compliant)	Likelihood ratio
Self-reported compliance (as a diagnostic test)	0–29%	14 (.246)	0 (0)	∞
	30–79%	7 (.123)	1 (.014)	8.8
	80–99%	12 (.211)	7 (.100)	2.1
	100%	24 (.421)	62 (.886)	0.48
		57 (1.00)	70 (1.00)	

classified as noncompliant if they reported any departure from recommended drug behavior [29].)

We carried this analysis one step further and calculated the likelihood ratios for each level of self-reporting. The results are shown in Table 8-5.

Once again, "asking the patient" emerges as a powerful diagnostic tool, and we can now compare this method of detecting the noncompliant patient with several others. Table 8-6 compares expensive but objective drug measurements in urine (Panel A) with the quicker but possibly "softer" method of asking the patient (Panel B). The result may surprise some readers.

Table 8-6 reveals that the quick patient interview may be as good as the slower (and often unavailable) drug level in detecting the noncompliant patient.

Table 8-6. Comparison of drug measurements in urine with asking the patient

Panel A

		Compliance by pill count	
		Low (< 80%)	High (≥ 80%)
Drug level in urine	Absent	22	7
	Present	18	46
		40	53

Panel B

		Compliance by pill count	
		Low (< 80%)	High (≥ 80%)
Self-reported compliance	<90%	20	5
	≥90%	20	48
		40	53

	Detection method	
Accuracy	Urine test	Self-report
Sensitivity	0.55	0.50
Specificity	0.87	0.91
Accuracy	0.73	0.73
Likelihood ratio (+)	4.16	4.80
Likelihood ratio (−)	0.51	0.55

Adapted from R. B. Haynes. Influence on Compliance. In K. C. Mezey (ed.), *Fixed Drug Combination: Rationale & Limitations*. London: Royal Society of Medicine/Academic Press, 1980.

If the answer is "yes" when a patient is asked if he has missed any pills, it is valid to assume an important amount of noncompliance, even if the patient qualifies his report by stating or implying that noncompliance is a very rare event ("maybe last Saturday") and only occurs under extenuating circumstances (such as going out in the evening). Those patients who admit to missing *any* pills usually have quite a low compliance. For example, we found that the average compliance among those who admitted missing *any* pills was 26%!

Combining the patient interview with failure to reach the treatment goal improves the prospects for detecting low compliance. When Inui classified as noncompliant patients who either admitted noncompliance or had diastolic pressures of 100 mm Hg or more, the sensitivity for detection of noncompliance (measured by home pill count) improved from 55% to 83%, albeit with a drop-off in specificity from 88% to 66%.

OVERVIEW

To summarize methods of detecting noncompliance: Clinical judgment is no better than flipping a coin, and searching for therapeutic effects or side effects often leads to mistakes. Pill counts (on a home visit, not at the clinic) and drug levels are accurate but expensive, and may not be available for most regimens in most settings. On the basis of our current knowledge, the approach to detecting the noncompliant patient that best combines accuracy and feasibility goes as follows: (a) seek out patients who have missed appointments or dropped out of care (for it is this group who usually have the lowest compliance); (b) in addition, focus on those patients who, despite vigorous treatment, have failed to reach the treatment target (the upper row of Table 8-2); (c) by a nonthreatening interview of patients who have not reached the treatment target (or, if readily available, by pill counts or direct measurements of drugs in their body fluids) identify the noncompliers (cell *a* of Table 8-2).

Having identified noncompliant patients, how do we help them take their medicine?

Prerequisites for Improving Low Compliance

Before we launch an often intensive and somctimes quite expensive program to improve a patient's compliance, we ought to satisfy ourselves that the prerequisites listed in Table 8-7 have been met.

Because most compliance-improving strategies are themselves interventions, and because the purpose of improving compliance is to enhance therapeutic benefit, we hold that compliance-improving strategies should be thought of as therapeutic maneuvers. As such, they ought to be subjected to the same vigorous scrutiny we apply to any treatment. The prerequisites set out in Table 8-7 are mostly self-evident. There would be no point in attempting to increase compliance with an incorrect or ineffective treatment—indeed it could add injury to insult for the patient.

Table 8-7. Logical and ethical prerequisites for any intervention to improve compliance

1. Disease diagnosis must be correct
2. Disease must be nontrivial
3. Therapy must be efficacious
4. Compliance intervention must be efficacious
5. Patient must be informed and willing

Adapted from R. J. Levine. Ethical Considerations in the Development and Application of Compliance Strategies for the Treatment of Hypertension. In R. B. Haynes, M. E. Mattson, and T. O. Engebretson, Jr. (eds.), *Patient Compliance to Prescribed Antihypertensive Medication Regimens*. Washington, D.C.: Government Printing Office, N.I.H., No. 80-2102, 1980.

Because the earlier parts of this book were devoted to making diagnoses and prognoses, and selecting efficacious treatments, we will assume that readers already know how to satisfy the first three prerequisites. By the same token, using a compliance-improving strategy that is useless is a waste of time for both patient and practitioner. We will return to sorting useful from useless strategies shortly.

The final prerequisite, that the patient be informed and willing to participate in the process, is a matter of ethics (and law) rather than logic. In most circumstances, patients have the right to refuse treatment and are protected from abuse and assault. All of the strategies that we will describe are designed for these circumstances and, for the most part, they are successful because they encourage active participation from the patient rather than gaining cooperation by coercion. There are, of course, situations such as psychosis or contagion in which patients pose such grave threats to themselves or others that local laws supersede our prerequisite of informed, willing consent. The strong-arm tactics that are sometimes applied in these circumstances are in sharp contrast to the more positive and facilitating procedures that follow. In fact, approximately 80% of noncompliant patients we have approached with offers to provide compliance-improving strategies have accepted our help willingly [25].

Strategies for Improving Low Compliance

We now return to the fourth prerequisite, that the compliance-improving strategy must be efficacious. To determine just which interventions merit this label, we will conducted a detailed overview. You may want to "cut to the chase" and skip the section below, Methods of Review. Otherwise, if you want to follow the review process along, you may want to check our approach against the criteria for critical appraisal of overviews set out in Chapter 12. We set the methods for the review out rather formally, as prescribed by Mulrow [48], though in a slightly different order.

METHODS OF REVIEW

Objective

We began the review by defining the question we were interested in as, "What is the efficacy of interventions that have been tested for improving patient compliance with appointments, referrals, and prescribed medications?"

Study Selection

Next we perused some relevant articles that we already knew about, to get a feel for the "lay of the land," particularly with respect to the strength of methods of testing interventions.* Then we set criteria designed to select the studies of highest quality from all on the topic. Many of the guides we applied in the previous chapter to the evaluation of claims that a treatment is efficacious can be applied to the assessment of compliance-improving strategies as well. The guides we

*In this particular instance, we were fortunate to have completed a review a decade ago when we were involved in research into this problem [24]. However, the review was quite out of date.

developed for reviewing the compliance literature are modified from these and appear in Table 8-8.

These criteria were intended to focus the review on studies that reported relevant endpoints (compliance and treatment outcome) in a scientifically acceptable fashion (randomized control group, at least 80% follow-up, statistical analysis, and protection against false-negative results). It can be argued that compliance is a phenomenon worthy of scientific interest in its own right and thus that the requirement for showing its relationship to treatment outcome is unnecessary. However, from a clinical perspective, improving compliance could be considered meddlesome if the treatment did not have to be taken in the recommended dose to achieve full effect, or it could even be considered unethical if the treatment was not efficacious but had adverse effects.

The readers' guides in Table 8-8 made our review of the growing literature on patient compliance efficient as well as effective. For example, our application of these guides as we prepared this chapter allowed us to cut the number of articles that we would review in detail from over 2000 to less than 30. (For different topics, the number of high-quality studies will vary from none to a great many. If there are no good studies, assuming that some information is likely to be better than none, the criteria can be relaxed to permit the best available studies in, even if none of them is close to perfection. If there are a large number of strong studies, the criteria can be tightened further.)

Data Sources

Having set the criteria for review, the next step was to round up all the literature published on compliance-improving strategies. To do this, we explored the following trails: (a) MEDLINE, using the medical subject heading PATIENT COMPLIANCE; (b) bibliographies of published articles on patient compliance; (c)

Table 8-8. Readers' guides for reviewing articles about compliance-improving strategies[a]

1. Was there randomly allocated a comparison group that did not receive the compliance-improving strategy?
2. Was there at least one valid measure of compliance?
3. Was there at least one measure of treatment outcome?
4. Were at least 80% of the participants followed to the end of the observation period?
5. For long term regimens, were the patients followed for at least 6 months?
6. Were both clinical and statistical significance considered?
   a. If a statistically significant effect on compliance was found, was it big enough to be worth the effort involved in applying the strategy?
   b. If no statistically significant effect on compliance was found, were there at least 50 patients in each group (intervention and control)?[b]

[a]Adapted from Haynes, R. B., Wang, E., and Da Mota Gomes, M. A critical review of interventions to improve compliance with prescribed medications. *Patient Educ. Counsel* 10: 155–66, 1987.

[b]This standard provides some protection against "false-negative" conclusions by ensuring a large enough number of subjects studied to detect a clinically-important benefit, in this case, an absolute difference of 25% in the proportion of patients found compliant with the regimen.

colleagues interested in the topic; and (d) Science Citation Index to collect articles that cited key studies. Collecting all the relevant articles is really "pick-and-shovel" work and it is impossible to be sure that you have completed the task. Basically, you just keep going until all routes are exhausted—and be prepared to incorporate new articles right up to the last moment.

Having pre-set criteria for acceptance into the detailed review helps a great deal, however. First, new articles can be screened quickly, excluding from further consideration studies that don't meet the criteria. Second, sticking to the criteria keeps you honest. If *all* articles that meet certain criteria are to be included, it becomes less likely that you will exclude an article because its results do not fit in with the others or with your own prejudices (and, if you do exclude, intentionally or unintentionally, articles that should be there, readers can detect what has happened).

Data Extraction

For studies that met all the selection criteria and demonstrated a statistically significant effect on compliance, we characterized the effect of the intervention by subtracting the percentage of patients judged compliant in the control group from the percentage compliant in the intervention group. If 70% were compliant in the intervention group and 50% of the controls, the effect size was (70% − 50% =) 20%. There are fancier ways of doing this, for example, using odds ratios [20, 40], but these are only needed for a formal "meta-analysis" which is perhaps most justified if there is disagreement among studies testing the same intervention, not the case here. The absolute percentage figure is easy to interpret: it is the number of people per hundred treated who are "rescued" from a noncompliant state by the intervention. Readers will recognize this as the father of the "number needed to treat" discussed in Chapter 7: inverting the figure (100 ÷ 20) gives the number of people receiving the intervention [5] needed to help one become compliant.

For the effect of the intervention on achievement of the therapeutic goal, we simply classified studies as showing a statistically significant effect or not. Because the studies involved many different medical disorders, clinical settings, methods of selecting patients, treatments, measures of treatment effects and so on, it did not make sense to us to try to look at effect sizes in a quantitative way.

Honorable Mention

Critics of the "ultra-rigorous" literature review argue that rigid application of arbitrary criteria trashes a lot of valuable information. We agree with this view, especially for specific types of compliance problems for which few or no studies met all criteria. There were, in fact, very few studies of interventions to increase the success of referrals, appointments, or compliance with short-term treatments that included measures of treatment outcomes. We therefore accommodated studies of these particular compliance problems that met all criteria *except* measurement of treatment outcome, or at least 6-month follow-up for long-term treatments, by giving them "Honorable Mention" in the comments after reviewing the studies that met all criteria. However, these studies are excluded from the tables. If there were not so many good studies in this field, it would make sense to relax the criteria to allow conclusions to be drawn (more tentatively) from a larger number of studies.

Data Synthesis

The "cream of the crop" studies that met our methodologic standards are summarized in Tables 8-9 to 8-13 and discussed here.

IMPROVING COMPLIANCE WITH REFERRAL AND SCREENING APPOINTMENTS

Persons found to have a disease through screening or case finding often require referral for further assessment and management. The only two studies of strategies for improving compliance with referral appointments that met all the guides are summarized in Table 8-9.

Hoehn-Saric and colleagues [28] counseled patients who were to be referred for psychiatric outpatient care about what to expect and how to gain the most from therapy. This counseling led to improvements in both attendance at appointments and cooperation at therapy sessions, and was followed by improvements in their clinical outcomes.

Fletcher and her colleagues [19] employed a special referral clerk who helped a random half of hypertensive patients discovered in an emergency room obtain convenient appointments and overcome logistical barriers such as lack of transportation and babysitting. The result was a 21% increase in attendance at the referral appointment compared with control patients who simply were advised to see their physicians. However, and this is the catch, a follow-up of these patients 5 months later revealed that the degree of blood pressure control was no better in the clerk-referred group, despite their higher rate of initial referral. The practical implication of this result is obvious: It does not make sense and wastes resources to assist a patient with one, early step along the path from detection to control when there is no demonstrable treatment benefit at the end of the trail. In this case, antihypertensive treatment and follow-up would need improvement before a referral service could be expected to improve the achievement of treatment targets.

Keeping this warning in mind, we found several randomized trials of inter-

Table 8-9. Improving compliance with referral appointments

Citation	Condition	Strategy	Effect on attendance (%)[a]	Effect on treatment outcome
Hoehn-Saric, Frank, Imber, et al. [28]	Psychiatric disorders	Preintake counseling	+ 20	Improved[b]
Fletcher, Appel, and Bourgois [19]	Hypertension	Special referral clerk	+ 21	No effect

[a]Figures derived by subtracting percentage of patients judged compliant in the control group from the percentage compliant in the intervention group; both figures reported are statistically significant ($P < .05$).
[b]Improvement statistically significant ($P < .05$).

ventions to improve referrals from one source of care to another and to improve adherence with recommendations for screening that merit "honorable mention": they fell short in study design only in that they did not assess the effect of the intervention on patient outcomes. Jones and her colleagues [31, 32] found that referral of patients from an emergency department for needed follow-up care could be improved by counseling the patients according to their perceptions ("health beliefs") about the benefits and costs of follow-up.

To increase hypertension screening, McDowell, Newell, and Rosser [42] tested three ways of encouraging patients in a large family practice to obtain a blood pressure check. Computer-generated reminders to physicians when patients were to visit for other purposes was the most cost-effective method, followed by a letter sent to patients, with phone calls to patients by nurses being least effective.

For cancer screening, randomized trials have shown that mailed invitations to breast cancer screening were more successful if they offered a specific appointment time (to be changed by telephone if necessary) rather than an open invitation [77]. Pierce and colleagues [55] found equal effectiveness from tagging patients' charts for the next visit to their physician (whatever the reason for the visit) and from a letter of invitation in improving screening rates for cervical cancer. Compliance with advice for colon cancer screening was increased by all three of the strategies: a talk from the physician or nurse, a reminder postcard or a reminder phone call, with the postcard being both most effective and lowest in cost [73]. Finally, again for colorectal cancer screening, Nichols and colleagues [52] found that invitation from a general practitioner during a routine visit was most effective (57%), followed by sending an appointment to the patient (49%), and sending a letter and a hemoccult test to the patient (38%). In this latter study, providing the patient with an educational pamphlet did not improve compliance. (Note that the efficacy of hemoccult testing for lowering morbidity and mortality from colon cancer remains uncertain.)

These studies demonstrate a number of ways to increase successful referral and screening appointments. Opportunistic screening (through flagging the patient's chart), letters with specific appointments, counseling, and special referral clerks were also effective. Unfortunately, only one study has shown that patients were better off as a result of their better compliance.

IMPROVING ATTENDANCE AT APPOINTMENTS

When we wrote this edition there were still no studies that documented whether strategies specifically designed to increase attendance at follow-up appointments resulted in improved treatment outcomes. In testing an intervention with broader objectives than just improving attendance, Smith and his colleagues [67, 68] reported an increase in attendance at scheduled visits for diabetics who received a complex intervention including a wallet card; a larger card with instructions giving symptoms that warrant calling the nurse or doctor; a booklet on diabetes care; a postcard reminder before each visit; a letter, followed by phone calls, after missed appointments; and a home visit if other methods had failed. Unfortunately, there were no differences in adverse outcomes (such as nonelective hospitalizations, emergency room visits, deaths, entry into dialysis programs, and so on) from any intervention.

There were a small number of "honorable mention" studies that met all the guides except for documenting treatment outcomes. Some found that attendance at scheduled appointments was increased by 15 to 20% by telephone [21, 66] or mail [21, 43, 66] reminders. There was no difference in the potency of telephone and mail reminders in these studies, but the latter were less expensive. It appeared, however, that the effect of reminders wore off as early as the second appointment [21], and one controlled trial found no deterioration in appointment keeping when mailed reminders were discontinued at a pediatric clinic [46].

In the absence of ironclad evidence, we offer the following two provisional conclusions: first, patients should be recalled if they miss an appointment; second, reminders before appointments have at least a short-term influence on attendance and can be used as needed. Whether patients who miss appointments are better off for having responded to one of these maneuvers remains to be demonstrated. Table 8-14 summarizes the positive findings.

IMPROVING COMPLIANCE WITH SHORT-TERM MEDICAL REGIMENS

Two studies met all the guides we posed, and they are summarized in Table 8-10.

Careful instruction on the need for taking all the tablets prescribed over a 10-day course of penicillin for streptococcal pharyngitis has improved both compliance and success in eradicating the bug [9]. Happily, this strategy was about as successful as giving patients a long-acting intramuscular injection of penicillin (ouch!).

What about simplifying the regimen? In the other well-designed study, there were modest but statistically significant improvements in compliance, and a clinically trivial but statistically significant improvement in one of several measures of respiratory function among asthmatics prescribed a twice-a-day theophylline preparation in comparison with the usual four-times-a-day schedule [74]. This particular strategy has potential for widespread application, although reducing the frequency of dosing probably does not have the large effect on compliance claimed in many pharmaceutical advertisements [23]. Three studies which met all review criteria except for the assessment of patient outcomes provide consistent support for a small benefit of reduced dosing frequency [2, 8, 71].

For some infections, an alternative solution might be to take advantage of the single, large, oral doses of medication that have proven as effective as longer courses of treatment for such conditions as uncomplicated urinary tract infections and some venereal diseases. However, care must be taken that the shorter treatment course is truly as efficacious. As Schwartz and colleagues have shown [63], a 7-day course of oral penicillin V for streptococcal pharyngitis is not as efficacious as a 10-day course for preventing relapses of pharyngitis. So the options for this particular disorder appear to be clear instructions for a 10-day course or a single, intramuscular injection, not a shortened oral course.

"Honorable mention" goes to some other interventions that have been shown to improve compliance but have not been tested for their power to improve treat-

Table 8-10. Improving compliance with short-term medications

Citation	Condition	Strategy	Compliance measure	Effect on compliance (%)[a]	Effect on treatment outcome[b]
Colcher and Bass [9]	Strep throat	1. Instruction by therapist	Urine bioassay	+ 22	Improved
		2. Intramuscular injection	Direct observation	+ 29	Improved
Tinkelman, Vanderpool, Carroell, et al. [74]	Asthma	Twice-a-day vs. four-a-day theophylline	Serum drug levels; pill count	+ 3.3	Improved

[a]Figures are derived by subtracting the percentage of patients judged compliant in the control group from the percentage compliant in the intervention group; all figures reported are statistically significant ($P < .05$).
[b]Improvement in outcomes is statistically significant in all studies.

ment outcomes. Compliance improvements have been shown following both written [35, 64] and verbal instructions [11] for short treatments. These reports suggest that it is unnecessary to convey an elaborate explanation of the illness and its treatment; it suffices to provide a simple but clear statement that the medication is to be taken until all that is prescribed has been consumed. Additional approaches that have been tested without documenting outcomes include pill calendars [11, 35], unit dose packaging [35], attempts by physicians or nurses to overcome medication and appointment scheduling difficulties and other compliance barriers [17, 18], and special pill containers with alarm devices [1]. These strategies hardly seem worth the effort, however, when one can do as well or better just through giving simpler instructions and reducing the frequency of dosing to the minimum required for efficacy. Furthermore, Cockburn and her coinvestigators found no additional benefit of written instruction or tailoring the medication schedule to the patient's usual activities when the medication prescription was for just once or twice a day [8]. The exact duration of effect of special instructions and pill packaging is not clear from these studies, but it appears reasonable to ascribe a "half-life" to the motivating effect of about 10 days to 2 weeks. This should not be confused with the effect of information programs on patient knowledge: information is frequently retained long after compliance has fallen off [24].

Finally, Maiman and her co-workers [38] found, in a randomized trial, that the compliance of pediatric patients with antibiotics for otitis media was improved if their pediatricians received tutorials and printed materials on understanding and improving compliance, or were sent the printed materials in the mail.

Achieving high, short-term compliance is relatively straightforward. Keep the regimen simple (single dose if possible, once or twice a day otherwise) and provide explicit instructions about how long to continue the treatment.

IMPROVING COMPLIANCE WITH LONG-TERM MEDICAL REGIMENS

If you currently see any ambulatory patients with chronic disorders for whom you have prescribed an ongoing medical treatment, what methods do you actually use to assure high compliance? If you use more than one method, do you apply them alone or in combination? Whether or not you currently see chronically ill ambulatory patients, what compliance maneuvers do you feel are effective? Write down your responses in the space below and then we will compare notes.

Compliance-improving strategies that I use	Alone or in combination?	Compliance-improving strategies that I think work

Logan [36, 37] asked similar questions of primary care physicians in Toronto, and focused on their management of hypertensive patients. Their responses are summarized in Table 8-11.

As shown in Table 8-11, (41% + 24% + 9% =) 74% of the Toronto physicians reported using one form or another of patient instruction ("explain risks/complications," "give them literature," "scare them") while less than one-third as many utilized what might be termed *behaviorally oriented strategies* (such as "frequent follow-ups" and "simplest possible dosage of drugs"). In the lower panel of the table we see that less than half of these physicians contacted patients who missed appointments and, of those who did, less than half contacted nonattenders routinely.

How do your own methods stack up against these? Do you use just instructional approaches like most Toronto doctors? Do you wait for nonattenders to contact you?

To find the truth about strategies to improve long-term compliance, we screened compliance-intervention studies with the same guides as before, plus a new one: Were the patients followed for at least 6 months? At the time that we wrote this book, 15 studies had been published that met all 6 guides. We will begin with the bad news and save the good news for last. Table 8-12 summarizes 7 randomized clinical trials that have exposed the futility of a variety of compliance strategies. Because these studies had sample sizes ranging from 115 to 1381, none was likely to have missed a clinically important benefit.

Table 8-11. What primary care practitioners in Toronto do to improve the compliance of their hypertensive patients

Actions taken to encourage patients to take their medication	Number of physicians (%)*
Explain risks/complications	31 (41)
Educate the patient/give them literature	18 (24)
Scare them	7 (9)
See the patient on a regular basis/frequent follow-ups	6 (8)
Pep talks/persuasion	5 (7)
Use simplest possible dosage of drugs	3 (4)
Try not to frighten the patient	3 (4)
Nothing	5 (7)
Other	7 (9)
Actions taken if patient does not appear for a prearranged appointment	
Wait for patient to make new appointment	41 (55)
Contact patient—sometimes	18 (24)
Contact patient—always	15 (20)
Other	1 (1)

*Figures add up to more than 100% because a small number of physicians reported using more than one action.

Adapted from A. G. Logan. *Investigation of Toronto General Practitioners' Treatment of Patients with Hypertension.* Toronto: Canadian Facts, 1978.

Table 8-12. Randomized trials demonstrating the futility of some strategies claimed to improve compliance with long-term medical regimens

Citation	Strategy	Compliance measure	Effect on compliance[a]	Effect on outcome[b]
Sackett, Haynes, Gibson, et al. [61]	Programmed teaching	Pill count	NS	NS
	Worksite care	Pill count	NS	NS
Shepard, Foster, Stason, et al. [65]	Self-monitoring	Attendance	NS for both compliance and outcome for all 3 measures for all 4 study groups	
	Nurse counseling	Dropouts		
	Tangible rewards	Interview		
	Peer group discussion			
Levine, Green, Deeds, et al. [33]	Counseling by health educators	Interview	NS	NS
		Weight loss	+ 21%	
		Attendance	NS	
Swain and Steckel [70]	Educational pamphlets	Dropouts	− 28%	NS
Johnson, Taylor, Sackett, et al. [30]	Home visits	Pill count	NS	NS
	Self-monitoring	Pill count	NS	NS
Spriet, Beiler, Dechorgnat, and Simon [69]	Unit dose packaging ± memory aid stickers	Pill count	NS	NS
Smith, Norton, Weinberger [67]	Wallet card	Attendance	+ 12%[c]	NS
	Written instructions			
	Postcard appointment reminders			
	Follow-up for missed appointments			

[a]Report as NS (nonsignificant) if effect not statistically significant; for significant effects figure derived by subtracting percentage of patients judged compliant in the control group from percentage compliant in intervention group.
[b]NS = no significant effect on therapeutic outcome.
[c]Calculated as a percentage increase in attended scheduled appointments

In the studies summarized in Table 8-12, all but one of the strategies were tested singly. Although it is clinically important to know that these simple methods are ineffective in isolation, some of them, as we shall see, became components of packages of interventions that did improve compliance. The first four studies tested approaches that instructed patients about their illnesses and the need for continued adherence to treatment [24, 33, 65, 70]. None of these studies found any influence on treatment outcome, and two of them found no influence even on compliance. A third documented improved weight loss but no change in pill taking or attendance [33] and the fourth found that educational pamphlets actually produced a substantial increase in dropouts [70]. We also unearthed 7 other "Honorable Mention" studies that concluded that instruction does not have a lasting influence on compliance [4, 6, 7, 13, 27, 39]. Of course, 11 studies are not really sufficient to test the infinite varieties of instructional content and format that are possible. Nevertheless, a consensus such as this is very rare in the medical literature and strikes us as sufficient to compel anyone who proposes an instructional program as a rational approach for gaining compliance with long-term treatments to test it in a proper randomized trial before adopting it or advocating its use by others.

These negative trials of instructional strategies should not be misinterpreted as a condemnation of either "patient education" (which nowadays goes far beyond instruction and includes all sorts of behavioral strategies) or of informing patients about their illnesses and their management. There are other reasons to instruct patients about their diseases: Patients cannot comply with a regimen if they do not know what it is; and they also need to be informed about their treatments for their safety. Finally, as we already have seen, instruction improves short-term compliance.

The important message in this body of evidence is that, for whatever reasons we decide to instruct our patients, we should not delude ourselves that this instruction will improve their long-term compliance (and must recognize that it may increase their risk of dropping out of care).

The final study in Table 8-12, by Smith and colleagues [67, 68], has already been mentioned in the section on attendance at appointments. No effect was observed on important treatment outcomes during the follow-up of the 859 diabetic patients in this investigation despite a multipronged intervention to increase attendance at scheduled appointments and improve the timeliness of patients reporting deteriorations in their health.

Four additional comments about Table 8-12 are in order. First, although the self-monitoring of blood pressure, blood sugar, weight, and other treatment outcomes has recently become popularized as a method of improving adherence to therapy, the second and fifth entries in this table [30, 65] found no benefit of self-monitoring as the sole compliance-improving strategy in hypertension. Second, although treatment at the worksite has also become popularized, it was not useful when it constituted just a change in the site where care was delivered [61]. Third, unit-dose packaging (regardless of whether it was accompanied by stickers that reminded patients about their regimen) was found to improve neither compliance nor blood pressure control in the only satisfactory study we have found [69]. An "honorable mention" study (which did assess outcomes (no effect) but reported only 3 months of follow-up) backs up this finding [3]. Finally, as yet, there is no magic bullet or cure for noncompliance: single interventions do not work.

Turning now to the good news, Table 8-13 summarizes nine trials that provide

Table 8-13. Randomized trials of successful compliance-improving strategies for long-term medical regimens

Citation	Strategy	Compliance measure	Effect on compliance*
Feinstein, Wood, Epstein, et al. [16]	Intramuscular injection and retrieval of dropouts	Attendance/ interview	+ 51%
Feinstein, Spagnuolo, Jonas, et al. [15]	Intramuscular injection and retrieval of dropouts	Attendance/ interview	+ 58%
Haynes, Sackett, Gibson, et al. [24]	Self-monitoring and cueing of positive reinforcement	Pill count	+ 21%
Levine, Green, Deeds, et al. [33]	Alone and in combination: counseling, family support, group discussions	Interview/ attendance	See text
Logan, Milne, Achber, et al. [37]	Nurse management at worksite and cueing, self-monitoring, reinforcement	Interview plus pill count	+ 19%
Nessman, Carnahan, and Nugent [51]	Self-monitoring and group discussion and management of drug protocol	Pill count Attendance	+ 19% + 15%
Swain and Steckel [70]	Contingency contracting and instruction pamphlets	Attendance	+ 28%
Takala, Niemela, Rosti, and Silvers [72]	Written instruction and feedback and recalls to nonattenders	Attendance	+ 15%
Pederson, McLean, Millingon [54]	Counseling and med container plus self-monitoring and mailed reminders	Prescription refills	+ 38%

*Figures derived by subtracting the percentage of patients judged compliant in the control group from the percentage compliant in the intervention group. All figures are statistically significant ($P < .05$) and all compliant improvements were associated with statistically significant improvements in treatment benefit.

a solid base for clinical policy and practice to improve compliance with long-term medical regimens.

The interventions listed in Table 8-13 are diverse, and we will discuss them individually. One highly effective method of limited applicability is to inject a long-acting medication parenterally, as in the prophylactic treatment of rheumatic fever [15, 16]. So long as the patient shows up for appointments, compliance with medications is guaranteed. Thus, to insure that the patient does attend, there must be an outreach service to retrieve nonattenders. A few other treatments can or must be given parenterally, such as fluphenazine for psychotic disorders [14] and insulin for diabetes [76], and investigation of them suggests that it is not so much the parenteral nature of the treatment as the supervision of its administration that is the key ingredient. On the other hand, the advent of implantable controlled-release devices [75] may minimize even the need for supervision.

Self-monitoring is another strategy that did not work well when tested alone [30, 65]. However, it has been part of several successful compound interventions that improve compliance in hypertension when included with positive reinforcement for improvements in compliance and blood pressure [24], nurse supervision at the worksite [36, 37], or group discussions combined with self-management of drug regimens [51].

A strategy that has received only limited testing but appears to hold promise, at least when combined with other methods, is soliciting and encouraging family support for the patient [33]. The attraction of this tactic is that it adds reinforcement for compliance into the patient's immediate environment and so may reduce the amount and cost of input required from clinicians. At the same time, some obvious potential dangers of this strategy require systematic study before it can be advocated. Family dynamics may be upset by making other family members responsible for, and giving them power over, the patient. Furthermore, other family members may be no more compliant than the patient and thus fail to follow through on their tasks!

Group discussions, in combination with other methods, provide another medium for enhancing compliance [33, 51]. One study reported long-lasting improvements in both attendance and medication compliance when the group discussions focused on self-help and included self-monitoring and even self-selection of medications from a standard protocol [51]. One difficulty identified by this latter study is its generalizability and overall impact; only about 10% of the noncompliant patients approached about this trial agreed to take part in it! The combination of counseling by a health educator, group discussions, and engendering social support through home visits improved compliance and blood pressures over a year [33] and, of special interest, a 5 year follow-up of the patients in this study revealed increased survival among patients assigned to the combined intervention group [49].

One conclusion from these positive trials is that the more attention is focused directly on the behaviors required in taking therapy as prescribed, the greater adherence will be. This general observation is given additional credence by the substantial success of a procedure called *contingency contracting* [70]. This involves the negotiation of a very brief contract at each visit in which patients agree, in writing, to perform some act that will assist them to achieve the treatment target, in return for which they will receive a suitable reward. For example, a patient might negotiate to lose 1 pound in return for having the next appointment scheduled at a more convenient time. Clearly, continued success depends on identifying a steady stream of both clinically significant compliance behaviors and rewards that are both affordable and legal. We'll try this one out on you in Chapter 14!

Pederson and colleagues [54] studied the value of a combination of maneuvers among epileptic patients, including self-monitoring, a special medication container, and mailed reminders to collect prescription refills and attend clinic appointments. There was a substantial increase in the proportion of patients who obtained prescription refills according to the prescribed schedule and a statistically significant reduction in the number of seizures in the intervention group, but not in the control subjects.

Several of the successful interventions discussed here are at best awkward and at worst too expensive for most clinical settings. Accordingly, Takala and colleagues [72] tested a highly practical three-step strategy in primary care. First, patients were given brief, written instructions about their regimens. Second, at each visit patients were given feedback about their treatment responses. Finally, any patients who missed an appointment were contacted, and a new appointment was scheduled. Both compliance and treatment responses improved.

These positive trials also revealed the lack of importance of two other features. First, no single type of health professional is essential. In fact, successful interventions have been executed by physicians, nurses, pharmacists, health educators, psychologists, and even one individual with no professional training at all. The common element is *what* is done (some sort of supervision aimed directly at the compliance problem), not *who* does it. Second, the provider and the patient must meet someplace, but it does not seem to matter where. Successful interventions have taken place in community health centers, general medical clinics, specialty clinics, pharmacies, worksites, and patients' homes.

Finally, all of the trials that continued to monitor compliance after an effective strategy was withdrawn documented a deterioration in compliance, often very rapid, back toward or to its prior low level. Permanent improvements in compliance appear to require permanent interventions.

Some Practical Conclusions

Although this chapter has distilled several thousand pages, we have still presented an enormous amount of information for you to digest. If we were to distill it further into a set of practical recommendations, what would they look like? Table 8-14 represents our best effort, but if we have accomplished our overriding objective of helping you become vigorous sceptics, you will pay it no more than a passing glance and will generate your own approach from the newer, better information that has accumulated in the time since we wrote this.

Although our review covered a lot of territory, it did not include interventions

Table 8-14. Some practical (but by now dated) conclusions

To detect low compliance
1. Watch for nonattenders
2. Watch for nonresponders
3. Ask the patient

To improve compliance
With referrals
1. Tell the patient what to expect
2. Help the patient make a convenient appointment

With appointments
1. Mail reminders (particularly if there is a long period between appointments)
2. Recall non-attenders if follow-up is important

With short-term treatments
1. Give simple, clear instructions (in writing, if possible)
2. Give injections rather than pills (when it makes sense)
3. Prescribe the minimum number of doses per day that will achieve the treatment target

With long-term treatments: (add at least two of the following)
4. Increase the supervision of noncompliers (e.g., more frequent visits; involve nurse, pharmacist, family)
5. Direct everybody's attention to the compliance problem (discussion, self-monitoring)
6. Encourage higher compliance—reminders
7. Reinforce good compliance when it occurs—recognize the patient's efforts to comply
8. Keep up compliance interventions as long as high compliance is desirable (it may be possible to titrate the "dose" of the strategy downwards at times).

to improve compliance with regimens that require substantial changes in behavior (such as cessation of bad habits and adoption of good ones). The success of maneuvers to increase compliance with such advice is generally less, but some progress is being made [5]. There are also some maneuvers that practitioners use in everyday practice to improve compliance that have not been tested in randomized clinical trials. For example, there may be several elements of the practitioner-patient relationship that affect compliance strongly, but there is no way to be sure until they are studied carefully.

In closing, we must not forget that there are circumstances when compliance is not in patients' interests, often for reasons best or only known to them; they will always maintain their right to refuse treatment. However, most noncompliance is unintentional and occurs through default or neglect, not active refusal. Patients can only realize the full benefits of efficacious treatments if we help them identify their low compliance and then help them overcome it.

Family Physicians' Estimates of Compliance Among Patients on Digoxin

The measures of performance for family physicians' estimates of compliance among patients on digoxin shown in Table 8-1 are as follows:

Prevalence (or pretest probability) of low compliance:

$$\frac{a + c}{a + b + c + d} = \frac{21}{71} = 30\%$$

Sensitivity of clinical judgment:

$$\frac{a}{a + c} = \frac{2}{21} = 10\%$$

Specificity of clinical judgment:

$$\frac{d}{b + d} = \frac{43}{50} = 86\%$$

Probability of low compliance when doctor predicted it (positive predictive value):

$$\frac{a}{a + b} = \frac{2}{9} = 22\%$$

Probability of high compliance when doctor predicted it (negative predictive value):

$$\frac{d}{c + d} = \frac{43}{62} = 69\%$$

Overall accuracy:

$$\frac{a + d}{a + b + c + d} = \frac{45}{71} = 63\%$$

Likelihood ratio for clinical judgment of low compliance:

$$\frac{a}{a + c} \div \frac{b}{b + d} = \frac{2}{21} \div \frac{7}{50} = .68$$

Likelihood ratio for clinical judgment of high compliance:

$$\frac{c}{a + c} \div \frac{d}{b + d} = \frac{19}{21} \div \frac{43}{50} = 1.05$$

References

1. Azrin, N. H. and Powel, J. Behavioral engineering: The use of response priming to improve prescribed self-medication. *J. Appl. Behav. Anal.* 2: 39, 1969.
2. Baird, M. G., Bentley-Taylor, M. M., Carruthers, S. G., et al. A study of the ef-

ficacy, tolerance and compliance of once-daily versus twice-daily metoprolol (Betaloc®) in hypertension. *Clin. Invest. Med.* 7: 95, 1984.
3. Becker, L. A., Glanz, K., Sobel, E., et al. A randomized trial of special packaging of antihypertensive medications. *J. Fam. Practice* 22: 357, 1986.
4. Bowen, R. G., Rich, R., and Schlotfeldt, R. M. Effects of organized instruction for patients with the diagnosis of diabetes mellitus. *Nurs. Res.* 10: 151, 1961.
5. Cameron, R., and Best, J. A. Promoting adherence to health behavior change interventions: recent findings from behavioral research. *Patient Educ. Counsel.* 10: 139, 1987.
6. Caplan, R. D., Robinson, E., French, J., et al. *Adhering to Medical Regimens: Pilot Experiments in Patient Education and Social Support.* Institute for Social Research, University of Michigan, Ann Arbor, 1976.
7. Clinite, J., and Kabat, H. Improving patient compliance. *J. Am. Pharm. Assoc.* 16: 74, 1976.
8. Cockburn, J., Reid, A. L., Bowman, J. A., and Sanson-Fisher, R. W. Effects of intervention on antibiotic compliance in general practice. *Med. J. Australia* 147: 324, 1987.
9. Colcher, I. S., and Bass, J. W. Penicillin treatment of streptococcal pharyngitis: A comparison of schedules and the role of specific counseling. *J.A.M.A.* 222: 657, 1972.
10. Cramer, J. A., Mattson, R. H., Prevey, M. L., et al. How often is medication taken as prescribed? A novel assessment technique. *J.A.M.A.* 261: 3273, 1989.
11. Dickey, F. F., Matter, M. E., and Chudzik, G. M. Pharmacist counselling increases drug regimen compliance. *Hospitals* 49: 85, 1975.
12. England, M. L., and Hershman, J. M. Serum TSH concentration as an aid to monitoring compliance with thyroid hormone in hypothyroidism. *Am. J. Med. Sci.* 292: 264, 1986.
13. Etzwiler, D. D., and Robb, J. R. Evaluation of programmed education among juvenile diabetics and their families. *Diabetes* 21: 967, 1972.
14. Falloon, I., Watt, D. C., and Shepard, M. A comparative controlled trial of pimozide and fluphenazine decanoate in a continuation therapy of schizophrenia. *Psychol. Med.* 8: 59, 1978.
15. Feinstein, A. R., Spagnuolo, M., Jonas, S., et al. Prophylaxis of recurrent rheumatic fever. *J.A.M.A.* 206: 565, 1968.
16. Feinstein, A. R., Wood, H. F., Epstein, J. A., et al. A controlled study of three methods of prophylaxis against streptococcal infection in a population of rheumatic children: II. Results of the first three years of the study, including methods for evaluating the maintenance of oral prophylaxis. *N. Engl. J. Med.* 260: 697, 1959.
17. Fink, D., Malloy, M. J., Cohen, M., et al. Effective patient care in the pediatric setting: A study of the acute care clinic. *Pediatrics* 43: 927, 1969.
18. Fink, D., Martin, F., Cohen, M., et al. The management specialist in effective pediatric ambulatory care. *Am. J. Public Health* 59: 527, 1969.
19. Fletcher, S., Appel, F., and Bourgois, M. Management of hypertension: Effect of improving patient compliance for follow-up care. *J.A.M.A.* 233: 242, 1975.
20. Gart, J. J. Point and interval estimation of the common odds ratio in the combination of 2 × 2 tables with fixed marginals. *Biometrika* 57: 471; 1970.
21. Gates, S. J., and Colburn, D. K. Lowering appointment failures in a neighborhood health center. *Med. Care* 14: 263, 1976.
22. Gilbert, J. R., Evans, C. E., Haynes, R. B., and Tugwell, P. Predicting compliance with a regimen of digoxin therapy in family practice. *Can. Med. Assoc. J.* 123: 119, 1980.
23. Haynes, R. B. Influence on Compliance. In K. C. Mezey (ed.), *Fixed Drug Combinations: Rationale and Limitations.* London: Royal Society of Medicine/Academic Press, 1980. Pp. 59–64.

24. Haynes, R. B., Sackett, D. L., Gibson, E. S., et al. Improvement in medication compliance in uncontrolled hypertension. *Lancet* 1: 1265, 1976.
25. Haynes, R. B., Taylor, D. W., and Sackett, D. L. *Compliance in Health Care*. Baltimore: Johns Hopkins, 1979.
26. Haynes, R. B., Taylor, D. W., Sackett, D. L., et al. Can simple clinical measurements detect patient noncompliance? *Hypertension* 2: 757, 1980.
27. Hecht, A. B. Improving medication compliance by teaching outpatients. *Nurs. Forum* 13: 112, 1974.
28. Hoehn-Saric, R., Frank, J., Imber, S., et al. Systematic preparation of patients for psychotherapy: I. Effects on therapy behavior and outcome. *J. Psychiatr. Res.* 2: 267, 1964.
29. Inui, T. S. Screening for noncompliance among patients with hypertension. Is self-report the best available measure? *Med. Care* 19: 1061, 1981.
30. Johnson, A. L., Taylor, D. W., Sackett, D. L., et al. Self-recording of blood pressure in management of hypertension. *Can. Med. Assoc. J.* 119: 1034, 1978.
31. Jones, S. L., Jones, P. K., and Katz, J. Health belief model intervention to increase compliance with emergency department patients. *Med. Care* 26: 1172, 1988.
32. Jones, S. L., Jones, P. K., and Katz, J. Compliance for low-back pain patients in the emergency department. *Spine* 13: 553, 1988.
33. Levine, D. M., Green, L. W., Deeds, S. G., et al. Health education for hypertensive patients. *J.A.M.A.* 241: 1700, 1979.
34. Levine, R. J. Ethical Considerations in the Development and Application of Compliance Strategies for the Treatment of Hypertension. In R. B. Haynes, M. E. Mattson, and T. O. Engebretson, Jr. (eds.), *Patient Compliance to Prescribed Antihypertensive Medication Regimens*. Washington, D.C.: Government Printing Office, N.I.H. No. 80–2102,1980.
35. Linkewich, J. A., Catalano, R. B., and Flack, H. L. The effect of packaging and instruction on outpatient compliance with medication regimens. *Drug Intell. Clin. Pharm.* 8: 10, 1974.
36. Logan, A. G. *Investigation of Toronto General Practitioners' Treatment of Patients with Hypertension*. Toronto: Canadian Facts, 1978.
37. Logan, A. G., Milne, B. J., Achber, C., et al. Worksite treatment of hypertension by specially trained nurses: A controlled trial. *Lancet* 2: 1175, 1979.
38. Maiman, L. A., Becker, M. H., Liptak, G. S., et al. Improving pediatricians' compliance-enhancing practices. *A.J.D.C.* 142: 773, 1988.
39. Malahy, B. The effect of instruction and labeling on the number of medication errors made by patients at home. *Am. J. Hosp. Pharm.* 23: 283, 1966.
40. Mantel, N., and Haenszel, W. Statistical aspects of the analysis of data from retrospective studies of disease. *J. Natl. Cancer Inst.* 22: 719, 1959.
41. Materson, B. J., Oster, J. R., Michael, U. F., et al. Dose response to chlorthalidone in patients with mild hypertension. Efficacy of a lower dose. *Clin. Pharmacol. Ther.* 24: 192, 1978.
42. McDowell, I., Newell, C., and Rosser, W. A randomized trial of computerized reminders for blood pressure screening in primary care. *Med. Care* 27: 297, 1989.
43. Meller, W., and Anderson, A. Medical compliance, the effect of appointment reminders on keeping appointments in a core city pediatric outpatient department. *Minn. Med.* 59: 625, 1976.
44. Mitchell, A., Haynes, R. B., Adsett, C. A., et al. Likelihood of remaining normotensive following antihypertensive drug withdrawal. *J. Gen. Intern. Med.* 4: 221, 1989.
45. Mollica, J. A. Monitoring compliance through analysis of drug and metabolite levels. *Controlled Clin. Trials* 5: 505, 1984.
46. Morse, D. L., Coulter, M. P., Nazarian, L. F., et al. Warning effectiveness of mailed reminders on reducing broken appointments. *Pediatrics* 68: 846, 1981.

47. Moulding, T., Onstad, G. D., and Sbarbaro, J. A. Supervision of outpatient drug therapy with the medication monitor. *Ann. Intern. Med.* 73: 559, 1970.
48. Mulrow, C. D., Thacker, S. B., Pugh, J. A. A proposal for more informative abstracts of review articles. *Ann. Intern. Med.* 108: 613, 1988.
49. Morisky, D. Five-year blood pressure control and mortality following health education for hypertensive patients. *Am. J. Public Health* 73: 153, 1983.
50. Nelson, A. A., Jr., Gold, B. H., Hutchinson, R. A., and Benezra, A. Drug default among schizophrenic patients. *Am. J. Hosp. Pharm.* 32: 1237, 1975.
51. Nessman, D. G., Carnahan, J. E., and Nugent, C. A. Increasing compliance. Patient-operated hypertension groups. *Arch. Intern. Med.* 140: 1427, 1980.
52. Nichols, S., Koch, E., Lallemand, R. C., et al. Randomised trial of compliance with screening for colorectal screening. *B.M.J.* 293: 107, 1986.
53. Norell, S. E. Monitoring compliance with pilocarpine therapy. *Am. J. Ophthalmol.* 92: 727, 1981.
54. Pederson, G. M., McLean, S., and Millingen, K. S. A randomized trial of strategies to improve patient compliance with anticonvulsant therapy. *Epilepsia* 25: 412, 1984.
55. Pierce, M., Luny, S., Palanisamy, A., et al. Prospective randomized trial of methods of call and recall for cervical cytology screening. *B.M.J.* 299: 160, 1989.
56. Roth, H. P. Measurement of compliance. *Patient Educ. Couns.* 10: 107, 1987.
57. Roth, H. P., and Berger, D. G. Studies on patient cooperation in ulcer treatment. *Gastroenterology* 38: 630, 1960.
58. Roth, H. P., and Caron, H. S. Accuracy of doctors' estimates and patients' statements on adherence to a drug regimen. *Clin. Pharmacol. Ther.* 23: 361, 1978.
59. Roth, H. P., Caron, H. S., and Hsi, B. P. Estimating a patient's cooperation with his regimen. *Am. J. Med. Sci.* 262: 269, 1971.
60. Sackett, D. L., and Gent, M. Controversy in counting and attributing events in clinical trials. *N. Engl. J. Med.* 301: 1410, 1979.
61. Sackett, D. L., Haynes, R. B., Gibson, E. S., et al. Randomized clinical trial of strategies for improving medication compliance in primary hypertension. *Lancet* 1: 1205, 1975.
62. Sackett, D. L., and Snow, J. C. The Magnitude of Compliance and Noncompliance. In R. B. Haynes, D. W. Taylor, and D. L. Sackett (eds.), *Compliance in Health Care*. Baltimore: Johns Hopkins, 1979. Pp. 11–22.
63. Schwartz, R. H., Wientzen, R. L., Pedreira, F., et al. Penicillin V for group A streptococcal pharyngotonsilitis, a randomized trial of seven versus ten day's therapy. *J.A.M.A.* 246: 1790, 1981.
64. Sharpe, T. R., and Mikeal, R. L. Patient compliance with antibiotic regimens. *Am. J. Hosp. Pharm.* 31: 479, 1974.
65. Shepard, D. S., Foster, S. B., Stason, W. B., et al. Cost-effectiveness of interventions to improve compliance with antihypertensive therapy. *Prev. Med.* 8: 229, 1979.
66. Shepard, D. S., and Moseley, T. A. Mailed versus telephoned appointment reminders to reduce broken appointments in a hospital outpatient department. *Med. Care* 14: 268, 1976.
67. Smith, D. M., Norton, J. A., Weinberger, M., et al. Increasing prescribed office visits: A controlled trial in patients with diabetes mellitus. *Med. Care* 24: 189, 1986.
68. Smith, D. M., Weinberger, M., and Katz, B. P. A controlled trial to increase office visits and reduce hospitalizations of diabetic patients. *J. Gen. Intern. Med.* 2: 232, 1987.
69. Spriet, A., Beiler, D., Dechorgnat, J., and Simon, P. Adherence of elderly patients to treatment with pentoxifylline. *Clin. Pharm. Ther.* 27: 1, 1980.
70. Swain, M. A., and Steckel, S. B. Influencing adherence among hypertensives. *Res. Nurs. Health* 4: 213, 1981.
71. Taggart, A. J., Johnston, G. D., and McDevitt, D. G. Does the frequency of daily dosage influence compliance with digoxin therapy? *Br. J. Clin. Pharmacol.* 1: 31, 1981.

72. Takala, J., Niemela, N., Rosti, J., and Sivers, K. Improving compliance with therapeutic regimens in hypertensive patients in a community health center. *Circulation* 59: 540, 1979.
73. Thompson, R. S., Michnich, M. E., Gray, J., et al. Maximizing compliance with hemoccult screening for colon cancer clinical practice. *Med. Care* 24: 904, 1986.
74. Tinkleman, D. G., Vanderpool, G. E., Carroll, M. S., et al. Compliance differences following administration of theophylline at six and twelve hour intervals. *Ann. Allergy* 44: 283, 1980.
75. Urquhart, J. Performance Requirements for Controlled-Release Dosage Forms: Therapeutic and Pharmacological Perspectives. In J. Urquhart (ed.), *Controlled-Release Pharmaceuticals.* Washington, D.C.: American Pharmaceutical Association, 1981. Pp. 1–48.
76. Watkins, J. D., Williams, T. F., Martin, D. A., et al. A study of diabetic patients at home. *Am. J. Publ. Health.* 57: 452, 1967.
77. Williams, E. M. I., and Vessey, M. P. Randomised trial of two strategies offering women mobile screening for breast cancer. *B.M.J.* 299: 158, 1989.
78. Wilson, D. M., Taylor, D. W., Gilbert, J. R., et al. A randomized trial of a family physician intervention for smoking cessation. *J.A.M.A.* 260: 1570, 1988.

9

Deciding Whether Your Treatment Has Done Harm

As this chapter was being rewritten, its authors were consulted:

1. To advise a general practitioner on whether captopril was a safe drug for a diabetic patient with proteinuria;*
2. To determine whether a patient's headache, nausea, diarrhea and visual symptoms were due to an antihypertensive multidrug regimen;
3. To rule on whether a rheumatoid patient's g-i bleed was caused by NSAIDs; and
4. To offer an opinion on whether fenoterol, a widely used bronchodilator, might be responsible for the deaths of some young asthmatics.

In each case, we were asked to pass judgment on whether a current or former therapy was doing harm; as well, we often were asked to suggest an alternative therapy† that would either reverse the harm or avoid its exacerbation.

Judgments of this sort must be made very frequently. At least 4% of medical admissions to acute general hospitals are claimed to be the result of adverse drug reactions, and four drugs were blamed for one-third of those occurring in the early 1970s (digoxin, aspirin, prednisone, and warfarin) [5, 6]. Reactions to diagnostic and therapeutic maneuvers are judged to befall an additional one-fifth to one-third of patients after they are admitted, and those who suffer them are likely to remain in the hospital more than 1 week longer than those who do not [30, 41].

On the other hand, if you have already read Chapter 2 it will come as no surprise to learn that even clinical pharmacologists disagree about whether a given patient has had an adverse drug reaction. For example, when three such clinicians reviewed 500 patients thought by their attending physicians to have suffered an adverse drug reaction, they disagreed on which drug was likely responsible in 36% of cases, on whether an adverse reaction really caused the admission in over half (57%) of cases, and on whether an adverse drug reaction contributed to death in over two-thirds (71%) of patients who died [21]. Moreover, the fact that an adverse reaction occurred *during* the administration of a drug provides incomplete evidence that it occurred *because* of the administration

*This example also raises the issue of keeping up to date, the subject of the next section of this book!
†Including, in the second example, an N-of-1 trial to really sort it out!

of the drug. In fact, when two clinical pharmacologists asked healthy university students and hospital staff who were not taking any medications whether they had experienced symptoms* often listed as side effects of drugs during the previous 72 hours, 81% said "yes" [33]. The median number of symptoms was two, and 7% reported six or more of them.

Faced with a problem that is pandemic yet controvertible, clinicians must equip themselves to answer two related questions:

1. Does this drug (or operation, or other treatment) cause that adverse effect in *some* patients? And, if so,
2. Did this drug (or operation, or other treatment) cause that adverse effect in *this particular* patient?

The remainder of this chapter will provide a framework for answering these two questions, and in doing so, it often will call upon the emerging field of pharmacoepidemiology [43].

Does This Drug (or Operation, or Other Treatment) Cause That Adverse Effect in Some Patients?

You can answer this question in two ways: You can borrow an answer worked out by someone else or you can generate your own. It makes sense to borrow the answer from someone else when it concerns a treatment that you rarely encounter and never prescribe yourself; you might as well accept the judgment of an acclaimed authority on the subject and save your precious reading time for other pursuits.

However, when the question concerns a drug (or operation, or other treatment) that you commonly prescribe or carry out, you ought to be able to answer the question for yourself. This involves tracking down and assessing the evidence (usually in the form of articles from biomedical journals) on whether the treatment causes the adverse effect. Because this assessment can be viewed as addressing a general question of *causation*, it therefore can benefit from what has been learned about asking and answering such questions in other fields. As it happens, there are some rules of evidence and readers' guides that can be applied to evidence on causation, and we will present them here. They are distilled from the work of a number of methodologists, most notably Austin Bradford Hill [14].

The application of these commonsense principles to the evidence presented in clinical articles (or other sources) can be distilled down to three readers' guides. They are of the same sorts as those you have already encountered when considering evidence about diagnostic tests, prognosis, and the beneficial effects of treatment. These guides are summarized in Table 9-1.

*The symptoms included rashes, hives, nightmares, sleepiness, dry mouth, diarrhea, headaches, nasal congestion, and the like.

Table 9-1. Readers' guides for determining etiology and causation

1. Is the study likely to provide a valid answer to the clinical question?
   a. Was the *type of study* the strongest that could have been performed under the circumstances?
   b. Were the opportunities for, and the determination of, *exposure* free from bias?
   c. Was the determination of *outcomes* (in a cohort study) or the distinction between *cases and controls* (in a case-control study) free from bias?

2. In reporting the *strength* of the association, were *both clinical and statistical significance* considered?
   a. If the relative risk/odds was statistically significantly greater than 1, was this increase clinically important?
   b. If the relative risk/odds was not statistically significantly greater than 1, was the study large enough to exclude a clinically important increased risk?

3. What happens when you apply *rules of evidence for causation*?
   a. Is the association *consistent* from study to study?
   b. Is the *temporal sequence* of exposure and outcome in the right direction?
   c. Is there a *dose-response gradient*?
   d. Does the association make *sense*?

First, clinicians can scan the Methods section of the article to see whether the study was likely to provide a valid answer to the clinical question. Second, readers can determine whether, in reporting the strength of the association between the treatment (exposure) and the adverse outcome, the authors considered both clinical and statistical significance. Third, you can apply a set of readers' guides to the report's findings. Let's go through each of these guides in greater detail.

IS THE STUDY LIKELY TO PROVIDE A VALID ANSWER TO THE CLINICAL QUESTION?

The issues here are three. First, *was the type of study the strongest that could have been performed under the circumstances*? Sometimes you can learn the basic method used in a study from its title; other times you must examine its abstract or methods. The first issue often can be resolved quickly, without having to read the Introduction or Discussion sections.

Suppose we were caring for a hypertensive man who developed impotence while taking thiazides, and therefore really wanted to find out whether thiazides caused impotence. What would be the strongest sort of study we could find in the clinical literature? Most of you, we hope, would start by looking for a true experiment in humans: a study in which hypertensive men would have been randomly allocated (by a system analagous to tossing a coin) to take thiazides or to take other drugs (ideally, if it were ethical, to placebos) and then followed to see how many in each group went on to become impotent.

Evidence from such a *randomized trial* is the soundest evidence we can ever obtain about causation (whether it concerns etiology, therapeutics, or any other

Table 9-2. A randomized trial

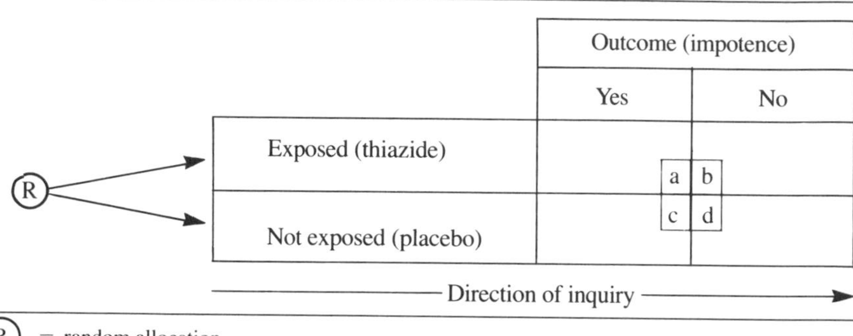

Ⓡ = random allocation.

causal issue), and the reasons for this have already been presented in Chapters 5 and 7. The basic architecture of the randomized trial is shown in Table 9-2.

As it happens, such strong evidence about whether thiazides (in this case, bendroflumethiazide) cause impotence (and several other symptoms) is available from the British Medical Research Council single-blind randomized trial of therapy in mild hypertension, and some of it is summarized in Table 9-3 [26].

The men in Table 9-3 all had sustained, untreated, fifth-phase diastolic blood pressures of 90 to 109 and were randomly allocated to receive a thiazide (bendroflumethiazide), a beta blocker (propranolol) or a placebo. Men randomized to the thiazide were 20 times as likely as men on placebo to be withdrawn from the trial because of impotence, and among those still on study drugs 2 years later, impotence was reported over twice as often by men on the thiazide than men on the placebo (both of these differences are statistically significant). This constitutes the strongest sort of evidence that at least this specific thiazide causes impotence.

Experiments sometimes have revealed quite dramatic, unexpected adverse reactions, even in clinical fields with long and proud traditions and records of subjecting treatments to randomized trials. For example, cardiologists had been doing randomized trials for decades when they tested encainide and flecainide against placebo in patients with asymptomatic or mildly symptomatic ventricular arrhythmias following myocardial infarction [7]. Despite all their prior experience and expertise, these cardiologists found themselves abruptly stopping the trial when it became clear that these drugs were increasing, not decreasing, the death rate among their patients.

Although the true experiment (randomized trial) would give us the most accurate (or valid) answer to a question of causation, and therefore represents the strongest method, we will not find it very often in our clinical reading. In the first place, of course, it is unethical to carry out randomized trials of agents suspected of harming those who are exposed to it. In many other cases it is not feasible to do a randomized trial to determine etiology, simply because of the numbers of patients required to demonstrate that a given adverse event is occurring more frequently in one treatment group than another. As it happens [36], to

Table 9-3. Evidence from a randomized trial about whether thiazides cause impotence

		Impotence	
		As a reason for withdrawal (rate/1000 patient years)	As a symptom at 2 years (prevalence)
Treatment group to which randomized	Bendroflumethiazide (5 mg bid)	20	23%
	Placebo	1	10%

Data from Medical Research Council Working Party. Adverse reactions to bendrofluazide and propranolol for the treatment of mild hypertension. *Lancet* 2:539, 1981.

be 95% confident of observing *one* (or more) adverse reactions to a drug, investigators need to follow *three times* the reciprocal of the true adverse reaction rate. This is, if the true rate is 1/1000 (which is roughly the rate at which patients on practolol developed eye damage), investigators would have to follow 3000 treated patients to be 95% confident of finding at least one such reaction.

Most new drugs are given to no more than 3000, and sometimes as few as 500, patients before they are put on the market [43]. From the foregoing, you can see that this number is sufficient to detect adverse reactions that occur between 1 and 6 times per thousand prescriptions. What if a serious adverse reaction occurred less often, affecting only 1 in 3000 patients who received it? Once again, you can see that you would need to carry out postmarketing surveillance on 9000 patients to be 95% confident of seeing at least one such adverse reaction.

Almost no randomized trials are large enough to detect even a few adverse reactions at these rates, and we are much more likely to encounter nonexperimental studies into the causation of the adverse effects of treatment. It's for this reason that this first issue considers the *circumstances* under which authors have had to work as well as the *strength* of the study design they employed.*

The next most powerful study method (the *cohort study*) would identify two groups (or cohorts) of patients, one cohort which did and the other which did not receive the treatment of interest. Such a study would then follow these two cohorts forward in time, counting the adverse events that occurred in each. In this case, the direction of inquiry is forward in time, as depicted in Table 9-4, which describes the British General Practitioners study of cohorts of patients who were and were not taking oral contraceptives [34].

*An occasional reader (and reviewer!) deduced that our first edition enshrined the randomized trial and trashed the case-control study as hopelessly flawed, thus adding to the "theater" that attends arguments about their relative merits [39]. We hope that this edition more clearly states our conviction that the cohort or case-control study often constitutes the only feasible approach to answering important questions about the risks of clinical interventions, and can generate results that are both valid and extremely useful.

Table 9-4. A cohort study

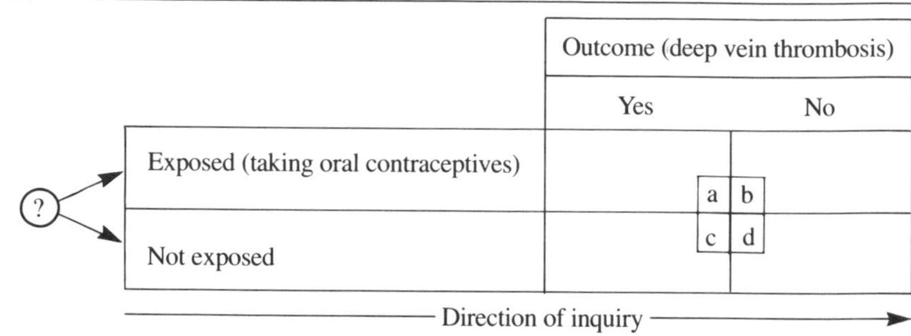

Outcome (deep vein thrombosis)
Yes
No
Exposed (taking oral contraceptives)
?
a
b
c
d
Not exposed
Direction of inquiry

The general practitioners following these patients diagnosed deep vein thrombosis in 41 of the oral contraceptive takers, but in only eight women who were not on oral contraceptive regimens, and calculated that the risk of deep vein thrombosis was almost six times as great among oral contraceptive takers. They therefore concluded that oral contraceptives cause deep vein thrombosis.

However, cohort studies of this sort are much weaker than randomized trials in establishing causation, and two reasons for this become clear when we consider who takes oral contraceptives and how one diagnoses deep vein thrombosis. First, because the clinician's decision to recommend, and the patient's decision to request or accept, oral contraceptives was not determined by random allocation, we have lost the guarantee (provided by randomization) that oral and nonoral contraceptive users are comparable. In fact, they are not; in the British study, oral contraceptive takers tended to be of higher parity, more likely to smoke, and less likely to have an important past history of diabetes, cerebrovascular disease, venous thromboembolism, or varicose veins. (Note that some of these characteristics increase, and others decrease, the risk of thromboembolism.)

Second, the hypothesis that oral contraceptives cause deep vein thrombosis was already well known at the start of the British study, and since oral contraceptive users had to see their physicians to have their prescriptions renewed, users had more frequent opportunities to be examined by unblinded physicians who already suspected that oral contraceptives cause deep vein thrombosis. These sources of potential bias [35] (the "diagnostic access" bias and the "diagnostic suspicion" bias) become all the more important when we realize that this study set down no objective criteria for what constituted deep vein thrombosis. Because less than half of patients with a clinical diagnosis of deep vein thrombosis can be shown, on objective testing by venography, actually to have this disorder [16], we would expect more deep vein thrombosis to be reported among oral contraceptive users even if the drug was innocent.

Our suspicion that cohort studies such as this one may not provide strong evidence about causation is boosted by the results of a randomized trial of oral versus nonoral contraceptives carried out among approximately 10,000 Puerto Rican women [23]. An initial list of 48 potential cases of thrombophlebitis was narrowed to 17 by a review panel of blinded internists (who excluded cases already present at entry that did not recur, postpartum thrombosis, and several cases that turned out to be lymphangitis, cellulitis, and the like). Of the 17 confirmed cases, nine occurred among women randomized to oral contraceptives and eight to women randomized to nonoral contraceptives. Accordingly, this randomized trial concluded (to the surprise of the investigators) that oral contraceptives carry a risk of thrombophlebitis somewhere between one-half to only twice that occurring when nonoral contraceptives are used (based on 95% confidence limits), not the sixfold risk generated in the cohort studies. We see, then, that we must view a nonexperimental study such as the cohort analytic study with caution.

A second type of nonexperimental study deserves even greater caution in interpretation, and this is the *case-control study.* In a case-control study, the investigator gathers "cases" of patients who already have suffered some adverse event and "controls" who have not. Both groups are then questioned (or their records examined) about whether they received the treatment of interest; if those patients who had the adverse outcome were more likely to have undergone the treatment, this would constitute some evidence, though not very strong, that the treatment might cause, or at least precipitate, the adverse outcome. So in this case the direction of inquiry is backwards in time, as shown in Table 9-5, representing a trio of studies that linked reserpine to breast cancer.

The September 21, 1974 issue of *The Lancet* delivered a bombshell in the form of three, back-to-back case-control studies that purported to show that reserpine, a drug then commonly used to treat hypertension, caused breast cancer [1, 3, 13]. Patients who had taken reserpine or its cousins had two to four times the risk of breast cancer as nonusers, and an accompanying editorial both concluded that the risks of rauwolfia outweighed its advantages and predicted "in the next few weeks most doctors must surely be reviewing their patients on these agents and reflecting on possible alternative treatments—or no treatment" [31]. Because reserpine was about the only adrenolytic drug approved for use in hypertension in the United States in those pre-beta blocker days, the concern among U.S. clinicians and their hypertensive patients was considerable, and the staunchness with which the investigators defended their conclusions in the

Table 9-5. A case control study

	Outcome (breast cancer)	
	Yes (cases)	No (controls)
Exposed (received reserpine)	a	b
Not exposed	c	d

◄—— Direction of inquiry ——

subsequent debate [4] only increased this burden of anxiety. Five years and eight more (mostly negative) investigations later, reserpine was exonerated. In fact, one of the consultants to the original study labeled it a "fluke" [44] and some of the original authors, in the best tradition of science, criticized both the execution of their earlier study and the fashion in which it was reported [38].

Why did we get this one wrong and precipitate so much controversy and suffering? Because scientists are still elucidating the proper methods for conducting case-control studies. For example, the original investigations of reserpine and breast cancer specifically excluded potential control subjects with cardiovascular diagnoses in order to render them "comparable" to the breast cancer cases, even though by doing so they excluded many hypertensive patients on reserpine. Critics found this exclusion "illogical and biased"; the investigators found their critics "naive." The resulting debate was good theater but only later did it address central methodologic issues in how case-control studies should be executed [10, 18].

By conducting case-control studies "after the fact," their investigators face a formidable series of potential biases [35]. It is because of this greater liability to bias that the case-control study is placed down near the weak end of the spectrum. Readers who want to learn more about these and other methodologic issues concerning case-control studies may benefit from reviewing the thick, theoretical "Bermuda Symposium" [18] or the thin, practical review for the clinician written by Hayden, Kramer, and Horwitz [12]. Those who want to pursue these issues at the highest level should consult the work of Miettinen [27].

If case-control studies are so liable to bias, why are there so many of them? The reasons are two. First, they are very easy to carry out and are becoming easier still as hospital records become computerized; one can execute literally hundreds of case-control studies at the push of a button simply by running all discharge diagnoses against all drug histories. We shall face more, not fewer, reserpine scares in the future.

The second reason that case-control studies will continue to be performed is that they constitute, at least for now, the only feasible method for studying rare and late adverse effects of drugs and other treatments. As we've already pointed out, randomized trials are neither big enough nor long enough to detect important but rare adverse effects. Until effective postmarketing surveillance systems become well established [19, 42, 43], we shall have to rely on case-control studies for most of our information on whether a given drug can cause a specific adverse reaction.

One final type of nonexperimental study deserves mention. This is the *case-series*, in which an investigator simply reports that one or more of his depressed patients developed arrhythmias while taking tricyclic antidepressants. No comparison group is included, and about all that the reader can conclude is that arrhythmias *can* (but not necessarily *must*) follow tricyclic antidepressant ingestion. This, after all, is what "spontaneous adverse drug reaction reports" are all about, and such case series, though often thought-provoking, are prone to overinterpretation, especially by their authors.* Because of their methodologic weakness, case series are best used to stimulate other, more powerful investigations. All too often, however, they provoke authoritarian (rather than authoritative) clinical advice about etiology, prevention, and therapy.

In summary, then, readers of reports purporting to show etiology or causation should begin by asking: Was the type of study the strongest that could have been performed under the circumstances? If the report at the top of the stack is a randomized trial, it constitutes the strongest possible evidence and usually can be trusted. If the strongest evidence you found comes from a cohort analytic study, although this evidence is usually weaker than that generated in a randomized trial, it is always preferred over a case-control study, and can sometimes be trusted. If the best you can find is a case-control study, you must recognize that this is a design that often has led to erroneous conclusions (such as the now discredited link between reserpine and breast cancer [38]); however, for some extremely rare disorders (especially rare adverse drug reactions) you may only have case-control studies to go by and may be forced, however reluctantly, to act upon their conclusions.

What if all you can find are one or more case-reports or a case-series? Unfortunately, it is not possible to tell whether any given case-series can, all by itself, be trusted on an issue of etiology or causation. The decision whether to use or ignore such evidence will be taken up at the end of this chapter.

The second of the three elements of this first readers' guide considers *whether the opportunities for, and the ascertainment of, exposure to the possibly harmful therapy were free from bias.* If you refer back to the British cohort study of oral contraceptives and thromboembolism, you'll be reminded that the opportunities were not free from bias: smoking women (at higher risk of thromboembolism) had less opportunity, while multiparous women (also at higher risk) had more opportunity, to receive oral contraceptives. What the net effect of these varying opportunities for exposure to the possibly harmful therapy would be, we can only estimate (and that's why the cohort study is lower on the study hierarchy than the randomized trial).

The case-control studies linking reserpine to breast cancer also excluded women with cardiovascular disease (precisely the group most likely to have received this antihypertensive drug) from the control group. This clearly led to a decreased opportunity for them to be exposed to reserpine, and could have produced the high relative risk observed in these studies where none existed (and that's why the case-control study is lower on the hierarchy than the cohort study).

In addition to reassuring yourself about equal opportunities for exposure, you also should seek reassurance that information about exposure to the possibly harmful therapy was obtained in a fashion that was protected from the influence of extraneous factors that might produce the appearance of an association where none existed. For example, the "catalog of biases" that one of us prepared [35] included an example in which investigators were trying to learn whether prior

*And especially if unconfirmed ones wind up official compendia of adverse drug reactions.

exposure to irradiation led to thyroid cancer in childhood [29, 32]. Routine questioning and record searching suggested that 28% of children in the first study, and none in the second, had prior irradiation. However, when the questioning and record searching were intensified, exposure to irradiation was reported in 47% of the former and 50% of the latter children. It is therefore clear that a less intense search for prior exposure among control subjects, coupled with a more intense search among cases, could create the appearance of an association where none, in truth, existed.

Good studies avoid or minimize these sorts of biases by using separate, objective sources of information (hospital or pharmacy records, and the like) about exposure, and by "blinding" their interviewers (and even their study subjects!) as to the precise question being tackled in the study. You'll often be able to find these safeguards described in the Methods sections of these reports.

The third element of this first readers' guide considers *whether the determination of outcomes (in cohort studies) or the distinction between cases and controls (in case-control studies) was free from bias.* The potential problem here is analogous to the previous one: If we search harder in only one of two groups that are being compared, spurious associations may appear where none exist, and small associations may be lost or exaggerated. Once again, a glance at that British study of oral contraceptives reminds us to wonder whether women on the pill might have been examined for thromboembolic complications with greater frequency and vigor than women using other forms of contraception. Moreover, when exposure to a treatment causes the *search for* a disorder, in addition to (or even rather than!) the disorder itself, the association between exposure and outcome will be spuriously elevated in both cohort and case-control studies. For example, Ralph Horwitz and Alvan Feinstein have documented how post-menopausal estrogens, by causing vaginal bleeding, increase the performance of diagnostic tests for endometrial cancer and "unmask" the disorder in its early stages [15]. As a result, when they compared endometrial cancer cases with both tumor registry controls and controls who also had undergone definitive diagnostic tests, the relative odds fell from 10:1 in the first instance to 2:1 in the second.*

Good studies avoid or minimize these sorts of biases by guaranteeing equally vigorous, objective searches for case-eligibility and outcomes, and by "blinding" their examiners, interviewers (and even their study subjects!) as to the precise question being tackled in the study. Again you'll often be able to find these safeguards described in the Methods sections of these reports.

IN REPORTING THE STRENGTH OF THE ASSOCIATION, WERE BOTH CLINICAL AND STATISTICAL SIGNIFICANCE CONSIDERED?

Strength here means the odds favoring the outcome of interest with, as opposed to without, exposure to the putative cause; the higher the odds, the greater the strength.

*This does not, of course, exonorate post-menopausal estrogens as a cause for endometrial cancer. It does, however, suggest that we may have overestimated their power for being such.

Different tactics for estimating the strength of association are used in different types of studies. In the randomized trial and cohort study (see Tables 9-2 and 9-4), patients who were and were not exposed to the putative cause are carefully followed up to find out whether they develop the adverse reaction or outcome. Thus, a cohort study of whether cimetidine causes impotence would compare the occurrence of impotence among ulcer patients who did and did not receive the drug. One reason that cohort studies (see Table 9-4) are methodologically attractive is because, like the randomized trial, they permit direct calculations of strength (relative risk) by comparing outcome rates in exposed and nonexposed persons:

$$\frac{a}{a + b} \div \frac{c}{c + d}$$

In the case-control study (see Table 9-5), in which patients with and without the outcome of interest (e.g., impotence) are selected and tracked backward to their prior exposure to the putative cause (e.g., cimetidine), strength (which in this case is called the "odds ratio") can only be indirectly estimated:

$$\frac{ad}{bc}$$

This calculation, though justified algebraically, is not intuitively obvious.

The results of causation studies usually are expressed as the "relative risk" (in randomized trials and cohort studies) or "relative odds" (in either cohort or case-control studies) of developing the adverse outcome with, as opposed to without, exposure to the possibly harmful treatment. If the treatment is innocent, and patients are no more likely to develop the adverse outcome on it than off it, the relative odds is 1.0. To the extent that the treatment is harmful, this measure rises above 1, and the accompanying P-value tells us the probability that we would have observed a relative odds this high or higher by chance alone. Another way of expressing this "statistical significance" would be the use of the confidence limits we introduced back in Chapters 6 and 7. Thus, in an article reporting that the relative risk of dying from asthma while on fenoterol was 1.55, the authors pointed out that the associated P-value was .03 and that the 95% confidence interval for this relative risk ran from 1.04 to 2.33 [8]. This result is statistically significant. Is it clinically significant as well? There are a few ways to address this latter question. First, we can simply look at the size of the relative odds: Because many of the biases that affect case-control and cohort studies can produce spurious relative risks of 2 or even 3, many methodologists would caution us not to get too excited until these values are exceeded.

On the other hand, a relative risk of 2 for a very common side effect can mean an awful lot of suffering, and we may want to invoke the same sort of thinking that developed the "number needed to be treated" (NNT) we introduced in Chapter 7. In this case, we could examine the article to see whether the authors calculated the number needed to be treated to produce one adverse outcome (or, if they provide us with the rates for adverse outcomes both on and off the treatment, we can calculate the NNT ourselves). For example, that randomized trial of bendroflumethiazide in mild hypertension documented that 23% of men on the active drug, as opposed to 10% of men on placebo, were impotent after 2 years of treatment [26]. That produces a relative risk of 2.3, which is elevated but perhaps not very impressive. On the other hand, the number of mildly hypertensive men one needs to treat with this drug for two years to produce one additional case of impotence is 1/(.23 − .10), or only about 8. To many of us, that latter expression is much more impressive. In interpreting NNTs for this purpose we should, of course, pay attention to the severity of the adverse outcome as well as its frequency.

A final measure of clinical significance expresses the proportion of adverse outcomes that are caused by the treatment and, therefore, the extent to which the adverse outcome would disappear if we withdrew the treatment. The authors of that paper on fenoterol and asthma deaths suggested that about 20% of asthma deaths, and 40% of the "excess" of asthma deaths that were occurring during the years of the study, could be due to this drug. We will meet this measure (the "attributable risk") again later under the readers' guide of "sense."

The preceding information will help us interpret articles reporting statistically significant increases in relative risks or relative odds. What if the results are not statistically significant? How do we know that these non-significant results aren't merely due to the study having been too small to have revealed a clinically important increased risk if it had occurred? The confidence interval and number needed to treat can help us here. Although the confidence interval will include 1.0 (that's why the result is not statistically significant), we still can examine the upper confidence limit. Is it still pretty low (say, less than 1.5), such that it wouldn't be clinically significant even if it were true? In that case, we can accept the study as a "true-negative" conclusion. If, on the other hand, the upper confidence limit extends into the clinically significant area, we may want to reserve judgment and look for additional articles on the subject. Similarly, we can examine the NNT to produce one adverse outcome and decide whether this is sufficiently small to cause us to reserve judgment and seek more information.

WHAT HAPPENS WHEN YOU APPLY RULES OF EVIDENCE FOR CAUSATION?

Having decided from the preceding text that the articles in hand warrant further consideration, you should then turn to their Results, Introductions and Discussions to see how their data fulfill the four commonsense rules of evidence that appear at the bottom of Table 9-1. They are discussed here in the order of their decreasing importance, and we have suggested the impact that each of them, as well as the second guide, should have on your causal decision in Table 9-6.

The strategies for interpreting clinical diagnostic tests that we described in Chapter 4 can be applied here as well. For example, some of these rules of evidence for causation (such as evidence from randomized trials) are much more accurate than others (such as evidence from case-control studies). Furthermore,

Table 9-6. Importance of individual guides and rules of evidence in making the causal decision

	Effect of test result on causal decision*		
	When test result is consistent with causation	When test result is neutral or inconclusive	When test result opposes causation
Strength of Association:			
From randomized trial	+ + + +	− − −	− − − −
From cohort study	+ + +	− −	− − −
From case-control study	+	0	−
Consistency	+ + +	− −	− − −
Temporal sequence	+ +	− −	− − − −
Gradient	+ +	−	− −
Sense	+ +	−	− −

*Meaning of symbols: + = causation supported; − = causation rejected; 0 = causal decision not affected. The number of +'s and −'s indicates the relative contribution of the diagnostic test to the causal decision.

many of them (such as temporality) are better for "ruling out" causation when they are negative than for "ruling it in" when they are positive. Finally, the test of "sensibility," although prominent in many articles, is low on the list because it has relatively low specificity; it is possible to "explain" almost any set of observations, and the risk of a "false-positive" conclusion about causation is substantial when these rules of evidence are applied in isolation. Let's consider the guides and rules of evidence for causation in greater detail:

Is the Association* Consistent *from Study to Study?
The repetitive demonstration, by different investigators using different research designs in different settings, of an association between exposure to the putative cause and the outcome of interest constitutes consistency. Thus, much of the credibility of the causal link between NSAIDs and gastrointestinal bleeding arises from the repeated demonstration of an association, by different investigators in different centers, using different research designs [11]. The best evidence about consistency often comes from meta-analyses, and we'll show you how to assess them in Chapter 13.

Is the* Temporal Sequence *of Exposure and Outcome in the Right Direction?
A consistent sequence of events of exposure to the putative cause, followed by the occurrence of the outcome of interest, is required for a positive test of temporality. When this test is positive, it supports a conclusion of causation. More important, when the temporal relation is found to go in the wrong direction, causation is ruled out: the putative cause is merely a consequence.

Although this rule looks easy to apply, often it is not. What if a second predisposing factor or a very early stage of the disorder itself is responsible both for exposure to the putative causal factor and for progression to the full-blown outcome? Such an explanation might apply to studies that have linked the use of illicit stimulant or depressant drugs to the subsequent diagnosis of psychosis or depression, respectively (25). Did the different illicit drugs cause specific forms of subsequently diagnosed mental illnesses, or did individuals with different subclinical but progressive mental illness seek out the specific drugs? This yardstick is understandably easier to apply to cohort than to case-control studies, since the latter address the association between "exposure" and "outcome" only after both have occurred.

Is There a* Dose-Response Gradient*?

The demonstration of an increasing risk or severity of the outcome in association with an increased "dose" or duration of exposure satisfies this rule. For example, in a report linking conjugated estrogens with endometrial carcinoma [45], the relative risk of developing endometrial cancer rose from 5.6 among those who used the drug less than 5 years to 7.2 among users for 5 to 6.9 years and, finally, to 13.9 among those who took conjugated estrogens for 7 or more years. Reverse gradients are useful, too. Indeed, some of the most compelling evidence on the link between cigarette smoking and lung cancer is the progressive decline in cancer risk that has been reported as previous smokers celebrate successive anniversaries of their last cigarette.

Does the Association Make* Sense*?

This guide has four elements. First, have plausible competing explanations for the association been ruled out? It is here that we should consider factors that might have caused a spurious association to have been generated. For example, good drugs for sick patients have three strikes against them before the study begins [37]: first, good but powerful drugs often are reserved for the most ill patients, leading to spurious guilt by association (the presence of life belts at scenes of drownings does not imply cause and effect); second, powerful drugs may encourage the clinicians who prescribe them to neglect other important elements of management that would keep patients from harm; third, complacent patients may overestimate the ability of "wonder" drugs to prevent or alleviate exacerbations of their illness, and may not seek additional care until it is too late.

The second element of "sense" inquires whether the results of the article are in harmony with our current understanding of the responses of cells, tissues, organs, and organisms to stimuli. It is with this yardstick that nonhuman experimental data should be measured (even though the mice, liver slices, or microbial cultures were randomly allocated to be exposed or not exposed to the putative cause). Although virtually any set of observations can be made biologically plausible (given the ingenuity of the human mind and the vastness of the supply of contradictory biologic facts), some biologic observations can be highly persuasive, such as finding an enteric-coated potassium chloride tablet at the site of a perforated small bowel [2]. Nonetheless, overinterpretation is a powerful temptation.

The third element of "sense" is satisfied when the article's results are in agreement with our current understanding of the distributions of causes and outcomes in man. This element is illustrated in the epidemic of primary pulmonary hypertension that swept through Switzerland in 1967 [9]. This disorder increased fifteenfold in one university clinic, and it was noted that many of its victims were obese. When local clinicians also noted that a new appetite-suppressing drug had been introduced a short time before, it dawned on them that the distribution of drug ingestion might match that for primary pulmonary hypertension. They were correct: In one center, it was discovered that almost 80% of the cases of primary pulmonary hypertension had taken the suspect drug. When it was withdrawn, the epidemic ceased.

Finally, the limitation of the association to a single putative cause and a single effect, although rarely encountered, adds to the "sense" of the association. Examples here are some of the highly characteristic disorders in which one, but virtually no other, drug (such as thalidomide) produces most examples of one, but no other, disorder (such as phocomelia).

When confronted by a question of causation, these three guides and four rules of evidence can be used to distill one's clinical reading and, with the assistance of judgments such as those shown in Table 9-6, to reach a causal conclusion. Moreover, when applied at the start of a literature search, these guides can also increase the efficiency of this search, by focusing your attention on those publications that will shed the strongest light on the causal question and by warning you against accepting plausible but biased conclusions.

Did This Drug (or Operation, or Other Treatment) Cause That Adverse Effect in This Particular Patient?

If the answer to the first question (Does this drug cause that adverse effect in some patients?), is "yes," we can then turn to the second question: Did this drug cause that adverse effect in this particular patient? It is in answering this second related question that the issue of whether our treatment has done harm becomes directly clinically relevant. Our answer will determine whether we stop, switch, or continue the treatment, and this answer will have tangible consequences for a patient in our care.

How should we answer this second question? Indeed, in the face of the previously noted disagreements, even among clinical pharmacologists, over whether a patient even has had an adverse drug reaction, how can we *begin* to answer this question?

In our judgment this second step calls for the adoption of a second set of guides for the individual case, and there are several to chose from [20, 22, 24, 28]. The one we've selected for this edition of the book is used by Mitchell Levine, a clinical pharmacologist who recently completed our clinical epidemiology graduate program [28]. We selected it because clinicians who apply it are likely to agree with each other (kappas .69 - .86), themselves (kappas .64 - .95), and with "experts" reviewing the same case-reports (kappas .75 to .91).*

This method generates a total score for ten questions that must be answered "yes," "no," or (thank heaven!) "don't know." The questions are shown in Table 9-7.

At each step, points can be added to (or subtracted from) a running total, and the final score (which could range from +13 to −4) indicates the probability that "this treatment caused that adverse effect in this particular patient":

≥ 9: It definitely did so
5 − 8: It probably did so
1 − 4: It possibly did so
≤ 0: It is doubtful that it did so

Question 1 in Table 9-7 concerns our previous general experience with the treatment and calls upon the guides and rules of evidence that sum to answer the first question posed in this chapter: *Does* this treatment conclusively cause that adverse effect in some patients?

Question 2 considers the temporal relation between treatment and adverse effect in the individual patient. Question 3 addresses one aspect of the "proof of the pudding": the effect of stopping (if possible) the drug ("dechallenge") or administering a specific antagonist, and Question 4 addresses the complementary question (to the brave) by asking what happens following rechallenge by the suspected drug. Question 5 seeks alternative explanations in the individual patient, and Question 6 proposes a single placebo period of the N-of-1 sort.

Question 7 seeks evidence of an overdose, and Question 8 is a reprise for Questions 3 and 4, replacing the all-or-none dosing with finer adjustments. Question 9 inquires after prior, similar episodes, and Question 10 seeks objective evidence for the adverse event.

In this way, the algorithm can be used to nail down adverse effects in the individual patient, and separate those due to specific treatments from those due to other causes. When the final score comes to 9 or more, you can be confident that the treatment caused the adverse effect and can act accordingly.

However, your subsequent actions may not always be clear, even when the score generated by using the algorithm is high. In some situations there may be other reasons to continue even an obviously guilty treatment, especially when it is the only effective one for the patient's illness.

Even after extensive reading, the application of all the readers' guides and rules of evidence for causation, and the application of this algorithm, you may remain uncertain about whether, for example, treatment A really causes adverse effect B in patient C. What do you do then, and how do you translate all of this deliberation into clinical action?

*Moreover, the reproducibility with the method we described in our first edition [22] is high ($r = .82$, $P < .001$).

Table 9-7. A scoring strategy for deciding whether this treatment caused that adverse effect in this particular patient

	Yes	No	Don't know
1. Are there previous *conclusive* reports on this reaction?	+1	0	0
2. Did the adverse event appear after the suspected drug was administered?	+2	−1	0
3. Did the adverse reaction improve when the drug was discontinued or a *specific* antagonist was administered?	+1	0	0
4. Did the adverse reaction reappear when the drug was readministered?	+2	−1	0
5. Are there alternative causes (other than the drug) that could on their own have caused the reaction?	−1	+2	0
6. Did the reaction reappear when a placebo was given?	−1	+1	0
7. Was the drug detected in the blood (or other fluids) in concentrations known to be toxic?	+1	0	0
8. Was the reaction more severe when the dose was increased, or less severe when the dose was decreased?	+1	0	0
9. Did the patient have a similar reaction to the same or similar drugs in *any* previous exposure?	+1	0	0
10. Was the adverse event confirmed by any objective evidence?	+1	0	0

We suggest, as shown in Figure 9-1, that this "decision for action" has two components.

The first component is our *certainty about causation*, based upon the application of the readers' guides and rules of evidence for causation to our clinical reading and the ten questions in the algorithm of Naranjo and colleagues [28] to our patient. The second component is our *consideration of the consequences of the alternative courses of action* that are open to us (recognizing that these courses of action include noninterference as well as maintaining the status quo). The ultimate decision for action results from the interplay of these two components.

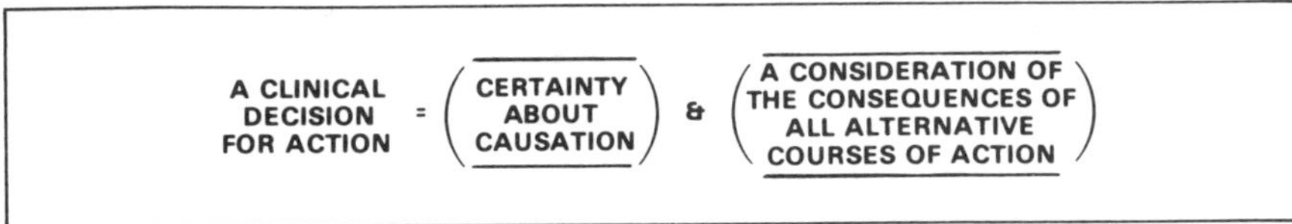

Figure 9-1. Components of a clinical decision for action.

In many situations both of these components push us toward the same action decision. If our certainty that drug A causes adverse reaction B in patient C is high (e.g., symptomatic increased airways resistance in a hypertensive challenged, dechallenged, and rechallenged with propranolol) and another course of action (e.g., thiazides) would be just as likely to achieve the treatment target, both components support an action decision to change the treatment (stop propranonol and start thiazides).

In other situations the two components push us in opposite directions and we must decide which component should take precedence. Consider a second example: The three reports indicting reserpine as a cause of breast cancer that appeared abruptly in 1974 precipitated a crisis in the management of hypertension. How were we to decide how to advise and treat patients whose high blood pressure was kept under control with this drug? The first component of this clinical decision considered the degree of certainty that reserpine did, indeed, cause breast cancer; it was never very great. On the other hand, the second component of this decision identified an alternative course of action that was highly attractive to many Canadian clinicians: switching appropriate patients from reserpine to propranolol. In this case, then, even a low degree of certainty about causation was attended by a clinical decision to take many patients off a drug because an alternative treatment was available.

By contrast to the reserpine case, the degree of certainty that oral contraceptives cause stroke and heart attack is much higher. Nonetheless, oral contraceptives remain in widespread use. Although the reasons behind this decision to continue oral contraceptive use in the face of growing evidence that they cause these disorders are complex, they include the effect of the second component of the decision: The consequences of alternative approaches to birth control may be judged even less desirable than the small but real risks of stroke or heart attack. And so the use of oral contraceptives continues (and, interestingly, the dose-response gradient is invoked to support the progressive reduction of certain of their hormonal constituents).

The diagnosis of causation is not simply arithmetic, and the strategies and tactics for making this judgment are still primitive. The guides, rules of evidence, and algorithm presented here are a start, however, and it is suggested that their use will improve the lot of patients whose clinicians are both willing and able to grapple with the emerging clinical evidence on the adverse effects of treatment.

Finally, we maintain that this approach to gathering and assessing evidence is of substantial educational value both to the clinicians who do it and to those they teach. Thus, the use of these guides and algorithm, particularly when clearly specified before a review of relevant data, will lead to more rational, albeit less colorful, discussions of causation in medicine.

References

1. Armstrong, B., Stevens, N., and Doll, R. Retrospective study of the association between use of rauwolfia derivatives and breast cancer in English women. *Lancet* 2: 672, 1974.
2. Baker, D. R., Schrader, W. H., and Hitchcock, C. R. Small-bowel ulceration apparently associated with thiazide and potassium therapy. *J. Am. Med. Assoc.* 190: 586, 1964.
3. Boston Collaborative Drug Surveillance Program. Reserpine and breast cancer. *Lancet* 2: 669, 1974.
4. Boston Collaborative Drug Surveillance Program. Rauwolfia derivatives and breast cancer. *Lancet* 2: 1315, 1974.
5. Boston Collaborative Drug Surveillance Program. Hospital admissions due to adverse drug reactions. *Arch. Intern. Med.* 134: 219, 1974.
6. Caranasos, G. J., Stewart, R. B., and Cluff, L. E. Drug-induced illness leading to hospitalization. *J.A.M.A.* 228: 713, 1974.
7. The Cardiac Arrhythmia Suppression Trial (CAST) Investigators. Special Report. Preliminary Report: Effect of encainide and flecainide on mortality in a randomized trial of arrhythmia suppression after myocardial infarction. *N. Engl. J. Med.* 321: 406,1989.
8. Crane, J., Pearce, N., Flatt, A., et al. Prescribed fenoterol and death from asthma in New Zealand, 1981–83: Case-control study. *Lancet* 1: 917, 1989.
9. Doll, R. Unwanted effects of drugs. *Br. Med. Bull.* 27: 25, 1971.
10. Feinstein, A. R. Clinical biostatistics: XX. The epidemiologic trohoc, the ablative risk ratio, and "retrospective" research. *Clin. Pharm. Ther.* 14: 291, 1973.
11. Gabriel, S. E., and Bombardier, C. NSAID-induced ulcers; an emerging epidemic? *J. Rheumatol.* 17: 1–4, 1990.
12. Hayden, G. F., Kramer, M. S., and Horowitz, R. I. The case-control study: A practical guide for the clinician. *J.A.M.A.* 247: 326, 1981.
13. Heinonen, O. P., Shapiro, S., Tuominen, L., and Turunen, M. I. Reserpine use in relation to breast cancer. *Lancet* 2: 675, 1974.
14. Hill, A. B. *Principles of Medical Statistics* (9th ed.). London: *Lancet,* 1971. P. 313.
15. Horwitz, R. I., and Feinstein, A. R. Alternative analytic methods for case-control studies of estrogens and endometrial cancer. *N. Engl. J. Med.* 299: 1089, 1978.
16. Hull, R., Hirsh, J., Sackett, D. L., et al. Combined use of leg scanning and impedance plethysmography in suspected venous thrombosis. An alternative to venography. *N. Engl. J. Med.* 296: 1497, 1977.
17. Hutchinson, T. A., Levinthal, J. M., Kramer, M. S., et al. An algorithm for the operational assessment of adverse drug reactions: II. Demonstration of reproducibility and validity. *J.A.M.A.* 242: 633, 1979.
18. Ibrahim, M. A. The case-control study: Consensus and controversy. *J. Chron. Dis.* 132: 1, 1979.
19. Inman, W. H .W. Postmarketing surveillance of adverse drug reactions in general practice: I: Search for new methods. *Br. Med. J.* 282: 1131, 1981.
20. Jones, J. Adverse drug reactions in the community health setting: Approaches to recognizing, counseling and reporting. *Family Community Health* 5: 58, 1982.
21. Koch-Weser, J., Sellers, E. M., and Zacest, R. The ambiguity of adverse drug reactions. *Eur. J. Clin. Pharmacol.* 11: 75, 1977.
22. Kramer, M. S., Leventhal, J. M., Hutchinson, T. A., and Feinstein, A. R. An al-

gorithm for the operational assessment of adverse drug reactions: I. Background, description, and instructions for use. *J.A.M.A* 242: 623, 1979.
23. La Haba, A. F., Curet, J. O., Pelegrina, I., and Bangdiwala, I. Thrombophlebitis among oral and nonoral contraceptive users. *Obstet. Gynecol.* 38: 259, 1971.
24. Lane, D. A., Kramer, M. S., Hutchinson, T. A., et al. The causality assessment of adverse drug reactions using a Bayesian approach. *Pharmaceut. Med.* 2: 265, 1987.
25. McLellan, A. T., Woody, G. E., and O'Brien, C.P. Development of psychiatric illness in drug abusers. *N. Engl. J. Med.* 301: 1310, 1979.
26. Medical Research Council Working Party. Adverse reactions to bendrofluazide and propranol for the treatment of mild hypertension. *Lancet* 2: 539, 1981.
27. Miettinen, O. S. *Theoretical Epidemiology: Principles of Occurrence Research in Medicine*. Toronto: Wiley, 1985.
28. Naranjo, C. A., Busto, U., Sellers, E. M., et al. A method for estimating the probability of adverse drug reactions. *Clin. Pharmacol. Ther.* 30: 239, 1981.
29. Nishiyama, R. H., Schmidt, R. W., and Batsakis, J. G. Carcinoma of the thyroid gland in children and adolescents. *J.A.M.A.* 181: 1034, 1962.
30. Ogilvie, R. I., and Ruedy, J. Adverse drug reactions during hospitalization. *Can. Med. Assoc. J.* 97: 1450, 1967.
31. Rauwolfia derivatives and cancer. *Lancet* (Editorial) 2: 701, 1974.
32. Raventos, A., Horn, R. C. Jr., and Ravdin, I. S.: Carcinoma of the thyroid gland in youth: A second look ten years later. *J. Clin. Endocr. Metab.* 22: 886, 1962.
33. Reidenberg, M. M., and Lowenthal, D.T. Adverse nondrug reactions. *N. Engl. J. Med.* 279: 678, 1968.
34. Royal College of General Practitioners. *Oral Contraceptives and Health: An Interim Report*. Tunbridge Wells: Pitman, 1974.
35. Sackett, D. L. Bias in analytic research. *J. Chron. Dis.* 32: 51, 1979.
36. Sackett, D. L., Haynes, R. B., Gent, M., and Taylor, D. W. Compliance. In W. H. W. Inman (ed.), *Monitoring for Drug Safety*. Lancaster: MTP, 1980.
37. Sackett, D. L., Shannon, H. S., and Browman, G. W. Fenoterol and fatal asthma. *Lancet* 1: 45, 1990.
38. Shapiro, S., and Sloan, D. Comment. *J. Chron. Dis.* 32: 105, 1979.
39. Should we case-control? (Editorial) *Lancet* 335: 1127, 1990.
40. Slone, D., Siskind, V., Heinonen, O. P., et al. Aspirin and congenital malformations. *Lancet* 1: 1373, 1976.
41. Steele, K., Gertman, P. M., Crescenzi, C., and Anderson, J. Iatrogenic illness on a general medical service at a university hospital. *N. Engl. J. Med.* 304: 638, 1981.
42. Strom, B. L. (ed.) *Pharmacoepidemiology*. New York: Churchill Livingstone, 1989.
43. Strom, B. L., and Tugwell, P. Pharmacoepidemiology: Current status, prospects, and problems. *Ann. Intern. Med.* 113: 179, 1990.
44. Vessey, M. P. Discussion in the case-control study: Consensus and controversy. *J. Chron. Dis.* 32: 109, 1979.
45. Ziel, H. K., and Finkle, W. D. Increased risk of endometrial carcinoma among users of conjugated estrogens. *N. Engl. J. Med.* 293: 1167, 1975.

III

Keeping Up to Date

10

Introduction: How to Review Your Own Performance

This final section may be the most important part of the book, for it presents strategies for combating clinical entropy.

To some extent this whole book, but especially this last section, is about strategies to keep you from becoming out of date. Keeping current in medicine is an awesome task, and it is made more, rather than less, difficult by the way that many medical journals and continuing medical education programs are operated. Accordingly, these last five chapters focus on helping you to master the practical assessment of your own clinical performance, the efficient use of a library (including your own), the quick but effective review of a clinical journal, and the judicious choice of continuing medical education programs. They have been designed to help you reject the irrelevant and nonsensical, avoid the hucksters, and spend the precious time you do have for keeping up in the most effective and efficient ways.

Distressing though it may be to contemplate, there is growing evidence that our effectiveness as clinicians, at least in some domains, begins to deteriorate as soon as we complete our clinical training. To be sure, our ability to execute the diagnostic strategy of pattern recognition improves with experience, and we become more efficient in our use of the hypothetico-deductive approach. We do not do so well in other areas, however.

Our factual knowledge of human biology deteriorates, both because we forget it and because we fail to learn new facts as they emerge. For example, when George Miller administered the freshman anatomy final written examination to upperclassmen (including one of this book's authors), house officers, and staff surgeons at the University of Illinois [50], everybody flunked it, raising questions about relevance as well as retention.

Our clinical skills may deteriorate as well, and this deterioriation may not simply be due to aging eyes and ears. As we described back in Chapter 2, one of our chief residents asked clinical clerks, residents, and attending physicians to examine the neck veins of a series of ICU patients and estimate their central venous pressure. When these estimates were compared with simultaneous readings from indwelling central lines, the correlations were highest for the clerks and lowest for the attending physicians. [8].

Furthermore, we fail to keep abreast of advances in diagnosis and therapy, and often continue to use the old (and sometimes ineffective) treatments we learned as trainees instead of newer, more effective ones. For example, several years ago our group carried out identical work-ups on 230 hypertensives and successfully referred every one of them, along with a copy of their work-up, to one of the 80 family physicians in and around Hamilton, Ontario [73]. The clinicians who saw these hypertensives started only two-thirds of them on antihypertensive drug regimens, permitting us to go back into our records and identify the predictors of the clinical decision to treat some, but not other, hypertensives. We found four such predictors. The first and most powerful predictor was the patient's diastolic blood pressure, as it should have been; the higher the diastolic pressure, the more likely that antihypertensive drugs would be prescribed. The second predictor, surprisingly enough, was the patient's age, with a greater reluctance to start treatment in the young. The fourth most powerful predictor was target organ damage; the more evidence of target organ damage, the more likely that drug therapy was begun. Again, this made good clinical sense.

However, the third predictor, and therefore more powerful than the presence of target organ damage, was the year of graduation from medical school of the physician to whom we had referred the patient! The more recent graduates were more likely to treat hypertension. The reports of the randomized trials that demonstrated the dramatic benefits of treating ever lower elevations of blood pressure were published midway through the era in which our clinicians had been trained. However, this new knowledge was either not disseminated to or not assimilated by those front-line clinicians who had already completed their training. As further proof of this, another one of us recently collaborated in a study of family physicians' knowledge about the modern management of hypertension. The correlation between the time since graduation from medical school and one's management knowledge was an awesome −.55; the greater the time since graduation, the more out-of-date the knowledge about the modern management of hypertension [13]. In other words, it appears that clinicians in our part of the world continue to make the same treatment decisions they learned from their teachers, and tend not to alter these decisions after they complete their training, even when subsequent evidence dictates that they should. Thus, although they may have been taught the best medical practice available at the time of their formal education, they apparently had not been taught how to decide when their medical practice became outdated and needed to be changed.

This last point is, in our view, the key to your continued effectiveness as a clinician: *learning how to decide when your current diagnostic and management maneuvers are no longer good enough and need to be changed.** This is also consistent with the finding that age was found to be a major predictor of inadequate performance in the 918 physicians assessed in the chart–audit peer-assessment program of physicians' office practices of the Ontario College of Physicians and Surgeons [47]. Interestingly, solo practice and lack of membership in the Canadian College of Family Practice were the other major predictors, suggesting that interaction with peers may also be important in providing insight into one's lack of keeping up-to-date with advances in patient management.

Our underlying assumption, once again, is that medicine is rational and so are you. That is, your clinical acts of diagnosis and management reflect your assessment of the evidence that this or that diagnostic test or treatment is valid and

*This admonition has additional meaning for clinical teachers. Not only must we keep up to date ourselves; we (both as instructors and as role models) also must help our students learn how to decide when their current diagnostic and management maneuvers are no longer good enough and need to be changed.

will do more good than harm. If this view of clinical practice is correct, then you should constantly be seeking evidence, not just conclusions or, worse still, authoritarian opinions. Just as your ability to achieve accurate diagnosis and efficacious therapy determines your clinical effectiveness today, it is your skills in self-assessment and in tracking down and assessing biomedical knowledge (most of which resides in the journals) that will more and more determine your clinical effectiveness tomorrow. This last part of the book will help you master these skills. We will start with the self-assessment of your own performance.

Performance Review

Most of the things you have learned so far in medical education, clinical training, continuing education, and even in the earlier sections of this book, constitute additions to your knowledge, skills, and (we hope!) your attitudes, as well. These attitudes, knowledge, and skills merge in what we call *clinical competence* [53]: the potential ability to evaluate and manage patients so that their health is maintained or improved. Thus, the written or oral examinations we undergo at various points in our careers measure our competence and decide whether our knowledge and skills are sufficient to turn us loose on patients (and other clinicians). To use an analogy (which we may regret later), competence may be likened to the potential energy (voltage) stored in a battery.

Mere competence is not enough. For patients to benefit, we have to apply our knowledge and skills to their problems; we need watts, not just volts. We (and others) shall call this application *clinical performance*.

Clinical performance has four determinants and we have pictured them in Figure 10-1.

As shown in Figure 10-1, clinical competency is a necessary precondition for correct clinical performance but is insufficient, all by itself, to guarantee that this correct performance will occur. For example, Patrick Ward and his colleagues [84] taught Minnesota medical students the knowledge and skills required for the rational ordering and interpreting of laboratory tests. They were able to document substantial gains in competence (measured by multiple-choice tests before and after the course) among those students who took this elective course. However, the subsequent clinical performance of the highly competent students who took this course was the same as that of the less competent students who did not take the course when assessed on the internal medicine service. On the pediatric service, on the other hand, these students did outperform those who did not take the course. The research team concluded that barriers (such as a lower priority for this knowledge and skill on the medical service) might explain their results, and the other determinants in Figure 10-1 may have come into play as well.

Robert Brook [4] has identified several other examples of the disparity between competence (volts) and performance (watts). Of several hundred studies documenting suboptimal clinical performance, many showed that simple, routine tasks (e.g., the recognition and treatment of hypertension, completing childhood immunizations, prescribing iron for anemia, screening children for visual

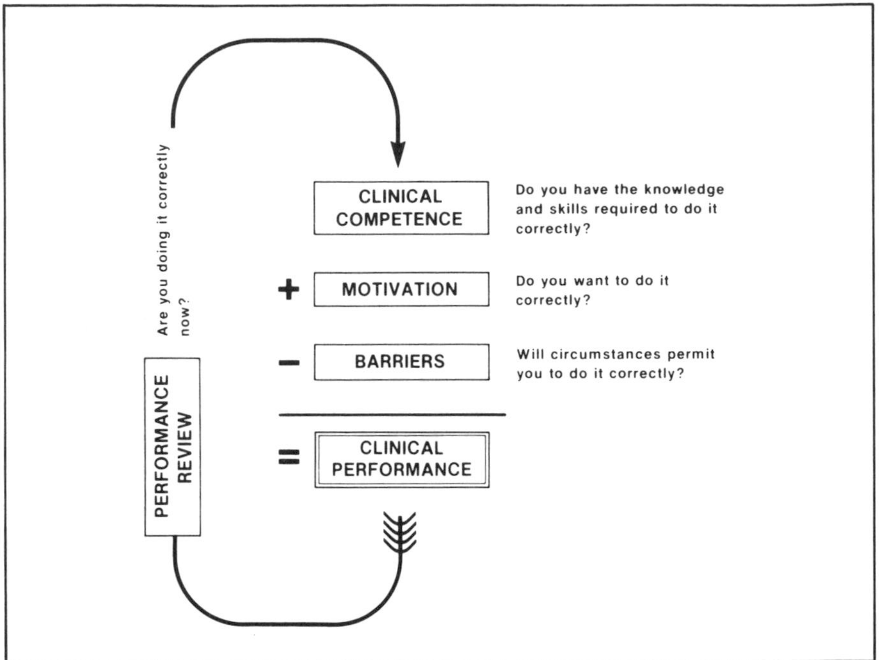

Figure 10-1. The determinants of clinical performance.

problems) are not performed consistently in most medical practices and health care systems, and that the successful completion of those routine activities depends much more upon the development of effective practice habits than on the acquisition of new knowledge. Robert Brook also has found that, at least in New Mexico, differences in apparent competency (e.g., the presence or absence of board certification) were not associated with differences in performance (e.g., the appropriate use of injectable antibiotics, vaccines, vitamins, gold, estrogens, iron, and the like) [3].

Another example of the discrepancy between clinical competence and clinical performance was described by Joseph Gonnella and his colleagues [21]. They began by verifying that 18 of 133 (14%) consecutive patients at a University of Illinois clinic had significant bacteriuria (back in 1970 when that was a "hot" topic), and that virtually all of them had what then was considered an indication for quantitative urine culture (signs, symptoms, previous treatment of urinary infection, or a history of catheterization, hypertension, or diabetes). When clinic physicians evaluated these same patients without realizing that they already had been screened for significant bacteriuria, less than half as many urinary tract infections were found; however, when these clinic physicians took a multiple-choice test and completed a management problem on urinary infection, most of them did well. Thus, these clinicians exhibited a disparity between competency and performance; once again they had the volts but not the watts, and those with the highest test scores were as likely to miss an infection as those with the lowest scores.

The second determinant of clinical performance shown in Figure 10-1, motivation, concerns the extent to which clinicians are positively inclined to put whatever clinical competence they have into practice. As with competence, motivation is necessary but insufficient, by itself, to guarantee proper clinical performance; motivation to do good to the patient who has aspirated his beefsteak will not dislodge the offending gobbet unless this motivation is coupled with the knowledge of why the patient may be choking plus the skill to perform an effective Heimlich maneuver. Robert Fox and his collaborators, in a unique study of changing and learning in the lives of a random sample of physicians, analyzed 775 reported changes in the medical practice of 340 physicians in Canada and the United States [66]. About a quarter (184) of these changes were in standards of performance (the other categories were financial well-being, personal well-being, stages in career, clinical environment, and regulations). The clinicians also were asked what had motivated these changes, and three factors were identified:

1. The discovery of an innovation or better way of practicing medicine motivated 54% of the changes. For example, an orthopedic surgeon acquired the skills for using cementless joint replacements, and a family physician began to incorporate risk factor questions on smoking.
2. Dissatisfaction with current procedures and outcomes motivated 28% of the changes. Examples have included embarrassment about inadequacy in assessing sexual problems, and dissatisfaction with one's success in controlling the symptoms of angina.
3. Finally, the desire to excel, an intrinsic component of living up to personal expectations of professional behavior, motivated 17% of the changes. For example, a family physician developed expertise in inserting IUDs because of the conviction that family physicians should be able to do this as part of providing "complete primary health care."

Enough said. These motivations shape our own practices, and we suspect that they influence yours as well. In spite of their power, our actual performance often fails to live up to our standards—we don't practice as well as we know how to practice. Why not?

The barriers to transforming clinical competence into clinical performance pictured in Figure 10-1 arise for a number of reasons. For example, your patient or your health system may not be able to afford to carry out efficacious maneuvers. Moreover, excessive patient loads, inadequate practice organization, and financial pressures all may restrict the time available for each patient and thus lower performance. In addition, the presence of "bad habits" (e.g., failing to measure blood pressure routinely in women on oral contraceptives [omission] or inappropriate prescribing of vitamins [commission]) and the absence of "good habits" (e.g., contacting hypertensive patients who miss appointments) can widen the gap between competence and performance.

Finally, our performance may be affected by subconscious barriers, such as our tendency to judge overweight patients as more nervous, less competent, and possessing poorer prognoses than leaner patients [11]. Added to this is our inclination to give different psychiatric diagnoses to patients from different social classes [25], races, or sexes [24], and to prescribe them different drugs and other treatments [32]; had George Washington been a commoner, he would have seen far fewer consultants and probably would not have been bled to death for his sore throat. Whether conscious or unconscious, these barriers prevent us from translating our clinical competence into the clinical performance that our patients need and deserve. All of us would benefit from knowing more about the unconscious barriers described by physicians such as John Eisenberg [11], and so would our patients. Systematic feedback from patients themselves or trainees can help identify and monitor such barriers [46].

Outside of this equation, but key to improving its sum, is *performance review:* feedback to clinicians on what they actually are doing, and how well they are doing it. Although this feedback obviously is crucial if we are to make our continuing education relevant both to our future clinical performance and to keeping up to date, most of us fail even to gather, much less critically appraise, evidence on our clinical performance. Accordingly, setting up and using a personal system for performance review will constitute both the body of this chapter and the starting point for the other chapters in this final section of the book.

PERFORMANCE REVIEW: CLINICAL SKILLS

The performance review of our clinical skills concentrates on the accuracy and precision of our histories and physicals. This is a good place to begin; the performance review of clinical skills can be done easily and quickly, and its execution tends to be fun.

The performance review of clinical skills begins by keeping a running account of the clinical impressions, conclusions, and predictions you make about your patients during your clinical examinations, but *prior to* the execution of confirmatory procedures (such as laboratory tests on blood or other fluids, biopsies, body imaging, consultations, operations, autopsies, or other definitive diagnostic tests). These impressions, conclusions, and predictions then are compared with the results of the confirmatory procedures.

It can be argued that this exercise is a waste of time: If you were going to order the confirmatory test anyway, why bother with that portion of the clinical exam? We think that the exercise is warranted for two reasons. First, the confirmatory test may take several days to be reported, and if your exam was accurate (or could become so), you would be that far ahead. Second, when the confirmatory test is expensive or uncomfortable, it would be nice to be able to forego it if your clinical examination could suffice.

It should be recognized at the outset, however, that this sort of performance review can only identify sins of commission; it cannot identify sins of omission in which you should have carried out a specific element of a clinical examination (and should have ordered the relevant confirmatory test) but didn't. The detection of this latter class of errors requires other strategies that will be discussed later in this chapter.

There are two methods for assessing your performance on the clinical examination, but because nobody we know (including ourselves!) still uses the "method of specifying probabilities" that we described in the first edition of this book, we'll confine this discussion to the "method of simple agreement." This method is illustrated in Table 10-1.

In Table 10-1, Patient A was judged to have gout on the basis of a history of pain in his foot and knee and the finding of red swollen foot and knee joints; this was confirmed on examination of the aspirated knee fluid. Similarly, the clinical impressions of atrial fibrillation in Patient B, breast cancer in Patient D, and anemia in Patient E were confirmed by subsequent, definitive diagnostic procedures. However, the pleural effusion in Patient C was missed on physical examination, and the impression of hyperthyroidism in Patient F was not confirmed by serum thyroid hormone levels. Thus, the extent of simple agreement between your clinical impressions and subsequent, definitive tests was four out of six, or 67%.

The method of simple agreement does tell us how we are doing in general terms and, if compared with a similar performance review carried out later, could give us a rough idea of whether we are making progress in reducing this type of clinical disagreement. Furthermore, this method could point out areas in which we might want to brush up our clinical skills (in this case, in the physical examination of the chest and in assessing the signs of hyperthyroidism).

However, as Alan Shapiro [75] has pointed out, the method of simple agreement has a major drawback: It treats clinical impressions as "all-or-none" judgments and fails to recognize that they are, with rare exceptions, contemplated (at least informally) in terms of probabilities (Patient A "probably has gout," Patient F " may have hyperthyroidism," and Patient B "almost certainly has atrial fibrillation"). For this reason Alan Shapiro proposed a more complex but much more useful method in which these probabilities are stated formally and then manipulated to generate a more clinically sensible index of performance. Despite firm resolve, however, none of us (or anyone we asked) actually carried it out faithfully.

The foregoing examples considered the *accuracy* of your clinical skills when compared with a confirmatory gold standard. If no gold standard is easily applied, or if the patient is to be examined repeatedly by you or other clinicians, your performance review can focus on the *precision* (consistency, reproducibility, or the likelihood that repeated exams of the same, unchanged patient would yield identical results) of your clinical skills.

In this case (and as described in Chapter 2) you and your colleagues would (re-)examine the patient "with an open mind"; that is, you would *not* read or discuss the findings of prior examinations before carrying out your own. Only in this fashion could you avoid observing falsely high degrees of precision due to the effects of expectation (when you know what you found on your previous examination) and friendship (when your colleague knows what you found on

Table 10-1. The method of simple agreement for assessing clinical impressions and predictions

	Clinical impression or prediction		Confirmation		Agreement*		
Patient	Evidence	Inference	Procedure	Result	Yes	No	
A	Pain and erythema in foot and knee	Gout	Synovial fluid analysis	Negatively birefringent crystals	√		
B	History of palpitations; irregularly irregular pulse	Atrial fibrillation	Electrocardiogram	Atrial fibrillation	√		
C	Percussion and auscultation normal	Normal chest examination	Chest x ray	Left pleural effusion		√	
D	Hard 2 cm lump in left breast; negative axillae	Breast cancer	Biopsy and surgical specimen	Breast cancer	√		
E	History of fatigue; pale mucosae and nail beds	Anemia	Hemoglobin determination	Low	√		
F	Anxious-looking, sweaty; fine tremor at rest	Hyperthyroid	Measure of serum thyroid hormone levels	Normal		√	
				Totals	4	2	6

*Simple agreement: 4/6 = 67%

your examination). Disagreements could be resolved through discussion or by means of a third, similarly "blinded" examination.

The results of these performance reviews will identify defects in the accuracy and precision of your clinical skills that need brushing up. You can then employ one or more of the strategies listed in Table 2-12 to correct these inaccuracies and inconsistencies.

However, before you go to all this trouble you should again consider our admonition from Chapter 2: Because efforts to improve the consistency and accuracy of your clinical examination will consume more of your time, and possibly that of your colleagues as well, you want to reserve this investment for those crucial items in a patient's history or physical examination that really are key determinants of the diagnosis. If the presence or absence of a specific sign or symptom adds nothing to the evaluation of a patient, why include it in your performance review, much less waste time raising the precision or accuracy with which you identify it?

Thus, the identification of inaccuracies or inconsistencies should also identify issues to be tracked down and appraised in the clinical literature; if you frequently miss a given physical sign, does it really matter? Is this sign, in fact, a key element in determining the diagnosis, prognosis, or treatment response? If so, you had better work on it. If, on the other hand, it is a finding of low importance, you may elect to drop it altogether from your clinical examination.

Your performance of bedside or "near-patient" laboratory tests is also worth checking out, especially before adopting them in your practice. For example, Hilborne and colleagues found that house officers were good at spinning hematocrits and identifying lymphocytosis and "left shifts" on blood smears, but often under-or overreported urinary sediments [30]. Significantly, although they found that house officers' proficiency in urinalysis correlated well with self-perceptions of their abilities, it was unrelated to the year of training! Nanji and coworkers showed that an acceptable level of precision can be achieved with blood chemistry desktop analyzers, and, equally important, identified these tests where the results are different from the routine laboratory (e,g., the serum creatinine differed by more than 10% on 34 out of 54 samples with one analyzer). Interestingly, the nurses in these practices were more adept than the physicians [52].

PERFORMANCE REVIEW: DIAGNOSIS AND MANAGEMENT

This type of performance review is more formidable and you will have to put much more thought into it before you begin. If you leap into this sort of performance review without careful planning, you may wind up wasting time and energy in the documentation of an expensive tap dance of flashy but nonproductive clinical procedures.

In general, performance reviews of diagnosis and management can focus either on the *outcomes* of this clinical care or on the *process* of the care itself [10]. There are advantages and drawbacks to each focus, and an effective performance review usually combines elements of both.

The outcome approach focuses on the end result that ought or ought not occur if our clinical performance has been appropriate. Thus, if our clinical performance with hypertensive patients is appropriate, they should exhibit good control of their blood pressure and should not develop the outcomes of stroke, heart failure, or degeneration of the eye or kidney. Performance reviews of this sort often set targets which, if they are not met, warrant attempts to discover why failures are occurring. For example, John Williamson and his colleagues [87] proposed that at least 50% of heart failure patients should become and remain symptom-free for at least 12 months if the clinical performance of their doctors was up to scratch; however, when 84% of them relapsed, a case-by-case review was carried out to identify gaps in clinical skills and knowledge. Similarly, Robert Kane has suggested that clinicians should specify the dates by which individual patients should show improvement or cure, with a review of all cases who fall behind schedule [36]. A group of senior U.S. academic health professionals have made a list of disorders in which the occurrence of a single case of disease or disability or a single untimely death should cause us to ask, "Why did this happen?" [72]. This list focuses primarily on preventive performance review (e.g., whooping cough, tetanus, bronchogenic carcinoma), but includes untimely deaths from treatable diseases (e.g., thyrotoxicosis, meningitis, asthma) to provide a therapeutic performance review as well.

Finally, the U.S. Department of Health and Human Services has initiated a "Medical Effectiveness" initiative that has as one of its components the search for substantial variations in outcomes among demographic and geographic groups (colloquially known by the buzz word/phrase "small area analyses") for patients in the Medicare and Medicaid system. Rates are prepared according to area (state, metropolitan, or rural) for hospital admissions, postadmission mortality, and population mortality for specific conditions (e.g., coronary revascularization, cholecystectomy, prostatectomy, myocardial infarction, congestive heart failure, and pulmonary disease). Once a major variation in outcomes is identified, a detailed investigation of the cause is implemented with further studies either retrospectively through auditing medical records or prospectively through observational analyses or randomized trials. Where changes in practice are indicated, feedback and education are implemented. The impact of this program is not yet known [71].

These outcome-oriented performance reviews sometimes produce dramatic results, and none of us requires a formal surveillance system to be jolted by a preventable death or complication in our own practice. On the other hand, there are three shortcomings to an outcome-oriented performance review that limit its usefulness:

1. When the bad outcomes of dangerous clinical actions are rare, we can get away with them. For example, many physicians would neither encounter fatal pulmonary embolism in their patients even if they confined postoperative patients to bed [34], nor aplastic anemia even though they treated patients with chloramphenicol who did not need it [83]. Thus, an outcome-based perfor-

mance review will fail to identify faulty performance when its adverse consequences, however devastating, are rare.

2. When the bad outcomes of bad performance are delayed, dangerous clinical acts can escape detection. For example, short-term performance reviews might terminate before the development of retinopathy in chloroquine-treated arthritics [31].
3. Finally, when unfavorable outcomes are the result of factors beyond the clinician's control, an outcome-based performance review will generate spurious conclusions about clinical performance. For example, death following a severe stroke is influenced far more by the severity of the initial brain damage than by anything that clinicians do once this damage has occurred, and a performance review based on outcomes in such a situation will blame the clinician for bad prognoses, not bad management. This third point is an important one, and is illustrated in Figure 10-2.

Figure 10-2. The determinants of the outcome of an illness.

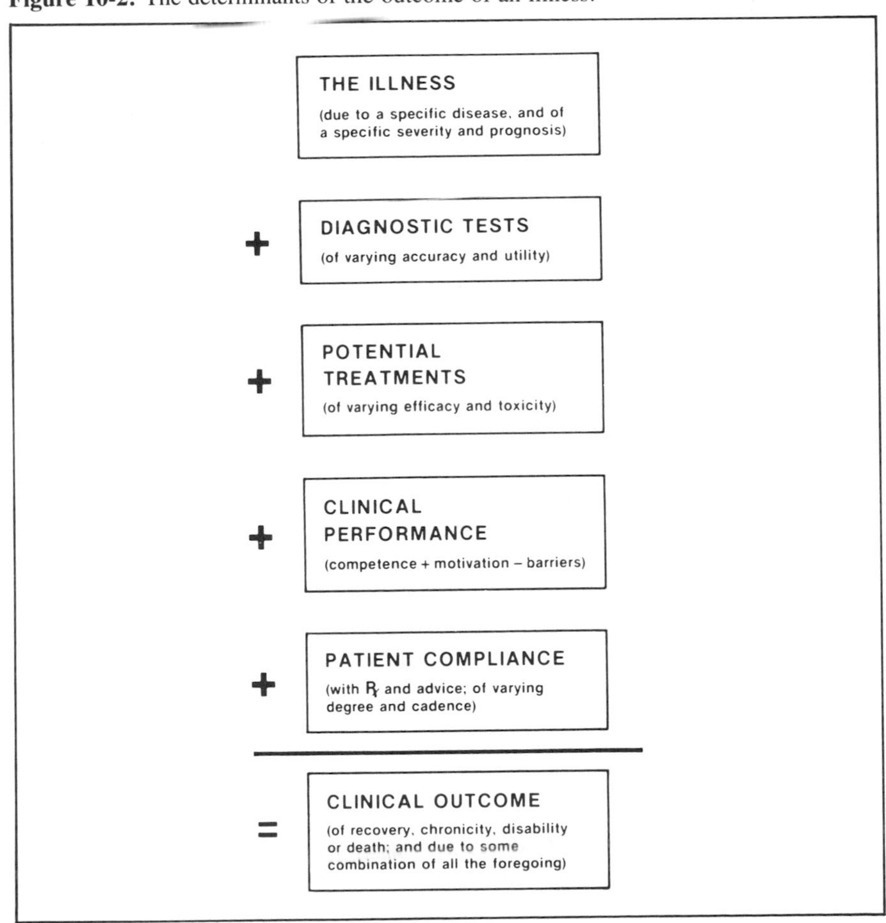

The determinants of the clinical outcome of an illness are five, and consist of:

1. The *illness* itself (due to a specific disease, and possessing a specific severity and a specific prognosis)
2. The *diagnostic tests* that might be used to identify the cause of the illness
3. The *potential treatments* that might be prescribed for the illness (including only watching and waiting for the patient to recover spontaneously, and possessed of varying degrees of efficacy)
4. The *clinical performance* of the clinician (on the basis of competence and motivation, tempered by whatever barriers that exist)
5. The degree of *patient compliance* with the diagnostic proposal, the treatment plan, and other advice offered by the clinician or anybody else

For this reason, you may not want to base all of your own performance review on clinical outcomes and may put at least some of your energy into keeping track of the *clinical performance* in caring for your patients. Others are even more enthusiastic about process-based performance review [5].

A process-based review of your clinical performance requires the development of a list of important clinical actions that ought to be carried out for the common conditions you see, followed by a periodic review of whether you (alone or with your peers) are actually carrying them out [82]. We have found it a humbling but educational experience to set process criteria for how we should evaluate and manage arthritis, hypertension, and stroke in our practices, and then to review our own performance in caring for such patients. For example, colleagues of ours got ten physicians to set criteria for how they should respond to given clinical situations and then sent actors trained to simulate these situations to these physicians' offices [56]. Between 30% to 45% of the recommended procedures were not performed, and 50% to 70% of the criteria were not recorded.

Does this sort of performance review really improve our clinical performance? If this substantial effort fails to result in improved performance, why (on earth) should we waste time executing it? Fortunately, there is increasing evidence of the efficacy of performance reviews and we will review it at the end of this chapter and in our final chapter on continuing medical education.

If you want to set up a process-based performance review, how do you decide which clinical processes constitute the "good quality" that should be measured and reported? By now it should come as no surprise to you to learn that we recommend a critical appraisal of the clinical literature to identify those clinical processes you ought to execute for the conditions you frequently encounter. To help you do this, we will recommend some simple guidelines that will help you avoid being overwhelmed by huge "laundry lists" that contain every conceivable act that anybody (especially a group of "experts") thinks you should carry out on patients with these illnesses. The six guides summarized in Table 10-2 will help you identify the best clinical processes to include in your performance review. These guides will also help you assess whether the methods used in the article to measure the clinical process will produce valid results that are relevant to your own practice.

Table 10-2. Readers' guides for articles about performance reviews

1. Did the study focus on what clinicians actually do?
2. Have the clinical acts under study been shown to do more good than harm? If not, is the article about a "process versus outcome" study that assembled an inception cohort, assured high compliance, included all relevant outcomes, and took prognosis into account?
3. Are the clinicians, patients, and setting similar to yours?
4. Were the clinical processes or acts measured in a clinically sensible fashion?
5. Were the clinical processes or acts measured in a scientifically credible fashion?
6. Were both clinical and statistical significance considered?

We will, as usual, consider the guides in turn:

Did the Study Focus on What Clinicians Actually Do?

Evaluations of the quality of clinical care can be classified into three categories, and we already have met the latter two of them. First, *clinical structure* studies simply tally the numbers and qualifications of health professionals and describe the administrative organization and physical facilities in which they work. If this tally satisfies some standard, however arbitrarily established, the clinical care provided is pronounced "high quality." Second, *clinical process* studies document the actions health professionals carry out as they manage patients; these actions sometimes are subdivided into technical processes (e.g., investigations carried out, physiologic monitoring executed, drugs prescribed) and interpersonal processes (e.g., patient education). Finally, *clinical outcome* studies of the quality of care document the end results of this care in terms of its effects on the patient's health (e.g., survival, symptoms, physical and psychosocial function); this is the "proof of the pudding."

Articles that focus only on structural descriptions do not deserve time from a busy clinical reader. We all know that impressive diplomas and credentials cannot guarantee clinical competency and that humble, unimpressive buildings can be the sites of excellent clinical care. By the same token, as we have already pointed out, the authors of articles that focus only on health outcomes may be fooling themselves if they assume that these outcomes are the exclusive consequences of the clinical processes executed earlier.

Thus, the most useful articles to read if you want to learn those clinical processes that you ought to carry out are articles that focus on what clinicians actually do. By restricting your selection of articles to those that report on clinical processes or actions that clinicians actually carry out, you already will have eliminated the large number of articles that focus exclusively on structure or outcome, or on processes that are not relevant to you as a clinician. In doing so, you also will increase the efficiency with which you use your scarce reading time.

One type of article especially worth tracking down and reading is the one that has the term *tracer condition* [37] or *indicator condition* [76] in its title or abstract. A tracer or indicator condition is an illness, clinical situation, or health state that either (a) should encourage clinical actions known to result in more good than harm when correctly applied (for example, high-dose aspirin in rheumatoid arthritis [43]) or (b) should discourage clinical actions known to result in more harm than good (for example, chloramphenicol for self-limited upper respiratory tract infections [83]).

Have the Clinical Acts Under Study Been Shown To Do More Good Than Harm?

This guide draws our attention to Chapters 3, 4, 5, 7, and 8 in which we described how to decide whether clinical maneuvers do more good than harm. To be sure, the clinical acts of prime importance will be therapeutic: prescribing therapies that help and avoiding therapies that harm. However, other clinical acts will also meet this guide, such as those acts of diagnosis that establish the need for therapy (doing the appropriate tests and avoiding the inappropriate ones), those acts of appropriate dose-setting and monitoring, those that detect and manage low compliance, and those that provide proper follow-up.

If you are confident that the clinical acts studied in the article really have been shown to do more good than harm, you are ready to go on to the next guide. If, however, this is not the case, then a modification of this second guide should be applied, as follows: *If the clinical acts have not been shown to do more good than harm, is the article about a "process versus outcome" study that assembled an inception cohort, assured high compliance, included all relevant outcomes, and took prognosis into account?*

This guide is quite a mouthful, but is really very straightforward. First, it states that you are wasting your precious reading time unless either the article is *about* clinical acts that do more good than harm or the article is *establishing whether* the clinical acts (or "processes") are linked to important clinical "outcomes." If neither of these apply, the article should join, in benign neglect, the mass of publications that merely count patients seen, tests performed and money spent.

Because "process versus outcome" studies contribute to our understanding of the integration of assessment, diagnosis, therapy, and patient compliance into patient care, you probably will want to read them. In doing so, there are four special features you should look for. First, the authors should have assembled an "inception cohort" of patients (consecutive patients identified at the first visit for a problem or diagnosis, or at the beginning of therapy). This is to ensure that patients who fail to continue attending the clinic or hospital are not lost to follow-up, especially when this failure is due to their developing a relevant outcome such as death or a severe disability that makes it impossible for them to answer questionnaires or attend follow-up clinics! For example, two widely quoted process versus outcome studies, one involving myocardial infarction [18] and the other hypertension [54], failed to generate inception cohorts and employed inclusion criteria that required patients to be "available for follow-up" or to come back to the clinic. As a result, they may have missed important patients and their outcomes, thus becoming highly susceptible to inaccurate conclusions.

Second, patient compliance needs to be taken into account in process versus outcome studies, since this is an essential link between the therapeutic actions of clinicians and the outcomes of their patients. The failure to take compliance into account has flawed several studies that concluded that there were no strong links between process and outcomes [2, 39, 40, 54, 70]. Other studies that took compliance into account have documented strong links between the process and outcomes of care for urinary tract infection, hypertension, iron deficiency anemia, and other conditions [27, 62, 78]. Thus, before we accept that no relationship exists between the processes and outcomes of care for a given condition, we should insist on documentation that the failure to observe a relationship was not merely due to low compliance.

Third, a process versus outcome study must examine all clinically relevant outcomes. Depending on the illness under study these might include death, improvement or deterioration in symptoms or in physical, emotional, or social function, or even the physiologic control of a risk factor for disease (when it is justified to substitute alterations in such risk factors for morbidity or mortality as in hypertension [33]), patient satisfaction, and the side effects of therapy. The methods for assessing these outcomes should be of acceptable accuracy, and to minimize bias their assessment should have been undertaken by an assessor who was blind to the details of the processes employed in the patients' management.

Finally, to isolate the effects of the clinical processes from those due to other determinants of outcome, it is necessary for process versus outcome studies to control for these other determinants of the clinical outcomes observed. As implied in Figure 10-2, sicker patients usually require more extensive assessment, monitoring, and intervention, but will nonetheless tend to have poor outcomes even when the quality of the care they receive is high. For this reason, an analysis that failed to control for this severity of illness would conclude that the greater the number of clinical processes carried out, the worse the outcome! As silly as it is, this conclusion has, in fact, been drawn in some process versus outcome studies.

Once satisfied that the processes executed by clinicians are, indeed, linked to the outcomes of their patients, you are ready to apply the next guide.

Are the Clinicians, Patients, and Setting Similar to Yours?

Information about the practice setting (primary, secondary, or tertiary care), the clinicians' training, certification, years of experience, and workload; and the source and types of patients involved will allow you to decide whether the results of the study would be applicable in your own practice. Moreover, the methods used to select the actual clinicians and patients for the study should be described, so that you can judge whether they are likely to be representative of the study site. For example, if only those clinicians who volunteered for a study were included, and they comprised less than 80% of eligible clinicians, it would not be wise to generalize their results either to those who did not volunteer or to clinicians in general.

Finally, the rules for what constitutes a case should be realistic. Thus, eligibility for inclusion in a study of an indicator condition should be based on an illness or complaint (e.g., sleep disturbance) rather than on a disease (e.g., depression), since the latter assumes a correct diagnostic process and misses those patients for whom the indicator condition was present but not diagnosed. Similarly, except for discrete emergencies, the definition of a "case" should allow the assessment of episodes of care that include follow-up visits when appropriate.

Since it is unlikely that any study setting will exactly replicate your own practice, you should consider this guideline from the perspective of asking yourself "Are the illnesses, the clinicians and their practices *so different* from the setting in which I am interested in quality of care, that I could *not* apply the study results?".

Were the Clinical Processes or Acts Measured in a Clinically Sensible Fashion?

The rules for measuring these clinical acts must be explicit, comprehensive, and flexible. First, the measurement criteria should be explicitly stated so that you can see if they make sense. This means that the actual criteria used must be available; ideally they will be included in the article, an appendix, a repository, or at least available from the author.

Second, the process criteria should be comprehensive. That is, they should include all the clinically important acts in the process of care (e.g., history taking, the physical examination, ordering laboratory tests, prescribing therapy, executing patient education, ordering a consultation, and the like) that should have been applied to all groups of patients (e.g., different age groups, different socioeconomic groups) about whom conclusions are desired. You cannot assume that just because a given clinician satisfied defined standards for performing the history, physical examination, and laboratory investigation, this same clinician necessarily met the other standards for drug management, patient education, and follow-up. Moreover, because of conflicting evidence over whether one can generalize from a clinician's performance with one type of patient problem to other types of patient problems [42, 59], it is necessary for authors to have evaluated all conditions about which they are drawing conclusions. Actually, a sizeable portion of most practices can be represented by a small array of health problems. By covering just these, a reasonable overview of an individual clinician's quality of care can, in fact, be obtained [26].

Finally, it is important to consider whether the process criteria used are flexible enough to allow for appropriate variations in management according to differing diagnostic probabilities, to differing severities of disease, and to the presence of complications. In many situations this is not necessary, and it would be acceptable to apply identical criteria to all patients (for example, criteria for having completed the immunization of all children by a defined age would be quite appropriate). On the other hand, you should expect and demand more sophisticated assessment methods when patients present with complex problems (e.g., emergency room patients with pleuritic chest pain) rather than clear cut diagnoses; similarly, flexible process criteria are appropriate for assessing the management of patients with different complications or levels of disease severity (such as in the management of chest pain due to acute myocardial infarction).

All too often, long and invariant "laundry" lists are applied to quite heterogeneous groups of patients. On the other hand, Jack Sibley's "indicator condition" approach (which stratifies patients by severity) [76] and Sheldon Greenfield's "criteria mapping" method (which has branching criteria to reflect sequential judgements) [22] provide ways of satisfying this guide, and articles should have incorporated methods such as these where needed. Some aspects of care may even need direct observation: When nurses' compliance with physicians' orders for close observation (determining vital signs more than once every 4 hours) was assessed by direct observation, the orders were carried out during only 23% of 284 nursing shifts [1]. No wonder, then, that two of us had to abandon a chart-based quality-of-care investigation among survivors of myocardial infarction when our pilot study revealed that only 25% of the key information recorded by nurse-observers ever got into the patients' charts. Moreover, our patients' recall was not accurate enough to fill in the gaps. As an alternative to direct observation, other successful studies have reviewed audiotapes to assess the quality of verbal interactions such as patient contracting [23].

Were the Clinical Processes or Acts Measured in a Scientifically Credible Fashion?

The method used to decide whether specific clinical actions were carried out must be both accurate and precise. Accuracy means that the method faithfully captures clinically important deficits or differences in the clinical process that really went on, and precision means that different examiners (including you!), applying the same method to the same cases, will draw the same conclusions about whether specific clinical processes were carried out.

A major limitation to the accuracy of the measurement of clinical processes by methods that rely on medical records is the inconsistency with which different clinicians record their clinical actions [60]. As a result it may be difficult or impossible to distinguish clinical acts not performed from clinical acts performed but not recorded. On the other hand, it can be (and is) argued that good clinical care necessitates good records, and important actions have to be recorded for recall, for communication with others, and for minimizing the clinical errors that arise from recording only conclusions and management decisions without the observations that led to them. Surprisingly, despite the faults of clinical records, several studies have shown that they can provide accurate, adequate data for a wide range of clinical processes; however, this accuracy is usually best achieved when explicit criteria have been restricted to bare essentials [22, 76]. Even so, relying on implicit clinical judgments about quality often fails to achieve consistency, even among "experts" [2]. To achieve precision, the criteria for acceptable quality of care must be explicit, and a high degree of interobserver agreement in applying the criteria should be documented in the article.

Finally, if a formal study of the impact of some educational maneuver on the quality of care is being assessed, the clinical process information should have been collected by individuals who were "blind" to the purpose of the study. This blinding is necessary to avoid bias due to the expectations of the abstractor who already knows the patient, the clinician, or the outcome. If logistics made complete blinding impossible, at least a sample of the observations should have been assessed in a blind fashion in order to obtain an estimate of bias.

Were Both Clinical and Statistical Significance Considered?

Many quality of care studies generate "grades" or "scores" for how well the desired clinical processes have been carried out. When you encounter such scores you should assure yourself that their construction and analysis make clinical sense and lead to conclusions that are both sensible and applicable in routine clinical care. In particular, you should beware of scores and analyses that simply add up the number of "right" things that were done, for such analyses can generate ludicrous conclusions. In such a study, for example, a clinician caring for a patient who vomited blood could take a thorough history (worth lots of points), execute a flawless series of diagnostic studies (lots more points), and then go back to bed with a reasonably high score while the patient exsanguinates for want of proper therapy.

Appropriate analyses are of two sorts. The first one is descriptive, and simply provides a table listing each clinical process and the proportion of cases in which it was executed. This descriptive analysis permits clinical readers to draw their own conclusions as well as to reflect on those drawn by the authors. The second sort of appropriate analysis establishes a minimum set of actions, *all* of which must be carried out for a case to have been handled with adequate quality of care. This analysis reflects the extent to which an entire set of clinical processes known or believed to affect clinical outcomes have been executed, and could be applied with profit to our earlier patient with hematemesis.

Finally, any conclusions about the quality of care provided in such articles should be backed up by tests of statistical significance. We would refer you back to Chapter 7, and will simply paraphrase the two questions on page 201:

1. If the difference in quality of care is statistically significant, is it clinically significant as well?
2. If the difference in quality of care is not statistically significant, was the study large enough to detect clinically significant differences in the quality of care if they had occurred?

The application of the foregoing guides will help you identify those illnesses (or presenting problems) upon which you could base your personal performance review. On this basis, you can identify the specific clinical processes you ought to both carry out and document in your records.

But how do you put such a plan into action in your own practice? How can you be sure that important clinical acts get recorded in your records? For those of you who keep detailed, complete records, the only challenge will be wading through them to get at the notations that document the performance of the key processes. The rest of us, whose records serve more to jog our memories than to document our actions, have a problem. If a process *is* recorded in one of our charts, all is well: we can be pretty confident that it was carried out. But what if our chart contains no entry about a process? How do we tell whether it wasn't done, on the one hand, or was done but wasn't recorded, on the other (especially when executing the process would not produce any other data, such as a laboratory report)?

In this latter case, if we are serious about carrying out performance reviews on ourselves we will have to begin by improving the documentation in our clinical records. Two approaches to improving our records deserve discussion: the "problem-oriented medical record" and the use of protocols or flow sheets.

The *problem-oriented medical record* (POMR), most eloquently described by Lawrence Weed [86], proposes that all data, assessments, and diagnostic or management plans be recorded in the medical record in association with the specific problem (a diagnosis, illness, sign, symptom, or abnormal lab result) to which they apply. If this rule is followed faithfully, most clinical acts will be recorded and the abstracting of a chart for performance review ought to be easier. Attractive as this proposal appears, a controlled comparison of the speed and accuracy of record review performed by Robert Fletcher found no difference between problem-oriented and traditional records [19]. The POMR's usefulness remains to be demonstrated in rigorous trials, and we agree with Alvan Feinstein, who attributes much of its apparent success to the enthusiasm and supervision with which it is introduced [16].*

The second approach is for those who want to carry out performance reviews but do not want to shift over to the problem-oriented medical record. This latter approach calls for introducing standard protocols or flow sheets for those clinical problems you want to scrutinize.

The adoption of protocols or flow sheets developed by others, or the generation of your own, is perhaps the easiest way to combine performance review and feedback strategy that encourages rather than interferes with good clinical practice. We use flow sheets for patient problems we encounter frequently, and the one that we use for hypertension is shown in Figures 10-3 and 10-4.

The similarity of these flow sheets to Figures 1-11 to 1-13 back in Chapter 1 that illustrate the "multiple branching" diagnostic strategy is no coincidence, for a flow sheet ought to represent an orderly set of rational actions that lead to the correct diagnosis and appropriate management. The elements of our hypertension flow sheets come from the recommendations generated by several Canadian Task Forces on hypertension [58] and serve both to to remind us about, and to document whether we carried out, certain diagnostic and management processes. Moreover, if we update these flow sheets when later Task Forces generate new recommendations, our practice will reflect advances in knowledge and we will avoid the stagnation that befalls many clinicians once they complete their training.

However, the hypertension flow sheet shown in Figure 10-3 fails to capture a key clinical process in the care of hypertension: the detection of the hypertensive patient. This detection calls for case finding whenever we see patients for any reason, and the performance review of this clinical process would require the

*Of course, the same thing could have been said for "critical appraisal" instruction until the recent spate of educational trials that are showing us when and where it does and doesn't actually work!

HYPERTENSION WORK-UP

RECORD OF INITIAL CLINICAL ASSESSMENT

EXAMINING PHYSICIAN ▶ ____

DATE OF EXAMINATION ▶ ____

Patient Name ▶

Address ▶

D.O.B. ▶

I.D. No. ▶

CLINICAL HISTORY

	DETAILS
TREATMENT FOR HYPERTENSION	PAST ☐ PRESENT ☐
TARGET ORGAN INVOLVEMENT	HEART ☐ KIDNEY ☐ BRAIN ☐
SECONDARY HYPERTENSION	ESTROGENS EXOGENOUS ☐ PREGNANCY ☐ FLANK PAIN/TRAUMA ☐ KIDNEY SURGERY ☐ PHEOCHROMOCYTOMA ☐ (Pounding headache *plus* sweating *plus* palpitations *plus* anxiousness) ENDOCRINE DISEASE ☐

PHYSICAL EXAMINATION

	DETAILS AND OTHER FINDINGS
BLOOD PRESSURE	SITTING (for diastolic use disappearance of sounds) R ARM ___/___ L ARM ___/___ Use arm with higher reading for follow-up Wt.____ Ht.____
FUNDUSCOPIC	ABNORMALITY PRESENT ☐
CARDIAC STATUS	PULSE Rate ____ Rhythm ____ HEART SOUNDS ____ Murmurs? LUNGS – Basal Rales ☐ Other signs of failure?
PERIPHERAL PULSES	Simultaneous radial and femoral Fullness ____ Timing ____
ABDOMEN	SUBCOSTAL BRUIT ☐
PITTING EDEMA	PRESENT ☐
EVIDENCE OF ENDOCRINE DISEASE	CUSHING'S ☐ THYROID ☐ ACROMEGALY ☐

INVESTIGATIONS

TEST	RESULTS AND DATE	TEST	RESULTS AND DATE
URINE DIPSTICK		CHEST X-RAY (If indicated)	
SERUM POTASSIUM		E.C.G. (If indicated)	
SERUM CREATININE			

Figure 10-3. A flow sheet for the evaluation of hypertension. (Reprinted with permission from C. E. Evans, M.D., McMaster University, Hamilton, Ontario, Canada.)

examination of an appropriate sample of our charts to see whether we were checking the blood pressure of all the patients we encountered. Thus, in this as in other presenting problems, the performance review has to examine multiple sources of information. For example, two of us recently collaborated in a randomized trial to find out whether providing an educational package that includes

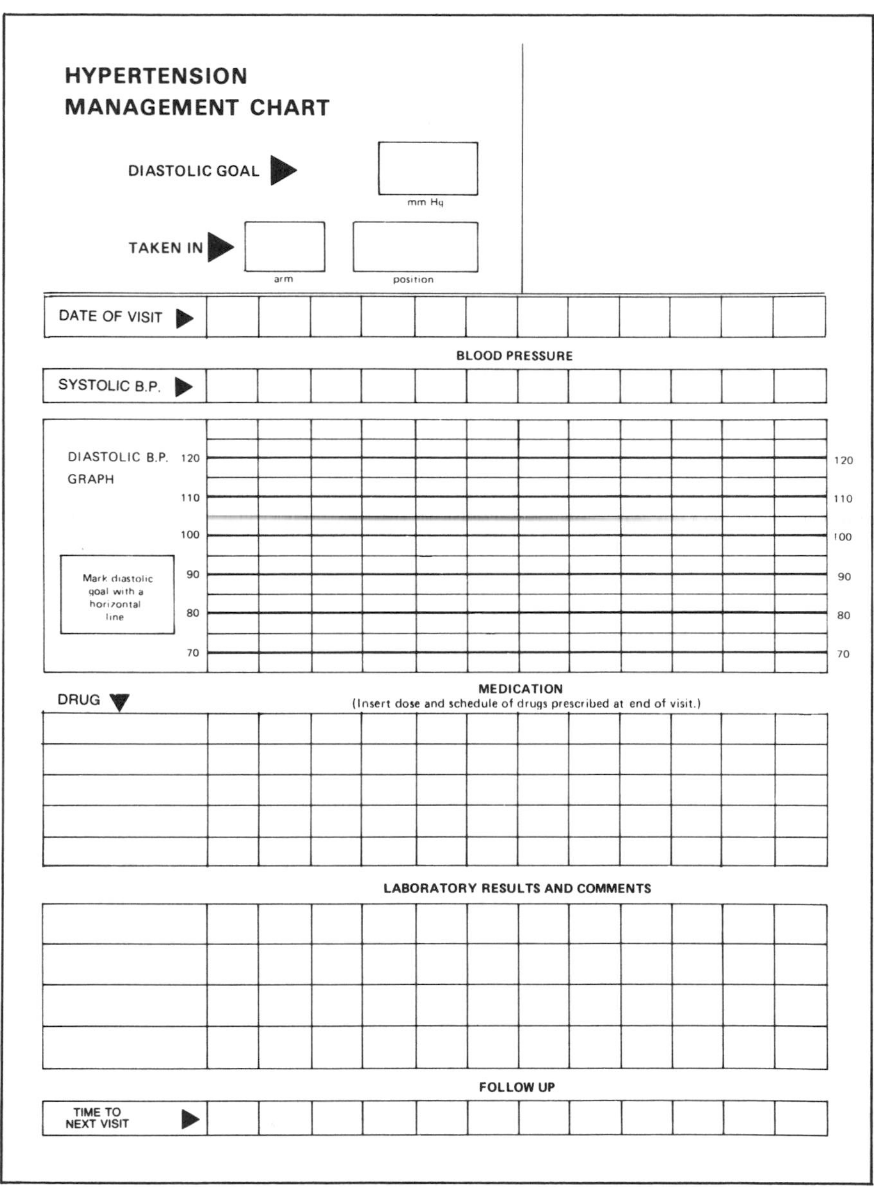

HYPERTENSION MANAGEMENT CHART

DIASTOLIC GOAL ▶ ______ mm Hg

TAKEN IN ▶ ______ arm ______ position

DATE OF VISIT ▶

BLOOD PRESSURE

SYSTOLIC B.P. ▶

DIASTOLIC B.P. GRAPH 120 110 100 90 80 70

Mark diastolic goal with a horizontal line

DRUG ▼

MEDICATION (Insert dose and schedule of drugs prescribed at end of visit.)

LABORATORY RESULTS AND COMMENTS

FOLLOW UP

TIME TO NEXT VISIT ▶

Figure 10-4. A flow sheet for the management of hypertension. (Reprinted with permission from C. E. Evans, M.D., McMaster University, Hamilton, Ontario, Canada.)

such flow sheets to half the physicians in two towns will improve the control of hypertension in their practices, compared to those of physicians who did not receive these educational packages and practice aids [14].

The foregoing sequence of identifying commonly encountered clinical problems, tracking down the clinical processes that have a real effect on the outcomes of these problems and, finally, incorporating these clinical processes into flow sheets that both remind and document these processes, will provide you with a very useful system of performance review. Moreover, if these flow sheets are updated to reflect advances in the diagnosis and management of these disorders, and if your reviews of your own performance continue to show that you are practicing up-to-date medicine, you have every reason to be enormously proud of your ability to keep abreast of advances in medicine. A very attractive attribute of this approach is the way it proceeds from advances in knowledge (gained through your clinical reading, discussions with consultants and other colleagues, or from more formal continuing education sessions) to revisions of a very practical flow sheet that both reminds you what to do with given patient problems and records whether you have done it, to an ongoing system of performance review that tells you whether you are practicing what you preach.

How might this performance review be initiated? We would suggest that clinicians begin by seizing "targets of opportunity" in the form of disorders or health states that they *know* are affected by clinical performance. Examples would be the proper use of antibiotics, the detection and treatment of hypertension, or immunization against certain infectious diseases. In the latter instances, the performance review could begin at once by scanning the charts of recent patients to see whether their immunization histories were ascertained or their blood pressures checked. They could then proceed to the "audit" of charts for the performance of specific clinical acts and patient outcomes.

Physicians in group practices have the advantage of already established working parties that could decide which performance to review and how to share the work. Moreover, those who use computer systems for patient accounts and scheduling possess a tool of great potential for performance review. If, for example, certain clinical procedures were both part of a performance review and constituted a compensable service (e.g., cervical cytology), the computerized account system would also monitor clinical performance.

The foregoing is nice, and is self-evidently effective, but it is also a lot of extra work. Is there solid evidence that it actually improves subsequent performance? Although we will discuss this in greater detail in Chapter 14, some initial comments are warranted here.

Flow sheets or algorithms have been shown in controlled trials to change physicians' actions: in caring for cardiac failure in family practice [85], the neonatal respiratory distress syndrome [89], burns in the emergency room (when combined with written feedback on performance) [41], and pneumonia, myocardial infarction, urinary infections, and gastrointestinal bleeding in community hospitals (when combined with individual feedback on deviations from protocol) [74]; in reducing the unnecessary performance of pelvimetry in community hospitals [6]; in executing the age-specific preventive procedures recommended by the Canadian Periodic Health Examination Task Force and the American Cancer Society [7]; and in helping smokers quit [88]. However, most of these trials looked only at the impact of these flow sheets and algorithms on the process of care; only the trial among clinicians caring for burn patients and the smoking cessation trial recorded improvements in clinical outcomes, and these were small.

Systematic written or verbal feedback of performance has also been shown in controlled trials to improve physician compliance with predetermined criteria for management of the following clinical problems: chronic obstructive lung disease in family practice (when combined with audiovisual programs and group meetings) [80]; hypertension, headache, otitis media and bronchitis in primary care [65, 20]; drug monitoring in community hospitals [38]; outpatients with various disorders cared for by residents and interns [64]; the proper use of prothrombin-time tests by residents [12]; preventive fluoride treatment by primary care residents [63]; the proper use of laboratory tests and diagnostic tests by hospital residents [45, 15, 46]; eight specific medical and pediatric conditions in an ambulatory care setting [61]; stool testing for occult blood by internists in an HMO* [89]; writing generic drug prescriptions [20]; and in the management of constipation and hazardous morbidity in nursing homes [51].

Automated performance review takes its extreme form in systems that feed back computer-generated performance scores. McDonald and his coworkers have shown in controlled studies that such computer-generated feedback can be successful in improving patient care for such conditions as hypertension and diabetes mellitus [48], and in reducing unneccessary test ordering [49]. Hershey showed that this type of feedback led to reduced prescription costs by residents [28, 29], and Studney has shown that this approach also is feasible in a private family practice setting [79].

Thus, there are a growing number of studies that show the potential of performance review, but most of them have only looked for changes in behavior, not outcomes, and have not been carried out in the randomized trial format.

Should paper-based or simulated/standardized clinical patient management problems be considered as an option for your performance review?

Geoff Norman has suggested a useful way of considering all this: the "Know-Can-Do" approach [55]. This variation on our earlier electricity/hydro model of volts and watts converts the former into "Know"—your theoretical knowledge which can be assessed on paper, as with a patient management problem. Watts are further divided into "Can"—your ability to manage a standardized clinical problem (such as a standardized/simulated patient) while being directly observed (the "fishbowl"), and "Do"—your performance in your day-to-day practice when no one is looking!

When we examine how well measures of "Know" and "Can" actually predict what we "Do," the results are not yet very encouraging. Thus, although the "Know" paper or simulated/standardized patient problems are popular in some academic settings, there is not yet sufficient evidence that these predict everyday performance. When Jones and his colleagues [35] reviewed 11 studies of the "Know-Do" link between written case simulations and actual clinical encounters, they concluded that the linkage was pretty weak. And, although clinicians respond similarly to simulated and standardized real patients in the same setting

*Applying Quality of Care criterion #2, we'd suggest that you consider whether the efficacy of occult blood testing is established. At the time that this edition was going to press, stool testing was producing earlier diagnosis of colorectal cancer but, as yet, no reduction in mortality from this disorder.

[55], a more recent study (not included in the previously cited review) by Rethans and his colleagues [69] found no relation between the way that 48 general practitioners managed a simulated patient with urinary tract infection who appeared at their offices and their own subsequent performance on a written case simulation of the same patient. Not only did they commit themselves to significantly more unnecessary and superfluous actions in the paper problem than in real life; they also carried out fewer of the most important actions (designated obligatory by a criteria-setting panel of their peers). Since "cueing" by presenting a written menu of options may be responsible for much of this bias, perhaps the new approaches now being developed will eliminate this and focus on the "obligatory actions" [57].

On the other hand, the evidence using multiple choice questions as a measure of "Know" is quite positive. The American Board of Emergency Medicine [77] examined the ability of two components of the specialty certification examination, a multiple-choice test and a structured oral examination, to predict performance in practice (assessed by chart review) 10 years later. The overall predictive validity was high, around .60. A similar study was conducted by Ramsay and the American Board of Internal Medicine [68], using their written multiple-choice certification examination and a peer assessment of practice performance 7 to 10 years later. The Pearson correlation coefficient was quite impressive, of the order of .53 to .59. However, it must be borne in mind that these competence measures are far removed from the "Do" of actual performance.

How about the use of simulated patients in a "fishbowl setting" such as a workshop or postgraduate course? Studies performed to date suggest that the "Can-Do" link may not be much stronger. Rethans [69] successfully introduced 4 standardized patients into the offices of 39 Dutch general practitioners and compared this "Do" with the "Can" that occurred when these same physicians worked up these same problems in a university fishbowl setting. Again, there was an increase in the number of actions taken in the fishbowl setting.

At present, the assessment of the clinical competence of an individual clinician appears to require a multiple measure approach. For example, the program that our university currently operates to help our province's licensing body assess physicians, whose charts suggest that they may have deficiencies in performance, has to be both lengthy and costly [57, 47]. The measurements include chart-stimulated recall (1–1.5 hours), a simulated office full of standardized patients (2–2.5 hours), a structured oral examination (1–1.5 hours), objective structured clinical examinations (1–1.5 hours), and multiple-choice questionnaires (1–1.5 hours). A moderately strong relationship among all the measures has been documented with the best discrimination provided by standardized patients and oral examination. It remains to be seen whether our current, costly approach can be pared down to be feasible for self-assessment. As we go to press, it is too early to know whether this intense assessment will be both valid and practical.

We regret not being able to provide more specific recommendations about which sorts of performance review to use and how to carry them out. However, because this field is still in its infancy and because we refuse to recommend any time-consuming maneuvers that have not been shown in proper experiments to do more good than harm, all we can do here is describe approaches that show the most promise. The role that these studies should play in selecting your personal approach to continuing medical education will be discussed further in Chapter 14.

Whatever means you employ, or are employed on you by others, your performance review will identify areas where you are out-of-date or otherwise falling short, and you will need to do something about it. This something usually begins with a trip, either in person or by computer, to the nearest medical library, often an intimidating place where what is findable is unlearnable and what is learnable is unfindable. We devote the next chapter to lessening this intimidation and to rendering the learnable findable.

References

1. Aidroos, N. Nurses' response to doctor's orders for close observation. *Can. J. Psychiatry* 31: 831, 1986.
2. Brook, R. H. *Quality of Care Assessment: A Comparison of Five Methods of Peer Review.* Washington: Government Printing Office. DHEW HRA-74–3100, 1973.
3. Brook, R. H., and Williams, K. N. Evaluation of the New Mexico peer review system, 1971 to 1973. *Med. Care* (Suppl.) 14: 1, 1976.
4. Brook, R. H., Williams, K. N., and Avery, S. B. Quality assurance today and tomorrow: Forecast for the future. *Ann. Intern. Med.* 85: 809, 1976.
5. Brown, C. R., and Uhl, H. S. M. Mandatory continuing education: Sense or nonsense. *J.A.M.A.* 213: 1660, 1970.
6. Chassin, M. R., and McCue, S. A Randomized Trial of Medical Quality Assurance. *J.A.M.A.* 256: 1012, 1986.
7. Cohen, D. I., Littenberg, B., Wetzel, C., and Neuhauser, D. V. B. Improved physician compliance with preventive medicine guidelines. *Med. Care* 20: 1040, 1982.
8. Cook, D. J. The clinical assessment of central venous pressure in the critically ill. *Amer. J. Med. Sci.* 299: 175, 1990.
9. Crowley, M. S., and Tillman, M. Performance audit in the selection and management of personnel in the physician's office laboratory. *Primary Care.* 13(4): 617, 1986.
10. Donabedian, S. Evaluating the quality of medical care. *Milbank Mem. Fund Q.* 44: 166, 1966.
11. Eisenberg, J. M. Sociologic influences on decision-making by clinicians. *Ann. Intern. Med.* 90: 957, 1979.
12. Eisenberg, J. M. An educational program to modify laboratory use by house staff. *J. Med. Educ.* 52: 578, 1977.
13. Evans, C. E., Haynes, R. B., Gilbert, J. R., et al. An educational package on hypertension for primary care physicians: Older physicians benefit most. *Can. Med. Assoc. J.* 130: 719, 1984.
14. Evans, C. E., Haynes, R. B., Birkett, N. J., et al. Does a mailed continuing education program improve physician performance? *J.A.M.A.* 255: 501, 1986.
15. Everett, G. D., deBlois, C. S., Chang, P., and Holets, T. Effect of cost education, cost audits, and faculty chart review on the use of laboratory services. *Arch. Int. Med.* 143: 942; 1983.
16. Feinstein, A. R. The problems of the "Problem-Oriented Medical Record." *Ann. Intern. Med.* 78: 751, 1973.

17. Fernow, L. C., Mackie, C., McGill, I., and Randal, M. The effect of problem oriented medical records in clinical management controlled for patient risk. *Med. Care* 16: 476, 1978.
18. Fessel, W. J., and VanBrunt, E. E. Assessing quality of care from the medical record. *N. Engl. J. Med.* 286: 134, 1972.
19. Fletcher, R. H. Auditing problem-oriented records and traditional records. *N. Eng. J. Med.* 290: 829, 1974.
20. Gehlbach, S. H., Wilkinson, W. E., Hammond, W. E., et al. Improving drug prescribing in a primary care practice. *Med.Care* 22: 193; 1984.
21. Gonnella, J. S., Goran, M. J., Williamson, J. W., et al. Evaluation of patient care: An approach. *J.A.M.A.* 21: 2040, 1970.
22. Greenfield, S., Lewis, C. E., Japlan, S. H., and Davidson, M. B. Peer review by criteria mapping. *Ann. Intern. Med.* 83: 761, 1975.
23. Greenfield, S., Kaplan, S. H., Ware, J. E., et al. Patients participation in medical care. *J. Gen. Intern. Med.* 3: 448, 1988.
24. Gross, H. S., Herbert, M. R., Knatternd, G. L., and Donner, L. The effects of race and sex on the variation of diagnosis disposition in a psychiatric emergency room. *J. Nerv. Ment. Dis.* 148: 638, 1969.
25. Haase, W. The Role of Socioeconomic Class and Examiner Class in Examiner Bias. In F. Riessman, J. Cohen, and A. Pearl (eds.), *Mental Health of the Poor.* New York: The Free Press, 1964.
26. Hamaty, D. Assessment of Performance in Ambulatory Care: Proceedings of a Conference. San Francisco: American Society of Internal Medicine, 1976.
27. Haynes, R. B., Gibson, E. S., Taylor, D. W., et al. Process versus outcome in hypertension: A positive result. *Circulation* 65: 28, 1982.
28. Hershey, C. O., Porter, D. K., Breslau, D., and Cohen, D. I. Influence of simple computerized feedback on prescription charges in an ambulatory clinic. *Med. Care* 24: 472, 1986.
29. Hersey, C. O., Goldberg, M. I., and Cohen, D. I. The effect of computerized feedback coupled with a newsletter upon outpatient prescribing charges. *Med. Care* 26: 88, 1988.
30. Hilborne, L. H., Wenger, N. S., and Oye, R. K. House officer performance of simple laboratory tests. *Clin. Res.* 38: 729A, 1990.
31. Hobbs, H. E., Sorsby, A., and Freedman, A. Retinopathy following chloroquine therapy. *Lancet* 2: 478, 1959.
32. Howie, J. G. Clinical judgment and antibiotic use in general practice. *Brit. Med. J.* 2: 1061, 1976.
33. Hypertension Detection and Follow-up Cooperative Group. Five year findings of the Hypertension Detection and Followup Program: I. Reduction in mortality of persons with high blood pressure including mild hypertension. *J.A.M.A.* 242: 2562, 1979.
34. International Multiple Centers Trial. Prevention of fatal postoperative pulmonary embolism by low doses of heparin. *Lancet* 2: 45, 1975.
35. Jones, T. V., Gerrity, M. S., and Earp, J., Written Case Simulations: Do they predict behavior? *J. Clin. Epidemiol.* 43: 805, 1990.
36. Kane, R. L., Gardner, J., Wright, A., et al. Relationship between process and outcome of acute episodes of care provided by different types of family practitioners. *J. Fam. Prac.* 6: 133, 1978.
37. Kessner, D. M., Kalk, C. B., and Singer, J. Assessing health quality: The case for tracers. *N. Engl. J. Med.* 288: 189, 1973.
38. Laxdal, O. E., Jennett, P. A., Wilson, T. W., et al. Improving physician performance by continuing medical education. *Can. Med. Assoc. J.* 118: 1051, 1978.
39. Lindsay, M. I., Jr., Hermans, P. E., Nobrega, F. T., et al. Quality of care assessment. I. Outpatient management of acute bacterial cystitis as the model. *Mayo Clin. Proc.* 51: 307, 1976.

40. Lindsay, M. I., Jr., Nobrega, F. T., Offord, K. P., et al. Quality of care assessment. II. Outpatient medical care following hospital dismissal after myocardial infarction. *Mayo Clin. Proc.* 52: 220, 1977.
41. Linn, B.S. Continuing medical education: Impact on emergency room burn care. *J.A.M.A.* 244: 556, 1980.
42. Lyons, T. F., and Payne, B. C. Interdiagnosis relationships of physician performance measures in hospitals. *Med. Care* 15: 475, 1977.
43. Mainland, I., and Sutcliffe, M. I. Aspirin in rheumatoid arthritis: A double blind trial. *Bull. Rheum. Dis.* 16: 388, 1965.
44. Martin, A. R., Wolfe, M. A., Thibodeau, L. A., et al. A trial of two strategies to modify the test-ordering behavior of medical residents. *N. Engl. J. Med.* 303: 1330, 1980.
45. Marton, K. K., Tul, V., Sox, H. C., Jr. Modifying test-ordering behavior in the outpatient medical clinic. A controlled trial to two educational interventions. *Arch. Intern. Med.* 145: 816, 1985.
46. Matthews, D. A., Sledge, W. H., and Lieberman, P. B. Evaluation of intern performance by medical inpatients. *Am. J. Med.* 83: 938, 1987.
47. McAuley, R. G., Paul, W. M., Morrison, G. H., et al. Results of 5 years of peer assessment of physicians office practices by the College of Physicians and Surgeons of Ontario. *Can. Med. Assoc. J.* 143: 1193, 1990.
48. McDonald, C. J. Use of a computer to detect and respond to clinical events: Its effect on clinical behavior. *Ann. Intern. Med.* 84: 162, 1976.
49. McDonald, C. J., Hin, S. L., Smith, D. M., et al. Reminders to physicians from an introspective computer medical record. *Ann. Intern. Med.* 100: 130, 1984.
50. Miller, G. E. Personal communication. 1982.
51. Mohide, E. A., Tugwell, P., Caulfield, P. A., et al. A randomized trial of quality assurance in nursing homes. *Med. Care* 26(6): 554, 1988.
52. Nanji, A., Poon, R., and Hinberg, I. Comparison of hospital staff performance when using desk top analysers for "near patient" testing. *J. Clin. Pathol.* 41: 223, 1988.
53. Neufeld, V. R., and Norman, G. R. *Assessing Clinical Competence: A Measurement Perspective*. New York: Springer, 1985.
54. Nobrega, F. T., Morrow, G. W., Smoldt, R. K., and Offord, K. P. Quality assessment in hypertension: analysis of process and outcome methods. *N. Engl. J. Med.* 296: 145, 1977.
55. Norman, G., Tugwell, P., and Feightner, J. W. A comparison of resident performance on real and simulated patients. *J. Med. Educ.* 57: 708, 1982.
56. Norman, G. R., Neufeld, V. R., Walsh, A., et al. Measuring physicians' performances by using simulated patients. *J. Med. Educ.* 60: 925, 1985.
57. Norman, G. Can an examination predict competence: The role of Recertification on Maintenance of Competence. *Ann. Roy. Coll. Phys. Surg. Canada,* 1991 In press.
58. Ontario Council of Health. *Hypertension. Report of the Task Force on Hypertension.* Toronto: Government Printing House, 1977.
59. Osborne, C. E. Interdiagnosis relationships of physician records in ambulatory child health care. *Med. Care* 15: 465, 1977.
60. Osborne, C. E., and Thompson, H. C. Criteria for examination of ambulatory child health care by chart audit development and testing of methodology. *Pediatrics* (Suppl.) 56: 625, 1975.
61. Palmer, R. H., Louis, T. A., Hsu, E. N., et al. A randomized controlled trial of quality assurance in sixteen ambulatory care practices. *Med. Care* 23: 751, 1985.
62. Payne, B. C., and Lyons, T. F. *Method for Estimating and Improving Ambulatory Medical Care. Final Report to the National Center for Health Services Research and Development.* Washington, D.C.: Government Printing Office, DHEW, 1978.
63. Pinkerton, R. E., Tinanoff, N., Williams, J. L., and Tapp, J. T. Resident physician performance in a continuing education format. *J.A.M.A.* 244: 2183, 1980.

64. Pozen, M. W., and Bonnet, P. D. Effectiveness of educational and administrative interventions in medical outpatient clinics. *Am. J. Publ. Health* 66: 151, 1976.
65. Putnam, W., and Curry, L. Patient care appraisal in the ambulatory setting: effectiveness as a continuing medical education tool. *Annu. Conf. Res. Med. Educ.* 19: 207, 1980.
66. Putnam, R. M., and Campbell, M. D. Changing learning in the lives of physicians. Fox, R. M., and Mazmanian, P. E. (eds.). New York: Putnam and Pirega, 1989. P. 79.
67. Putnam, R. W., and Curry, L. Physicians' participation in establishing criteria for hypertension management in the office: Will patient outcomes be improved? *Can. Med. Assoc. J.* 140: 806, 1989.
68. Ramsey, P. G., Carline, J. D., Inui, T. S., et al. Predictive validity of certification by the American Board of Internal Medicine. *Ann. Intern. Med.* 110: 719, 1989.
69. Rethans, J. J. E., and Van Boven, C. P. A. Simulated patients in general practice: A different look at the consultation. *Br. Med. J.* 294: 809, 1987.
70. Romm, F. J., Hotha, B. S., and Mayo, F. Correlates to outcomes in patients with congestive cardiac failures. *Med. Care* 14: 765, 1976.
71. Roper, W. L., Winkenwerde, W., Hackbarth, G. M., and Krakauer, H. Effectiveness in Health Care: An initiative to evaluate and improve medical practice. *N. Eng. J. Med.* 319: 1197, 1988
72. Rutstein, D. D., Berenbert, W., Chalmers, T. C., et al. Measuring the quality of medical care. A clinical method. *N. Engl. J. Med.* 294: 582, 1976.
73. Sackett, D. L., Haynes, R. B., Gibson, E. S., et al. Hypertension control, compliance and science. *Am. Heart J.* 296: 297, 1977.
74. Sanazaro, P. J., and Worth, R. M. Concurrent quality assurance in hospital care. Report of a study by private initiative in PSRO. *N. Engl. J. Med.* 298: 171, 1978.
75. Shapiro, A. R. The evaluation of clinical predictors. A method and initial application. *N. Engl. J. Med.* 296: 1509, 1977.
76. Sibley, J. C., Spitzer, W. O., Rudnick, K. V., et al. Quality of care appraisal in primary care: A quantitative method. *Ann. Intern. Med.* 83: 46, 1975.
77. Solomon, D. J., Reinhart, M. J., Bridgeham, R. G., et al. An assessment of an oral examination format for evaluating clinical competence in emergency medicine. *Acad. Med.* 65: S43, 1990.
78. Starfield, B., and Scheff, D. Effectiveness of pediatric care: The relationship between process and outcome. *Pediatrics* 49: 547, 1972.
79. Studney, D. R., and Kunstaetter, A. R. Experience with a Costar Quality Assurance Program in Private Practice. In *Proceedings of the 5th Annual Symposium in Computer Applications in Medical Care.* Washington, D.C.: IEEE Computing Society Press, 1981. P. 205–8.
80. Terry, P. B., Wang, V. L., Flynn, B. S., et al. A continuing medical education program in chronic obstructive pulmonary diseases: Design and outcome. *Am. Rev. Respir. Dis.* 123: 42, 1981.
81. Tierney, W. M., Miller, M. E., and McDonald, C. J. The effect on test ordering of informing physicians of the charges for outpatient diagnostic tests. *N. Engl. J. Med.* 322: 1499, 1990.
82. Tugwell, P. A methodological perspective on process measures of the quality of medical care. *J. Clin. Inves. Med.* 2: 113, 1979.
83. Wallerstein, R. V., Condit, P. K., Kasper, C. K., et al. Statewide study of chloramphenicol therapy and fatal aplastic anemia. *J.A.M.A.* 208: 2445, 1969.
84. Ward, P. C. J., Narris, I. B., Borke, M. A., and Horwitz, C. Symptomatic instruction in interpretive aspects of laboratory medicine. *J. Med. Educ.* 51: 648, 1976.
85. Watkins, C. J. Medical audit in general practice: Fact or fantasy? *J. Roy. Coll. Gen. Practit.* 31: 141, 1981.
86. Weed, L. L. *Medical Records, Medical Education, and Patient Care* (5th ed). Cleveland: Case Western Reserve Press, 1971.

87. Williamson, J. W. Evaluating quality of patient care: a strategy relating outcome and process assessment. *J.A.M.A.* 218: 564, 1971.
88. Wilson, D. M., Taylor, D. W., Gilbert, J. R., et al. A randomized trial of a family physician intervention for smoking cessation. *J.A.M.A.* 260: 1570, 1988.
89. Winickoff, R. N., Coltin, K. L., Morgan, M. M., et al. Improving physician performance through peer comparison feedback. *Med. Care* 22: 527, 1984.
90. Wirtschafter, D. D., Sumners, J., Colvin, E., et al. Continuing medical education: An assessment of impact upon neonatal care in community hospitals. *Annu. Conf. Res. Med. Educ.* 18: 252, 1979.

11

Tracking Down the Evidence to Solve Clinical Problems

In this chapter, we'll describe means of rapidly retrieving information and published studies on the current, pressing problems that confront you in your clinical practice. In doing so, we will expand on previous articles from our group on this topic [15, 16]. In Chapter 12, we will describe regular surveillance of the literature to keep up to date with advances in medical care.

To benefit your patient, the retrieval technique you use must find the best article(s) published on the problem or find summaries verifiably based on such evidence. To be practical, the process must be quick enough that patients who are sick won't be kept waiting. You can achieve both these aims if you make expert use of both traditional and modern information resources. There are many possible ways of doing this and we will describe several in current use. But you will need to develop your own system, depending on your local information resources, the state of the information services in your own clinical field, and your local access to information specialists.*

To illustrate these search strategies, we'll begin with some patient problems that also may pinpoint gaps in your own knowledge. These patient problems demonstrate several points. First, they cover the gamut of the prognosis, diagnosis, and treatment of disease. Second, they span the range of our own familiarity, from the prognosis of cardiac enlargement (where we felt quite knowledgeable but discovered, as is often the case, we were mistaken), to a problem in management of a perinatal disorder (about which we knew nothing and wanted to determine if our information routes and resources could hold up under the challenge of great ignorance), to establishing the diagnosis of deep venous thrombosis and pulmonary embolus (to illustrate the use of a new type of compendium of diagnostic test characteristics). All these questions arose from our clinical practices or personal experiences and thus are "take 'em as they come" problems, the solution of which shows the joys and frustrations of current information resources. Because of these varied features, we hope you will work through each problem even if the clinical topic is not of direct interest to you, so you can try the techniques for your own areas of clinical practice.

Here are the problems in more detail:

Problem 1: The prognosis of cardiomegaly. You are an internist and see a 59-year-old woman for the first time. You find that she has had hypertension for many years, not always well controlled, and now has a blood pressure of 152/94 mm Hg on hydrochlorothiazide 50 mg per day. She has no symptoms or clinical signs of complications of her hypertension but a recent chest x-ray report

*We are indebted to many information specialists who helped in our struggles to master information resources and technology. Although the list is too long to mention everyone, the people who merit special mention include Ann McKibbon and Cindy Walker at McMaster, Rose Marie Woodsmall at the National Library of Medicine, and Ken Warren with the Maxwell Foundation.

from her medical record shows mild cardiomegaly (cardiothoracic ratio, .52). The patient asks you what the enlarged heart means for her future. She states that she would like a pretty exact answer, as she is considering early retirement. You lack exact knowledge of the prognostic implications of cardiomegaly and tell her that you will discuss this on her next visit, at which time you will recheck her blood pressure. (Recalling the information in Chapter 8 on compliance, you ask her if she has taken all her pills during the last week. She says that she may have missed one when she was out last weekend but usually takes them all. You ask her to be sure to take them all until the next visit.)

How would you go about finding solid evidence that would help this woman with her problem? Take a moment to write down the routes you would usually use and any others that you would like to try. Try them out before you review what we have done.

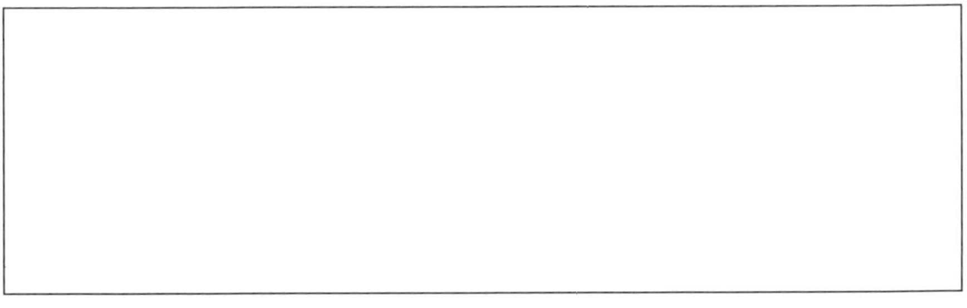

Problem 2: Are corticosteroids beneficial in preterm delivery? You are working in a primary-care setting and your patient (or spouse, sister, cousin, niece, or next door neighbor, if you don't see obstetrical patients) is in her thirty-second week of pregnancy when labor pains begin. You are not an obstetrician, so you refer her for care. You look in on her the next day and the labor pains are intermittent despite tocolytic therapy. You notice that there is no order for corticosteroid to help with fetal lung maturity, should the baby deliver prematurely. You are not up-to-date on the value of corticosteroids for preventing respiratory distress syndrome and don't want to butt in, at least not without learning more.

Again, write down how you would go about finding the evidence to solve this problem.

Problem 3. Assessing the likelihood of deep venous thrombosis and pulmonary embolism in a complicated patient. A 59-year-old male patient presents to the

Emergency Department complaining of right-sided, pleuritic chest pain. He has been in bed for three days with a severe bout of the "flu," with fever and chills, muscle aches, a runny nose, and the infection now seems to be heading for his chest, though he has had little coughing and no sputum. He has a past history of duodenal ulceration with hemorrhage 9 months ago; he has had no recent symptoms, but admits to taking some aspirin for his flu. On examination, the patient's temperature is 37.9°C and heart rate 88 beats per minute. He has inflamed nasal passages with excess, clear secretions, a reddened throat with no exudates, some tenderness on palpation over the area of pleuritic pain at the mid-right lateral chest and no other remarkable findings. An electrocardiogram shows evidence of an old inferior myocardial infarction with no acute changes. The hemoglobin is normal, the white count is 11,000 with 78% neutrophils, and other laboratory tests are normal. A chest x ray shows no evidence of acute disease. Your hospital has begun screening for deep venous thrombosis (DVT) of the legs using impedance plethysmography (IPG) and this is positive on the right leg, suggesting that there may be a clot in his leg, increasing the likelihood that his chest pain might be due to pulmonary embolism.

Normally, you would anticoagulate the patient at this point, but his past history of gastrointestinal hemorrhage gives you pause. Also, you know that the IPG is quite good for detecting DVT and less good as a screening test for PE, but you've forgotten just how accurate it is. How do you locate the pretest likelihood of DVT or PE, the operating characteristics of IPG, and thus determine the posttest likelihood of DVT and PE for this patient?

Getting Started

There are some quick moves you can employ as an opening gambit in any information search:

1. Ask an expert to cite a specific reference (unless you want to abdicate your own critical appraisal role, ask the expert *where* to find the answer, not *what* the answer is!).
2. Check your personal library to see whether the information is already at hand in a textbook, journal, or reprint file.
3. Visit a hospital, medical society, or medical school library if there is one close by.

4. Do an electronic literature search on your home or office computer (skip the experts and the textbooks and go right to the source).
5. Consult a specialized print or electronic database.

Either of the first two moves can serve you well and we will include them in our explorations. However, if you keep your critical appraisal standards high, you will find that the payoff from these two routes, although quick, is often inaccurate or, if once accurate, now out-of-date. Unfortunately, it's seldom possible to determine when either of these problems arises without looking further. Accordingly, although these moves can be very useful sometimes, you often will need to go beyond them, particularly for clinical problems that you frequently encounter for which you had better be the expert. If you have very easy access to a medical library, particularly one with a professional library staff, step 3 would be a great place to start. Unfortunately, even if you work in a building with an excellent library, it can be difficult to find the time to go to it, find what you need, and return to what you were doing quickly enough to keep up with the pressing events of the day. That's where the fourth step comes in (and is often the place to start, rather than end): plug your personal computer into the electronic universe and do on-line literature and information searches from wherever there is a telephone line. Finally, while the opportunities are still limited, the fifth step offers a short cut if someone else has done the work of assembling and updating evidence with high standards for basing clinical recommendations on solid evidence.

PROBLEM 1. PROGNOSIS OF CARDIOMEGALY (AND BEST TREATMENT TO PREVENT COMPLICATIONS)

Ask an Expert

As a first step, you get a "hallway" consultation from a cardiologist, who indicates that the prognosis depends on the etiology of the cardiomegaly and that, if hypertension is the cause and she has never had symptoms of congestive heart failure, the prognosis is good and will improve if the blood pressure is well controlled. He can't give you an exact figure for her prognosis, particularly as he hasn't assessed her, and can't cite a recent reference on this issue. He would put her on an ACE inhibitor if she needs more medication because there has been a study showing that enalapril saves lives in congestive heart failure. He thinks the enalapril study was in a recent issue of the *American Journal of Cardiology.*

Check your Personal Library

You suspect that a textbook of cardiology might have the information you need on prognosis of cardiomegaly but won't be up-to-date enough for the study of enalapril if this study was published in the past year. In any event, you don't have a textbook of cardiology but do have three of the major texts in internal medicine, a 1988 Cecil* [4], a 1987 Harrison's* [14], and a Scientific American

*These were the most current editions at the time this chapter was prepared in 1990. The twelfth edition of Harrison's textbook was published in 1991.

Medicine [28], which is updated monthly. You suspect that they won't have much information on prognosis—that would be too much detail to expect for general medical texts—but might provide comments on, and citations for, the enalapril study.

Cecil's textbook contains a description of heart size and the measurement of cardiothoracic ratio, with the ominous but unreferenced and not particularly illuminating statement, "Cardiac enlargement is the single most important observation in the suspect cardiac patient." The book devotes two pages to vasodilator therapy for heart failure, including a penultimate paragraph on captopril. It indicates, "A study designed to examine the issue of survival has not yet been completed" (p. 235). Enalapril is not mentioned. The section concludes with an annotated citation of an article on a placebo-controlled trial of captopril in refractory congestive heart failure, ". . . demonstrating improved clinical state and exercise tolerance."

Harrison's text doesn't provide any information about the relationship of heart size to prognosis. Captopril and enalapril appear in a table of vasodilators, and are mentioned in two sentences, neither of which indicate any effect on survival. The bibliography for the section includes a 1982 reference to captopril and a 1985 article on enalapril (the title alludes to effects on exercise tolerance in congestive heart failure but contains no indication of the type of investigation, if any).

Scientific American *Medicine* also lacks information on the prognostic implications of increased cardiothoracic ratio. On management of congestive heart failure, the text states, "Randomized trials have shown that survival has been improved by the combination of hydralazine and isosorbide dinitrate [7, 23] and by enalapril [8]. A review of 28 randomized, placebo-controlled trials found only the angiotensin converting enzyme inhibitors associated with both enhanced survival and improved functional status" [23].

None of these books provided useful information about the prognosis of patients with cardiomegaly, not surprising for general texts. For congestive heart failure, all said something about vasodilator therapy but there are some obvious differences in the style and timeliness of their remarks. Cecil's and Harrison's textbooks do not cite references in the text but provide a few, annotated references at the end of each section. Scientific American *Medicine* does cite specific references for many of its declarations. Moreover, the content and references of Cecil's and Harrison's texts were out of date for this problem at the time when it came up in early 1990 (Harrison's has since published a new version). Even though the landmark trial reporting increased survival of patients with severe congestive heart failure on enalapril was published in 1987, it was not cited in either of these traditional texts. Scientific American *Medicine* did have it and more—a meta-analysis of randomized, placebo-controlled vasodilator trials published in 1988.

Does that mean that the authors of Cecil's and Harrison's are out of date? No. Indeed, from the statement in the text quoted above, the author in Cecil's obviously knew of the trial even before its publication. The problem is not one of authors but of deadlines. New editions of Cecil's and Harrison's appear only once every few years and there can be a considerable delay between the date when an author prepares his chapter and the actual date of publication, followed by the aging of each edition once it hits the bookshelves. Scientific American *Medicine* is designed to overcome this problem. Also, because the reason for updating a section tends to be important new evidence rather than arbitrary press deadlines, evidence is given prominence in updates, each of which comes with a brief review of the highlights of the update (*Bulletin*), a list of new citations, a new index, and new pages to be inserted in the text.*

While much of the information in medicine does not become obsolete so quickly as that for therapy, the most important reason for consulting a textbook is to help treat the patient. Traditional textbook publication processes simply cannot compete with the approach adopted by Scientific American *Medicine* and its offspring, on pre- and post-operative care, *Care of the Surgical Patient* [1], which is updated twice a year.

At this point, you don't have anything in hand that you can apply the guidelines for critical appraisal to. You could accept the information in Scientific American *Medicine* at face value or look for the articles cited there in the journals you keep on hand or in your reprint file. Unfortunately, none of the texts had useful information on the prognosis of cardiomegaly and you will certainly have to look elsewhere for this. Furthermore, while the leads in Scientific American *Medicine* are very helpful, you will still need to check the original articles to determine key details about the patients who were studied (to see if the results can be extrapolated to your patient), how the treatment was prescribed, and the adverse effects observed. You may also want to determine if Scientific American *Medicine* really is up-to-date.

Do an Electronic Literature Search

At this point, we divide you into the "haves" and the "have nots" of the modern era of information access. Do you do on-line or CD-ROM searches of the medical literature on a personal computer in your office or home, or in your hospital wards or clinics? If your answer is "yes," tag along: we'll show you some new wrinkles, including how to work critical appraisal into information searches.

If your answer is "no," then you are part of a vanishing breed of information Luddites.† In our surveys of first-year medical students at McMaster during 1987, 1988, and 1989, personal-computer access rose from 29% to 49%, modem use by those with computers rose from 17% to 50%, and use of CD-ROM MEDLINE in the library rose from 64% to 88%. During the same period, faculty use of MEDLINE on their own computers rose from 6% to 34% [18]. Perhaps we can convince you to look into electronic access to the literature in the examples that follow.

*Insertion of new pages and removal of old is the bane of this approach to keeping up-to-date. If you can hire someone to do this (your secretary or offspring), you will enjoy the publication a lot more. Fortunately, this problem is solved with the new compact disc version, CONSULT™, for which the whole disc is replaced (see product list at the end of this chapter). Alas, this means less frequent (quarterly) updates and a higher price tag.

†The Luddites were a group of workers in the early 1800s who chose to destroy rather than employ the labor-saving machines of the industrial revolution.

We will use GRATEFUL MED software to search the MEDLINE medical literature database for this search. As a testimony to the importance of the MEDLINE service and the astonishing rise in its popularity with clinicians during the past few years, there are now over 20 combinations of computer access routes to MEDLINE (software front ends, CD-ROMs, and on-line vendors). We will enumerate the ones we know about later. GRATEFUL MED (GM) is a very inexpensive software program from the National Library of Medicine, created to help clinicians search MEDLINE without having to know much about on-line searching. It has been so successful that, within 3 years of its availability, over half of all MEDLINE searches were being done through it. Searches mediated through librarians continued at a relatively constant rate during this period; the increase was due to clinical "end users" like us, without expertise in searching, doing searches through GRATEFUL MED. The basics are pretty straightforward, and can be learned in an hour or two. Here is a blow-by-blow account.

1. *Define the clinical question.* The first step in doing a computer search of MEDLINE is to define clearly the question you want answered. It can be expensive, frustrating, and embarrassing to discover, while the computer dollars are adding up, that you had not thought through the problem clearly enough to organize a search for relevant articles or, while you thought you were using the correct indexing (Medical Subject Heading or "MeSH") terms, the ones you've sent to the MEDLINE computer result in "NP" (no postings) messages. So the first step is to write out the exact clinical question you want answered, and do so in the most specific terms possible. In this case, we want to answer the following question: "What is the effect on survival of increased cardiothoracic ratio on x ray?"
2. *Decide whether to search for specific authors or titles.* Figure 11-1 illustrates a GRATEFUL MED input screen and the search we formulated for this question. We didn't put anything on the AUTHOR/NAME line on the form screen because we didn't know in advance the names of authors of good articles on the subject.* Also, we didn't use the TITLE WORDS line because it limits retrieval of articles to those that have specific words in their titles (such as "cardiothoracic" and "prognosis"). Trying to choose the words authors and editors might have put in the titles of articles is a guessing game at best, unless you are looking for a specific author or article.
3. *Let the search program help you find the best subject words.* The first SUBJECT WORDS line in Figure 11-1 has the phrase EXPLODE CARDIOMEGALY. This intriguing juxtaposition of MEDLINE and medical jargon isn't as dangerous as it sounds. It took a little bit of fiddling to get to it, however. We typed in CARDIOTHORACIC to begin with, then, as noted on the GM screen, pressed the F10 key. This brought up the screen in Figure 11-2, an alphabetical list of the medical subject headings (MeSH) that staff

*Sometimes we do know the names of specific authors, but usually we use author searches to find out what visitors to our institution are up to so we can pick their brains, try to sound intelligent, or ask them obstreperous questions.

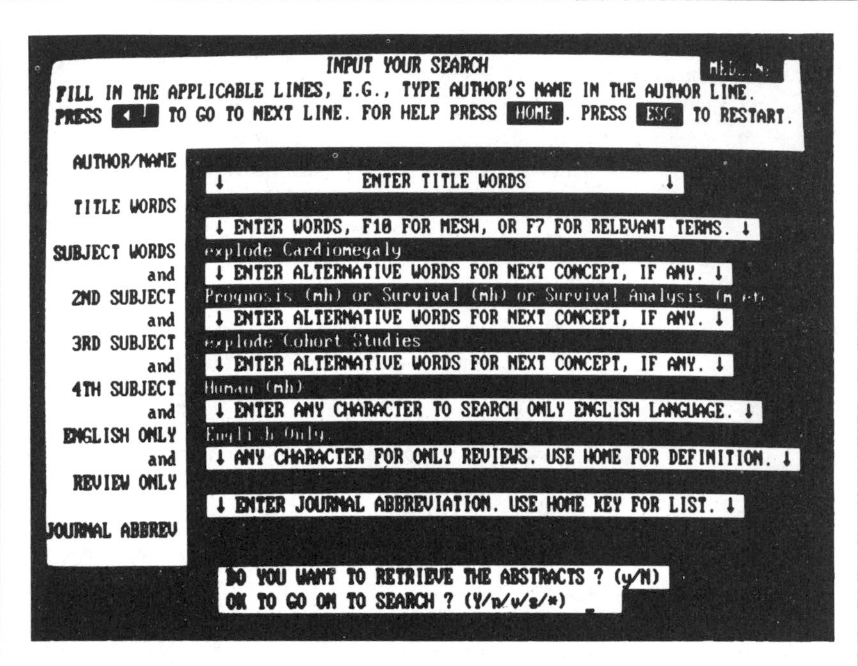

Figure 11-1. A MEDLINE search on a personal computer with GRATEFUL MED software. (Print supplied by R. B. Haynes.)

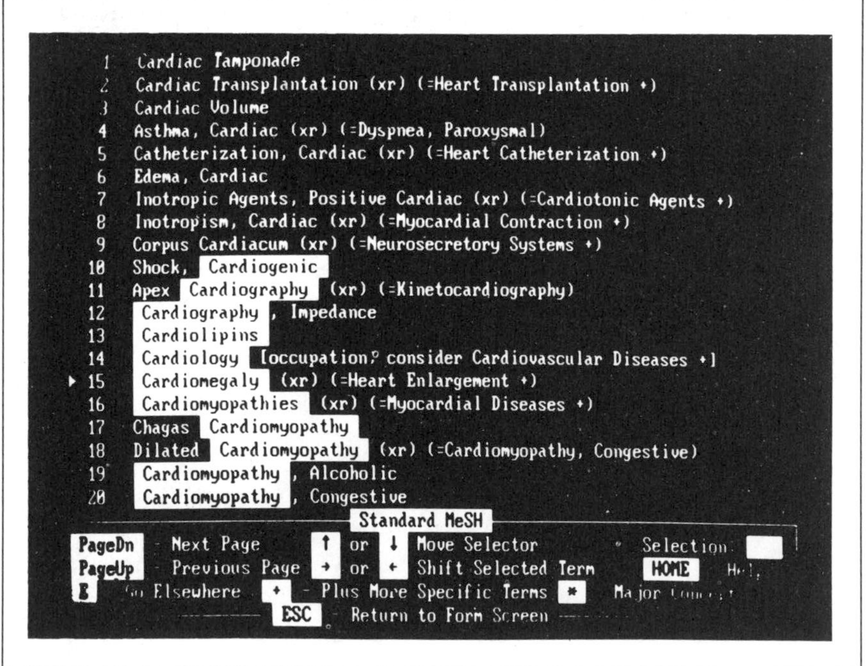

Figure 11-2. The medical subject heading screen from GRATEFUL MED for cardiomegaly. (Print supplied by R. B. Haynes.)

at the National Library of Medicine (NLM) use when indexing the features and contents of articles as they are being entered into the MEDLINE computer.* As it happens, cardiothoracic isn't a MeSH term so the software leaves us in its alphabetic vicinity. Then we had to think of a synonym. We spied CARDIOMEGALY close by, went to it, and found that it was cross-referenced to HEART ENLARGEMENT+. The + sign is important: it means that HEART ENLARGEMENT has one or more subheadings under it. Indexers at the NLM are trained to use the most specific terms possible when they index concepts—heart enlargement won't do if the article is actually about congestive cardiomyopathy, a more specific entity than heart enlargement. If you want articles on congestive cardiomyopathy, you will need to use either this specific term or explode heart enlargement (or explode cardiomegaly which is cross-referenced to heart enlargement), which retrieves articles that have been indexed as *either* heart enlargement or congestive cardiomyopathy. On the other hand, because this particular patient doesn't have congestive cardiomyopathy, the results of the search might have fewer irrelevant articles if we use just the term cardiomegaly or heart enlargement. In general, it is better to explode every term that can be exploded, as it is easy to discard inappropriate citations and there is a high risk of missing appropriate articles that have been indexed more specifically. This is particularly so with GM as the software indicates only whether there are more specific terms under a heading, not what those terms are.†

4. *Narrow the search*. The next step is to narrow the search by combining EXPLODE CARDIOMEGALY with terms that get at prognosis. To do this, we move to the second line, and type in the prognosis terms. This maneuver of typing on the next line automatically combines whatever we put on the first line with whatever we put on the second. This results in a search for only those articles that are about both the concept on subject line 1 AND the concept on line 2. As you can imagine, this is a powerful tactic for excluding articles that are about cardiomegaly or prognosis, but not both. We will illustrate just how powerful shortly.

   In choosing a term for prognosis, we must be careful. MeSH has many terms that might do, including prognosis and survival. Indexers have some freedom in which terms they apply and the best we can do is try to include all the terms they might have used. In this case, we typed PROGN (as the first few letters of prognosis), hit F10, picked up the term, PROGNOSIS, then, staying in this part of the software program, used the E FOR ELSE-

*Indexers at the National Library of Medicine are well-trained information specialists. For major articles in important journals, they select from 5 to 15 index terms (called MeSH headings) to describe the content of the article and the type of subjects, research features, and so on. All of these terms can be searched on the computer, along with words in the title and abstracts of the articles. Authors and specific journals can also be "searched."

†If you want to get around this problem, you can purchase the Medical Subject Heading books from the National Technical Information Service (see the Books section in the Appendix at the end of this chapter). However, these are the size of telephone books (and about as user- and environment-friendly).

WHERE option (see the bottom of Figure 11-2) to explore other possibilities. We started with SURVIVAL and hit an alphabetic strand of related terms, including SURVIVAL ANALYSIS and SURVIVAL RATE, so we picked them all.

There are other options here. We could have added COMPLICATIONS or MORTALITY as a subheading, for example, but didn't think of these at the time. They did appear in the MeSH headings for the articles we retrieved, so we could have added them to supplement the search for a second iteration. GRATEFUL MED identifies such terms automatically when the search is complete, so presumably we don't need to worry about getting the search perfect the first time. But why should we have to guess what an indexer will use among all these options, anyway? Surely, survival, survival rate, and mortality sound similar enough that if you pick one you ought to get them all. However, when we checked, we found that the term SURVIVAL has a meaning that doesn't quite match the intent of our search: "continuance of life or existence under adverse conditions; includes methods and philosophy of survival; survival after disasters, plane crashes, shipwrecks, etc. Triumph of the individual or group against the hazards of a hostile environment."* Including this term in our search didn't have much effect because we "ORed" it with a number of other more relevant terms, but, if we had "ANDed" it, we would have been in trouble because the retrieval would have been limited to studies of cardiomegaly in which there had been a disaster or triumph of some sort. At least partly because of the complexity of MEDLINE, our studies have shown, on a given topic, no two searchers do exactly the same search or get more than a portion of the same articles, even when they are experts at searching [17]. We aren't certain how important this problem is because the literature on most topics is quite redundant, with many articles on the same topic. In this instance, using other, related terms didn't make much difference to the success of the search because the same key article came up with or without them. In general, it seems safe, effective, but messy, to "OR" together all the terms from MeSH that you can think of that indexers might use for a concept.

5. *Add a critical appraisal quality filter*. The next step in Figure 11-1 brings critical appraisal into the fray. Some articles on the prognosis of cardiomegaly could be editorials or letters to the editor or case reports, and so on. While all of these may be of some value, the best articles are likely to be those in which cohorts of people with newly diagnosed enlarged hearts are followed to determine their fate. The indexing in MEDLINE is not precise enough to provide exactly what we want, but it does have terms that are useful in identifying different types of studies. The ones we know about

*You can check the definitions of MeSH terms by looking them up in the MESH file of MEDLINE. If you use GRATEFUL MED, use DIRECT from the ACTION screen to get on to MEDLINE, then type FILE MESH at the USER: prompt; then, in the MESH file, type the name of the term you want defined (e.g., SURVIVAL). If it is a MeSH term, MEDLINE will indicate that there is one posting for the term. Then type PRINT FULL to get the definition.

Table 11-1. Selected medical subject headings that indicate research methodology* (MeSH 1990)

- Epidemiologic methods
  - Data collection
    - Health surveys†
    - Interviews
    - Nutrition assessment†
    - Questionnaires
    - Records†
    - Registries
    - Vital statistics†
  - Statistics
    - Actuarial analysis
    - Analysis of variance†
    - Cluster analysis†
    - Confidence intervals
    - Data interpretation, statistical
    - Discriminant analysis
    - Factor analysis, statistical
    - Models, statistical†
    - Monte Carlo method
    - Probability†
    - Regression analysis†
    - Statistical distributions (nonmesh)†
    - Stochastic processes†
    - Survival analysis
  - Study characteristics (nonmesh)
    - Analytic studies (epidemiology) (nonmesh)
      - Case-control studies
        - Retrospective studies
      - Cohort studies
        - Longitudinal studies
          - Follow-up studies
          - Prospective studies
      - Cross-sectional studies
        - HIV Seroprevalence
    - Clinical trials
      - Multicenter studies
      - Randomized controlled trials
    - Feasibility studies
    - Intervention studies
    - Pilot projects
    - Sampling studies
  - Study design (nonmesh)
    - Double-blind method
    - Meta-analysis
    - Random allocation
    - Reproducibility of results
    - Sensitivity and specificity (epid.)
      - Predictive value of tests
      - ROC Curve
    - Seroepidemiologic methods
    - Single-blind method
- Evaluation studies
  - Clinical trials
    - Multicenter studies
    - Randomized controlled trials
  - Drug evaluation
  - Drug screening
    - Drug screening assays, antitumor
      - Subrenal capsule assay
      - Tumor stem cell assay
  - Product surveillance, postmarketing
  - Program evaluation
  - Reproducibility of results

*'†' denotes further specific MeSH terms not listed here

appear in Table 11-1. We added one to the third subject line, EXPLODE COHORT STUDIES. This restricts the articles retrieved to those that are not only about the prognosis of heart enlargement, but have been also indexed as COHORT STUDIES OR LONGITUDINAL STUDIES OR FOLLOW-UP STUDIES,* the latter two terms being indented under COHORT STUDIES (see Table 11-1).

We will take a peek at this point to see the powerful effect of combining terms. If we were to look through the citations under each of the headings we have chosen so far (explode cardiomegaly, explode cohort studies, and the collection of prognosis terms), we would be swamped. As shown in the

*No doubt the indexers at the National Library of Medicine know the difference between these terms. But for practical purposes, it seems to us that one would have been enough.

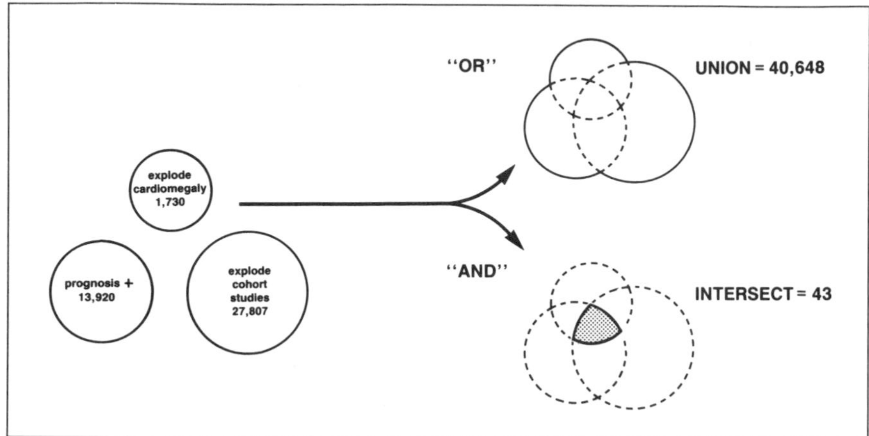

Figure 11-3. Numbers of articles identified by some different ways of combining terms. (Print supplied by R. B. Haynes.)

left side of Figure 11-3, even the smallest of them, EXP CARDIOMEGALY, has 1730 entries.*

On MEDLINE, we can combine the terms in various ways. In the upper right part of the Figure 11-3, we see the results of collecting all the citations under EXP CARDIOMEGALY OR EXP COHORT STUDIES OR (the collected) PROGNOSIS (terms). The *union* of these terms is an avalanche of over 40,000 citations! Another way to combine the terms is to ask MEDLINE to give us the citations listed under EXP CARDIOMEGALY AND EXP COHORT STUDIES AND (the collected) PROGNOSIS (terms). The delightful result of the *intersect* of these terms is just 43 articles. Thank goodness that computers excel at such mindless, repetitive tasks!

6. *Limit the search by species and language.* Using the remaining lines, we restricted the search further to include studies that have humans in them and to articles published in English: 26 of the articles qualify.
7. *Decide whether to restrict the types of articles and journals.* For the next two lines of the form, although we didn't do this, we could have restricted the search further by requesting only reviews and by specifying only certain journals. The latter is useful for indicating titles of a set of journals you want to review regularly; you can create a special file for this once and use it thereafter without retyping the journal abbreviations. You can also specify the "core" clinical journal subset of MEDLINE by typing AIM (the abbreviation for Abridged Index Medicus). This restricts the search to a subset of about 300 journals chosen by the National Library of Medicine as being the

*If we were to look in *Index Medicus*, the print version of MEDLINE, we wouldn't see this many citations because, for a given term, *Index Medicus* cites only articles for which this is a major topic. On average, an article would be listed under only 1 to 3 terms in *Index Medicus*, but would have 5 to 15 terms in MEDLINE—a fivefold increase in ways to retrieve an article, plus opportunities for rapidly narrowing searches to articles that meet multiple criteria.

most relevant for clinical practice. As this is only about 10 percent of all the journals in MEDLINE and as the literature on a given topic can be scattered unpredictably over a larger number of journals, it is difficult to know whether this restriction does more good than harm.

8. *Decide whether to retrieve abstracts*. We then press **ENTER** and GM asks: "DO YOU WANT TO RETRIEVE THE ABSTRACTS (y/N)?" The default here is N or no but we usually respond y as in this case. It costs a little more to retrieve the abstracts and it may be reasonable to forgo them if you do not quite know how to search for articles on an unfamiliar topic—on such fishing expeditions, taking a look at some titles may be an inexpensive way to see if you are in the right pond. However, abstracts have much more information than titles, and save you time and mistakes when deciding which articles to procure in full text form.
9. *Decide whether to revise, review, or save the search strategy, or to forgo retrieval of the indexing terms*. GM then asks if it is: "OK TO GO ON TO SEARCH (Y/n/v/s/*)?". The default is Y. To revise the search, press *n* and the cursor will return to the top of the screen to permit editing. To view the search as it will be submitted to MEDLINE (translated by GM to suit the MEDLINE computer), hit v. This is a useful step that we routinely use. GRATEFUL MED doesn't print the search strategy when it prints the search retrieval and we can't recall, from one minute to the next, exactly what terms we used. By using the view option and pressing the **PRINT SCREEN** key on the computer, the search strategy appears at the top of the printout. The s stands for save: If you want to use the same search later (for example, for a monthly update—see Chapter 12), or store a record of your search strategies, use this option. Finally, '*' tells the MEDLINE computer that you don't want to retrieve the indexing terms with the citations that meet your criteria. This saves a little time and reduces the search costs a little, but disables the feature of GM that indicates which indexing terms were most prominent in the articles retrieved (including MORTALITY and COMPLICATIONS in our example). We recommend retrieving the MeSH terms under most circumstances, but they are not needed for a monthly update search, for example.

It has taken pages of text to get us this far, and if you don't already do your own searching, you might be wondering if this is really a skill you need to acquire. In fact, when we tested the use and usefulness of GRATEFUL MED and MEDLINE in our hospital wards and clinics, we found that novices are able to perform basic searches after 2 to 3 hours of instruction and practice [17], and over 80% indicated that they preferred doing their own searches rather than having a librarian do them. In this study we also found that clinicians with some experience in searching retrieve as many relevant citations as trained librarians, although the librarians still have the edge in eliminating irrelevant citations from their search retrievals.

Although it did take some time for us to describe how the search was formulated, the "real time" to set up the search to this point was less than

3 minutes. To determine whether it was worth it, this cost, and the ones that follow, must be compared with the benefits of running the search.

10. *Let the search program take over.* We let GM run the search. It connects our computer through its modem with the MEDLINE computer in Bethesda, Maryland. As we watch the screen, the search is performed, yielding 21 citations that meet all the criteria we specified. The citations, abstracts, and MeSH headings are transferred to our computer. The process, at a rather busy time for the MEDLINE computer (about 10 A.M. Eastern Standard Time), takes 7 minutes and costs $3.64 for use of the MEDLINE file plus a telecommunications charge of $.70. (The total charge would be less than $2 if conducted from the United States, in off-peak hours, and from an educational institution with a 50% discount.)
11. *Review the results.* GM takes us through the citations. One clearly has the best credentials: Rautaharju and colleagues [27] compared ECG and two radiologic measures of heart size, including cardiothoracic ratio, with survival of 1807 men and 2143 women followed for 5 to 12 years. Applying the criteria that appear in Figure 12-2 for studies of prognosis, the abstract isn't clear on the source of the subjects, whether they were an inception cohort, or the success of follow-up, but does indicate that survival rates were significantly related to each of the 3 measures of cardiac size, and the rates were adjusted for various extraneous prognostic factors.
12. *Decide whether to revise the search, go back through previous years, or retrieve the full text articles from one or more of the citations.* So far, our information quest has taken us about 10 minutes, with a direct cost of about $5. At this point, we have at least one good citation and some options. We can extend the same search into previous years: The first search on MEDLINE takes us back only about 2 years, but we can extend this as far back as 1966 when the program asks if we want to do so. Second, if we feel that we may have missed something and can think of a way to modify the search to capture it, we can edit the search and rerun it on the current (most recent 2 years) file. Finally, if satisfied with the search results, we will need the full text of the articles that suit our purposes if we are to proceed further.

The article that appeared to be best was published in the *American Journal of Cardiology* so we sit tight at the computer and request it from a second on-line database: BRS Colleague. This service has over 80 full-text journals in electronic form,* including the one we want. We request the appropriate article by specifying the full text file (JOUR), the specific journal by its Colleague four-letter abbreviation (AJCA), the lead author (RAUTAHARJU), and any two (important) words in the title of the article (e.g., VENTRICULAR and CARDIAC). Four minutes later, the complete text of the article has been transferred to our

*Colleague has a number of databases including MEDLINE, a full-text textbook file and full text journals. We prefer the NLM MEDLINE service, because it costs less and we have become attached to the off-line features of GRATEFUL MED, but NLM doesn't have a full text journal service.

computer at a charge of just under $3.* This provides all the information we need for critical appraisal: the study population was randomly selected to represent the U.S. population; over 90% of the cohort were followed; exposure and outcome variables were reproducibly measured; and there was adjustment for extraneous prognostic factors.

Alas, some of the key information in the article is contained in tables and figures that are not available in the electronic version. Thus, some 15 minutes into our search, we must pause to retrieve the full text article from the library, from our own collection, or from Colleague, which has a clipping service ($10 per article for regular mail, more for fax or courier). Such is the state of current on-line full text databases.

When we do acquire the article, we see that our patient's cardiothoracic ratio (CTR) of 52% exceeds the mean value for white females, whether normotensive or hypertensive (44% and 48%, respectively). Figure 3 in this article shows that, with a CTR in the highest quintile, she has about a 20% chance of dying from cardiovascular disease during the next 12 years. Of course, this also means that she has an 80% chance of surviving this fate.

In addition, as we were told on our initial foray into Scientific American *Medicine,* her risk of developing congestive heart failure may be reduced by better control of her hypertension. As for what might be the best drug to improve her hypertensive control, the studies documenting the survival benefits of ACE inhibitors for congestive heart failure lead to an obvious nomination. However, we haven't reviewed the original articles as yet and don't know whether the citations in Scientific American *Medicine* accurately reflect current knowledge. This is easy to check with another computer search. To do this, we loaded the following terms into GRATEFUL MED: EXPLODE HEART FAILURE, CONGESTIVE AND MORTALITY (SH†) AND DRUG THERAPY (SH) AND EXPLODE RESEARCH DESIGN. The last phrase, EXPLODE RESEARCH DESIGN, permits electronic critical appraisal. This restricts the search to articles that have been indexed as involving RANDOM ALLOCATION OR DOUBLE-BLIND METHOD OR META-ANALYSIS. The search yielded 13 references, cost $1.86, and retrieved additional reports by the authors of the definitive enalapril study [19, 20, 29], the review by Mulrow and her colleagues [23], and some additional studies [22, 24] and reviews [11, 26] of the use of ACE inhibitors for congestive heart failure. These provide some additional useful information on adverse effects and the range of benefit, with no studies showing a survival benefit among patients with asymptomatic or mild congestive heart failure. However, these reports also illustrate the enormous amount of overlap in the literature and confirm that the information in Scientific American *Medicine*

*BRS Colleague charges $32 per hour in the United States (+ $6 per hour for telecommunications in Canada) from 6 A.M. to 6 P.M. ($22 per hour at other times), and the search took .067 decimal hours when we performed it by stacking commands in our own computer to reduce the cost of entering requests while connected to the Colleague computer.

†(sh) means subheading. Subheadings modify major search concepts by restricting their focus to specific issues, such as treatment by drugs, as in this case.

American *Medicine* remains up to date. Parenthetically, the review article by Mulrow and her coworkers [23] is an excellent example of the new breed of systematic review studies that can be critically appraised (see Figure 12-2 for criteria).

What do you tell the patient and what do you do for her? In almost all situations, no matter how good the evidence, there remains a gap between what we know to be true and what we need to know. To be truthful, we could tell the patient that people like her in a study of heart size and survival had a 20% chance of dying over the next 12 years and that lowering her blood pressure more might lower this risk. However, we are not quite sure how long she has had the enlargement of her heart and, therefore, don't know how well this prognosis fits her. On the other hand, what to tell *this* patient depends also on her personality, need for information, and desire to be involved in decisions concerning her care [3], her circumstances (is she the main breadwinner of her family?), and other important but not easily quantified matters. Having accurate information on prognosis does not let us off the hook for taking into account these important "intangibles." Rather, it expands the options for what we can tell the patient and firms up some of them.

How was this information actually used for this patient? On the repeat visit, her blood pressure was still elevated at 160/98 mm Hg, despite her insistence that she had taken all the pills. She was told that, while an exact probability couldn't be determined for her, based on the experiences of people like her, there was a better than 80% chance that she would live at least 12 years, well beyond the usual date of retirement at age 65 years, and that this chance could be increased by keeping her blood pressure well controlled. Thus, she could retire early if she wished, but did not need to do so because of poor health. She was switched from hydrochlorothiazide to enalapril, more because the former wasn't adequate at its current recommended highest dose than because of the success of enalapril for congestive heart failure (which the patient didn't have). Her blood pressure became well controlled when the dose of enalapril was increased to 10 mg per day on a subsequent visit.

Use of MEDLINE Searching to help solve clinical problems raises some important issues for health professionals attempting to remain competent. First, should clinicians be responsible for tracking down and examining recent publications of health care studies? It would be nice to think that our periodic continuing-education activities would be enough to keep us up to date. Unfortunately, it is clear that formal continuing education courses don't meet this challenge. Traditional textbooks are also unable to keep up with new information, although books that renew themselves regularly and cite their sources may be adequate for the topics they cover—there are, however, very few such books. One can, of course, refer patients with unfamiliar problems to (other) specialists, but, unless we are to give up practice entirely, we must keep up with new evidence concerning the types of problems for which we consider ourselves competent care providers.

Second, should all clinicians learn to perform MEDLINE searches on their own? Yes! MEDLINE provides the best access to the medical literature because of the large number of journals it covers and the ease of accessing appropriate articles through the use of index terms and words that appear in their titles or abstracts. Can you learn to become a competent MEDLINE searcher? Certainly! You can learn on your own using the manual from the National Library of Medicine [30] or from the excellent manual for GRATEFUL MED or from introductory courses provided by most health sciences libraries or by vendors such as Dialog and Colleague. While the method we prefer is to access the MEDLINE file through GRATEFUL MED software, and full text journal access through Colleague, there are over 20 routes to the MEDLINE database at present including on-line services (BRS Colleague, Dialog, and PaperChase) and compact disc services (CD Plus, Compact Cambridge, Dialog on Disc, EBSCO, Silver Platter, and Aries Knowledge Finder). There is also software, Pro-Search^{TM}, that permits searching the many databases on Dialog and BRS with a single search strategy. We are currently evaluating these services for effectiveness and efficiency and, by the time you read this book, we may have had an opportunity to publish our results. If interested, you ought to be able to find our report using any one of these access routes by doing an author search (the command on MEDLINE would be HAYNES RB (AU)).

You won't have the time to do MEDLINE searches for each problem that arises. In our recent investigation [17], when self-service MEDLINE searching was made available in clinics and wards of our hospital, clinicians used this service between once and twice a week on average. Whether or not this is optimal, exploration of one to two important clinical problems per week translates into increasingly impressive numbers over a month, year, and practice lifetime.

PROBLEM 2: ARE CORTICOSTEROIDS BENEFICIAL IN PRETERM DELIVERY?

You wander down to the hospital library and ask the librarian if there are any special resources for obstetrical care. A sunny smile lights his face as he indicates that the Chief of Obstetrics for the hospital had recently insisted they purchase a computer program, the Oxford Database of Perinatal Trials (ODPT)[5]. He leads you to a computer station near the reference desk and suggests that you type ODPT, press **ENTER** and just follow the instructions on the screen.

The menus appear to flow in an intuitive fashion and you indicate SELECT OVERVIEWS from the first menu. From the next menu that pops up, you select 2. PRETERM LABOUR AND DELIVERY. Another menu indicates various interventions, and you select CORTICOSTEROIDS PRIOR TO PRETERM DELIVERY. You then direct the program to DISPLAY SELECTION and examine the overview details. You direct the output to the printer and an 11-page overview churns out [12]. The printout includes the author of the overview, a contact address and telephone, the date of the most recent update, measures of outcome, a table of contents, a brief overview summary, and several tables summarizing the results of 12 randomized trials published up to, and including, the current year. The tables classify results for various endpoints including the effect of corticosteroids on the occurrence of respiratory distress syndrome (RDS) overall; RDS following optimal treatment; RDS following delivery in less than 24 hours or in more than 7 days; RDS in babies less than 31 weeks or in babies greater than 34 weeks gestation; RDS in male babies and female babies; and a bibliography. Browsing through the tables, you see that the numbers of experimental and control subjects are given along with the number of events and an odds ratio with 95% confidence intervals. The odds ratio for respiratory distress syndrome, overall, is .49 (95% CI .41–.60) indicating a reduction in the odds of respiratory distress of over 50%.

A brief overview statement neatly summarizes the results of the trials and indicates that ". . . treatment with antenatal corticosteroids is associated with a substantial reduction of risk of respiratory distress syndrome." It indicates that the reduction is greatest when the baby is delivered more than 24 hours but less than 7 days after starting treatment and that babies delivered after 34 weeks may also benefit, but confidence limits are wide. Adverse effects have not been documented but the studies are not conclusive in this respect.

You are delighted at having such a clear display of the evidence. Your suspicion is confirmed that corticosteroids would be indicated in this situation. While you don't manage complicated obstetrical cases in your own practice, you would certainly be happy to have such a program on your office computer to help sort out such patients for referral. You ask the librarian where you can obtain it and how much it costs, and he indicates that it is a bit pricey at $895. When you wince, he indicates that there are two paper offspring of the electronic version. The first, by Iain Chalmers, Murray Enkin, and Marc Keirse [6], is a two-volume edition that includes tables and text for the obstetrical trials registered in ODPT, including 1989. (A companion volume for the newborn is in preparation.) The second print version, by Murray Enkin, Marc Keirse, and Iain Chalmers [9] is just 320 pages long and summarizes the results of the obstetrical trials in paperback form for just $19.95. It does not contain tables of evidence, as in the software or the large print volume, but it is "hard-wired" to their conclusions in a faithful and concise fashion. You make a note of the latter so that you can purchase it. You marvel that such a resource could be developed and provided in such complementary forms—and hope that enough people and institutions will purchase the three formats to keep the production going.

Leaving the library, you run into your patient's obstetrician who indicates that she is on the way to the ward. You inquire gently about whether corticosteroids would be indicated for the fetus in this situation. The obstetrician states that they usually are and that she will look into this on her visit.

PROBLEM 3. ASSESSING THE LIKELIHOOD OF DEEP VENOUS THROMBOSIS AND PULMONARY EMBOLISM IN A COMPLICATED PATIENT

To start, you may want to approach a consultant or look yourself into the sensitivity and specificity of IPG for deep venous thrombosis and for pulmonary embolism. We took the latter route and looked at a new textbook, by Kuhns, Thornbury, and Fryback [21], that provides quantitative information concerning diagnostic imaging procedures as well as information on pretest and posttest likelihoods. This book is a compendium of abstracts from the recent scientific literature concerning diagnostic procedures, arranged according to body system, and pretest probabilities organized according to specific disorders. It concludes with a section on how to search the medical literature for imaging data. The book also provides a slide rule that allows easy conversion from pretest to posttest likelihoods for specified sensitivities and specificities for positive and negative tests and a thoughtful and informative section on the relationship of diagnostic certainty to treatment.

For our patient, we first looked in the index of this book for *impedance plethysmography,* but found no entry. Disappointed but not deterred, we looked for *thrombosis, venous* and found numerous entries. Turning to the pages for the entry *deep,* we found several pages on thrombophlebitis and deep venous thrombosis. This part of the book is organized like a series of file cards with many tables and a brief discussion of studies selected for information on specific tests. The entry on page 389 concerning IPG briefly describes the technique of the procedure, and detailed information on a large study comparing IPG with venography. The pretest probability for the series is given as 22% among patients referred for possible DVT. The sensitivity and specificity of IPG are given as 92% and 99%, respectively, for proximal DVT and 93% and 97% for all veins in the legs.* As we're also concerned about pulmonary embolism, we looked up the entry for this and found a cornucopia of information about the value of various elements of history and physical examination (none of these features being very discriminating), and information about the sensitivity and specificity of ventilation-perfusion scanning for pulmonary embolism as well as the sensitivity and specificity of venography and IPG for pulmonary embolism. For IPG, the sensitivity and specificity for pulmonary embolism are 57% and 77%, respectively.

Applying these figures to our patient, and assuming that our patient is similar to others who are referred for suspected DVT (that is, a pretest likelihood of DVT of 22% as indicated in the text), the positive IPG increases the likelihood of DVT to about 96%. The text does not provide a pretest probability of pulmonary embolism among those with clinically suspected pulmonary embolism, presumably because most such patients receive anticoagulation without going on to V-P scans or angiography. On clinical grounds, including the positive IPG, if we assign our patient a pretest likelihood of, say, 50% for pulmonary embolism, the posttest likelihood becomes about 70%. In any event, exact probability is academic at this point because the treatment for proximal deep vein thrombosis and pulmonary embolism is the same. Nevertheless, an important problem for this patient is his prior history of bleeding duodenal ulcer. Heparinization under such circumstances would certainly be risky for the patient. One would want to consider a Greenfield filter as an alternative to heparinization, but the insertion of this device is uncomfortable for the patient and a bit risky. You would certainly want to be very sure of the diagnosis of DVT in this case, and venography

*The section also provides information on charges for procedures, radiation dosages when applicable, mortality for procedures (for example, 1/15,000–1/93,000 for venography) and comments concerning the methodology and results of the major studies cited.

would be indicated to establish the existence and location of clots. Time to do a search on the risks of anticoagulation in such patients or to call in a consultant. Our own medical center is a mecca for thromboembologists, and the IPG technician had already tipped off the thrombo consultant on call, so we followed the line of least resistance in this case. (After confirming the presence of extensive proximal DVT by venography, the consultant recommended, and the patient accepted, a Greenfield filter.)

This problem raises the thorny issue of where pretest likelihoods come from. It would be nice to think that our clinical acumen was adequate for establishing the baseline probability of various diagnoses for patients on the basis of their initial clinical findings, but, particularly for generalists, often our expertise is not up to the task [2, 10]. Fortunately, the book provides useful information on this for many disorders.

The availability of a resource such as the book by Kuhns and his colleagues [21] is certainly heartening in this era when we are struggling to connect evidence with individual patient management without always having to resort to original sources. There are other resources, too. For problems in internal medicine, Paul Griner and his colleagues [13] have produced a book on over 40 common problems and Robert Panzer and others [25] have produced a companion software program that provides sensitivities and specificities for many clinical findings and diagnostic tests pertinent to these problems, as well as a variety of options for performing calculations to convert pretest likelihoods into posttest probabilities. Paul Griner and company are working on a new edition of their book, to be entitled *Diagnostic Strategies for Common Medical Problems,* which will be published by the American College of Physicians. It will likely be out by the time you read this chapter. We have listed a number of similar resources in the appendix to this chapter.

Reprise

By the time you read this chapter, much of the information provided here on the prognosis of cardiomegaly, the best treatment for congestive heart failure, the value of corticosteroids in preterm delivery, and the diagnosis of deep venous thrombosis will be out of date. That is precisely the point of this chapter: Information on matters of health care must be sought by means that capture new developments as they occur.

It can be challenging to find review and original evidence that is both valid and exactly on target for a clinical problem you must solve. Application of information technology puts you in contact with evidence sooner, and application of the common sense principles of critical appraisal allows you to cut away the irrelevant and the invalid. Electronic resources, such as MEDLINE, *Oxford Database of Perinatal Trials* [5] and CLINDX [25], and texts such as *Effective Care in Pregnancy and Childbirth* [6] and its paperback summary [9], *Clinical Diagnosis and the Laboratory* [13], *Decision Making in Imaging* [21], and the others listed in the appendix at the end of this chapter, will make life easier for all of us.

There are also a multitude of on-line search services in addition to MEDLINE, including EMBASE (the on-line version of *Excerpta Medica,* the European literature database for the health sciences), BIOSIS (a product of Biosciences Information Services of Philadelphia which focuses on basic biologic research), SCISEARCH (the on-line version of *Science Citation Index*), PSYCHINFO (which includes citations from the literature of psychology and the social sciences), and ERIC (which contains information from the field of education). There are also many more specialized electronic databases, including CANCERLIT, AIDSLINE, HEALTHLINE, TOXLINE, AVLINE, and ENVIROLINE, available through the National Library of Medicine.

Searching for Answers to Problems Versus Surveying the Literature Regularly

Most clinicians report that they keep up to date by reading journals. Regular critical surveillance of a number of journals for articles of great clinical pertinence and high scientific merit, as we discuss in Chapter 12, is necessary if you are to become aware in a timely way of important advances in health care while avoiding false leads. Surveillance, however, can't satisfy all your information needs. First, in surveillance, you will need to cover a broad range of topics, even if you are working in a quite specialized field, and thus can't afford to do so in depth. Second, there's no guarantee that a patient will present with the problems covered in your surveillance before you've forgotten about the advance or the advance has been superseded. Third, you will have to retrieve and review the information on the advance for details before you try to apply it (there's no point in trying to memorize these details when you first read them unless you encounter the problem very frequently in your practice). Fourth, even the best studies in the literature, those that pass all your screening criteria for keeping up to date, will seldom be definitive or comprehensive enough to deal with most clinical situations. These are reasons why a good part of the time you set aside each week for keeping on top of medical knowledge should be spent in an activity that is even more important than surveillance—searching for the answers to problems as they confront you in clinical practice.

Appendix. An Annotated List of Medical Information Products Described in the Chapter*

SOFTWARE PROVIDING ACCESS TO MEDLINE

GRATEFUL MED. Software for searching the National Library of Medicine MEDLARS databases directly. Available from the National Technical Information Service, 5285 Port Royal Road, Springfield VA 22161. (Send advance payment of $29.95 plus $3.00 for shipping; specify IBM-PC or Apple Macintosh.)

*There are far too many information sources to do justice to them all. The resources listed here are selected because we have some working knowledge of them.

Pro-Search™. Software for standardizing searches of the on-line Dialog and BRS databases. Available for IBM-PC and compatibles and for Macintosh, from Personal Bibliographic Software, Inc., 525 Avis Drive, Suite 10, Ann Arbor, MI 48108 (Tel: 313-996-1580. Fax: 313-996-4672) and from ISI, 3501 Market Street, Philadelphia, PA 19104 (800-336-4474, operator #75). Price about $300 (Depends when you look and which price list you look at!).

MEDLINE VENDORS

BRS Colleague and BRS After Dark, Dialog and Knowledge Index, and MEDLARS (National Library of Medicine)—see information at the end of Chapter 12.

PaperChase: Division of Computer Medicine, Beth Israel Hospital, 330 Brookline Ave, Boston, MA 02215 (617-735-5610).

SOFTWARE FOR CRITICAL APPRAISAL OF THE MEDICAL LITERATURE

Roaten, S. LITEVAL 3.0. (S. Roaten, Jr., 1600 Providence Drive, Waco, Texas 76707). This program guides the reader through critical appraisal criteria, documenting their application to a specific article and producing a permanent copy that can be appended to the article. The software can be obtained from Dr. Roaten for $25.

COMPUTERIZED DATABASES

Oxford Database of Perinatal Trials. Oxford Electronic Publishing. Oxford University Press, Walton Street, Oxford. Contains details and overviews of over 5000 trials in perinatal care. Available for IBM PC's and compatibles. $895 plus $10 shipping and handling in US: Oxford University Press, 200 Madison Avenue, New York, NY 10016, attention: Marketing Director for Science and Medical Books. £495 in England from Oxford Electronic Publishing, Oxford University Press, Walton Street, Oxford, OX2 6DP, UK (Tel.: 0865 56767, ext. 4278. Fax: 56646).

Panzer, R. J., Schoch, D. R., and Sammann, H. W. *Clinical Diagnosis and the Laboratory: Computer Supplement.* A computer companion for the book by Griner et al. (see below); runs on IBM and compatibles and costs about $50. Available from Paragon Computer Projects, Inc., 92 Sleepy Hollow Lane, Rochester, NY 14618.

Scientific American *Medicine* CONSULT is Scientific American *Medicine* on a compact disc. Hardware requirements: IBM PC/XT, AT, or PS/2 or compatible; 640K memory with 530K free (560K free if a VGA adapter is used); CD-ROM drive with Microsoft CD-ROM Extensions installed; 100Kb free disk space (hard or floppy disk); optional: VGA monitor and adapter (needed to view graphics). Price in 1990: $375 for individuals, $595 for institutions. Hardware purchase option: Hitachi 1503S CD-ROM drive with controller card, interface cable, and Microsoft CD-ROM extensions: for IBM XT/AT or compatible, $635; IBM PS/2 or compatible, $727. Available from Scientific American *Medicine,* 415 Madison Avenue, New York, NY 10017 (800-345-8112).

BOOKS

Chalmers, I., Enkin, M., and Keirse, M. J. N. C. (eds.). *Effective Care in Pregnancy and Childbirth* (vols. 1 and 2). Oxford: Oxford University Press, 1989. Contains information, tables, and overviews from the *Oxford Database of Perinatal Trials* (1520 pages with 575 illustrations). Available from Oxford University Press for £225 in UK, $400 elsewhere.

Enkin, M., Keirse, M. J. N. C., and Chalmers, I. (eds.). *A Guide to Effective Care in Pregnancy and Childbirth.* Oxford: Oxford University Press, 1989. Faithfully summarized version of the Oxford Database of Perinatal Trials, without tables or illustrations (320 pages) $39.95, cloth; $19.95, paper.

Scientific American *Medicine* (annual subscription fee in USA and Canada, $265) and *Care of the Surgical Patient* ($235) are available from Scientific American *Medicine,* 415 Madison Avenue, New York, NY 10017 (800-345-8112).

Medical Subject Headings—Tree Structures. Available from the National Technical Information Service, 5285 Port Royal Road, Springfield, VA 22161.

The Basics of Searching MEDLINE: A Guide for the Health Professional. Bethesda, MD: National Library of Medicine, 1985. Available from the National Technical Information Service, 5285 Port Royal Road, Springfield, VA 22161.

McNeil, B.J., Abrams, H.L. (eds). *Brigham and Women's Hospital Handbook of Diagnostic Imaging.* Boston: Little, Brown, 1986. A rational and empirically supported approach to diagnostic imaging procedures based on the nature of the clinical problem rather than the type of procedure.

Sox, H. C., Jr. (ed.). *Common Diagnostic Tests. Use and Interpretation.* Philadelphia: American College of Physicians, 1987. A product of the Clinical Efficacy Assessment Project of the American College of Physicians and Surgeons, this is a compendium of the articles that appeared in the *Annals of Internal Medicine* on common diagnostic tests and therapeutic interventions from the beginning of the project up to 1987. (The series continues in the *Annals.*)

References

1. American College of Surgeons. *Care of the Surgical Patient.* New York: Scientific American. Updated semi-annually.
2. Anderson, R. E., Hill, R. B., and Key, C. R. The sensitivity and specificity of clinical diagnostics during five decades. *J.A.M.A.* 261: 1610, 1989.
3. Brody, D. S., Miller, S. M., Lerman, C. E., et al. The relationship between patients' satisfaction with their physicians and perceptions about interventions they desired and received. *Med. Care* 27: 1027, 1989.
4. *Cecil Textbook of Medicine* (18th ed.) Wyngaarden, J. B., and Smith, L. H., Jr. (eds.). Philadelphia: Saunders, 1988.
5. Chalmers, I., (ed.). *Oxford Database of Perinatal Trials.* Version 1.0, Disk Issue 2. Oxford: Oxford University Press, August 1989.
6. Chalmers, I., Enkin, M., and Keirse, M. J. N. C. (eds.). *Effective Care in Pregnancy and Childbirth* (vols. 1 and 2). Oxford: Oxford University Press, 1989.
7. Cohn, J. N., Archibald, D. G., Ziesche, S., et al. Effect of vasodilator therapy on mortality in chronic congestive heart failure: Results of a Veterans Administration Cooperative Study. *N. Engl. J. Med.* 314: 1547, 1986.
8. Effects of enalapril on mortality in severe congestive heart failure: Results of the Cooperative North Scandinavian Enalapril Survival Study (CONSENSUS). The CONSENSUS Trial Study Group. *N. Engl. J. Med.* 316: 1429, 1987.
9. Enkin, M., Keirse, M. J. N. C., and Chalmers, I. *A Guide to Effective Care in Pregnancy and Childbirth.* Oxford: Oxford University Press, 1989.

10. Feightner, J. W., Norman, G. R., and Haynes, R. B. The reliability of likelihood estimates by physicians (abstract). *Clin. Research* 30: 298A, 1982.
11. Furberg, C. D. and Yusuf, S. Effect of drug therapy on survival in chronic congestive heart failure. *Am. J. Cardiol.* 62: 41A–45A, 1988.
12. Grant, A. M. (ed.). Corticosteroids prior to preterm delivery. In: I. Chalmers (ed.). *Oxford Database of Perinatal trials.* Version 1.0, Disk Issue 2. Oxford: Oxford University Press, August 1989.
13. Griner, P. F., Panzer, R. J., and Greenland, P. *Clinical Diagnosis and the Laboratory: Logical Strategies for Common Medical Problems.* Chicago: Year Book Medical Publishers, 1986.
14. *Harrison's Principles of Internal Medicine* (11th ed.). New York: McGraw-Hill, 1987.
15. Haynes, R. B., McKibbon, K. A., Fitzgerald, D., et al. How to keep up with the medical literature: IV. Using the literature to solve clinical problems. *Ann. Intern. Med.* 105: 636, 1986.
16. Haynes, R. B., McKibbon, K. A., Fitzgerald, D., et al. How to keep up with the medical literature: V. Access by personal computer to the medical literature. *Ann. Intern. Med.* 105: 810, 1986.
17. Haynes, R. B., McKibbon, K. A., Walker, C. J., et al. A study of the use and usefulness of online access to MEDLINE in clinical settings. *Ann. Intern. Med.* 112: 78, 1990.
18. Haynes, R.B., McKibbon, K.A., Walker, C.J., and Ramsden, M.F. Rapid evolution of microcomputer use in a faculty of health sciences. *Can. Med. Assoc. J.* 144: 24, 1991.
19. Kjekshus, J., and Swedberg, K. Tolerability of enalapril in congestive heart failure. *Am. J. Cardiol.* 62: 67A, 1988.
20. Kjekshus, J., and Swedberg, K. Enalapril for congestive heart failure. *Am. J. Cardiol.* 63: 26D, 1989.
21. Kuhns, L. R., Thornbury, J. R., and Fryback, D. G. *Decision Making in Imaging.* Chicago: Yearbook Medical Publishers, 1989.
22. Magnani, B. Converting enzyme inhibition and heart failure. *Am. J. Med.* 84: 87, 1988.
23. Mulrow, C. D., Mulrow, J. P., Lin, W. D., et al. Relative efficacy of vasodilator therapy in chronic congestive heart failure: Implications of randomized trials. *J. A. M. A.* 259: 3422, 1988.
24. Newman, T. J., Maskin, C. S., Dennick, L. G., et al. Effects of captopril on survival in patients with heart failure. *Am. J. Med.* 84: 140, 1988.
25. Panzer, R. J., Schoch, D. R., and Sammann, H. W. *Clinical Diagnosis and the Laboratory: Computer Supplement.* Paragon Computer Projects, Inc., 92 Sleepy Hollow Lane, Rochester, NY 14618.
26. Rahimtoola, S. H. The pharmacologic treatment of chronic congestive heart failure. *Circulation* 80: 693, 1989.
27. Rautaharju, P. M., LaCroix, A. Z., Savage, D. D., et al. Electrocardiographic estimate of left ventricular mass versus radiographic cardiac size and the risk of cardiovascular disease mortality in the epidemiologic follow-up study of the First National Health and Nutrition Examination Survey. *Am. J. Cardiol.* 62: 59, 1988.
28. Rubenstein, E., and Federman, D. D., (ed.). Scientific American *Medicine.* New York: Scientific American, 1989.
29. Swedberg, K., and Kjekshus, J. Effects of enalapril on mortality in severe congestive heart failure: results of the Cooperative North Scandinavian Enalapril Study (CONSENSUS). *Am. J. Cardiol.* 62: 60A, 1988.
30. *The Basics of Searching MEDLINE: A Guide for the Health Professional.* Bethesda, Maryland: National Library of Medicine; 1985.

12

Surveying the Medical Literature to Keep Up to Date

In Chapter 10, we reported the dating of one's knowledge of current clinical recommendations and of validated procedures that begins as soon as one completes formal professional education. We've come to call this phenomenon the "slippery slope of declining clinical competence." Searching for the solutions to clinical problems as they arise will certainly give us some grip on this slope, as we discussed in Chapter 11. However, this will help only for the problems that we perceive and act on. There is another difficulty. As we suggested back in Chapter 6, "It ain't what we don't know that gets us into trouble. It's what we do know that ain't so." If we don't review new knowledge regularly, we won't know when what we know "ain't so" any longer. We need skills and habits that are complementary to tracking down solutions that permit us to survey the medical literature efficiently and extract just the evidence that is new and directly pertinent to our patients. Unfortunately, it is more difficult to find the time to keep up with new knowledge when we are beyond our formal training and caught up in the hurly burly of clinical practice.

It is easy to blame this dilemma on the rate of advance in medical knowledge in general. This is a cop-out. Although medical knowledge is expanding rapidly, the new information that each of us needs is only a tiny fraction of the whole. We need just the information based on truly sound studies that are directly pertinent to the patients we serve. But how are we to find that fraction? The path to this information is fouled by articles written and published for reasons that have nothing to do with our reasons for reading them* and by the extraordinary volume of articles reporting studies that are on topic but preliminary or poorly done. Fortunately, we can organize the muddle for ourselves by understanding its nature and by taking advantage of good new information technology and good old clinical epidemiology. In this chapter, we will deal with perusing the literature on a regular basis ("maintenance").

We'll concentrate on the medical journal literature as the prime source of information for keeping up to date. The journal literature has several key features that warrant this status of "prime source." First, refereed announcements of new findings appear initially in the medical literature. Second, journal articles reporting studies give both methods and results in sufficient detail for the reader to assess the validity of the findings and, as important, their applicability to the reader's own practice. Third, the medical literature is indexed fairly extensively

*We read clinical articles mainly to get usable information; their authors often write them to get tenure, fame, and fortune, including justifying past and future research grants. The reasons for founding and continuing journals are, from a clinical perspective, sometimes even daffier and include the vanity of would-be editors and the chauvinism and profit motives of research and clinical societies.

and is available electronically (in citation and, increasingly, in full-text form), so that it is accessible from our homes and offices without the need to maintain a large personal library or file system or to visit the library.

Understanding the Muddle of the Medical Literature

Before starting with strategies for keeping up to date, it's worthwhile getting a feel for the "lay of the land" of the biomedical literature from the perspective of clinical practice [3]. Biomedical journals, including "clinical" journals, serve, first and foremost, as communication channels from scientists to scientists. The vast majority of studies that are published are not directly pertinent to clinical practice because their participants are not human (laboratory studies) or they are preliminary studies among humans, not designed to give a definitive answer to a medical question so much as to determine whether it would be worthwhile to pursue a definitive answer. (Rarely, the results of preliminary studies are so clear-cut that no further studies are needed—for example, there has never been a randomized trial of the effects of smoking on health, and such a trial would be unethical now because studies of smoking, using less direct methods of testing causal relationships, have been so consistent and the relationship so strong.) Often these preliminary studies are highly pertinent to the *problems* of our patients (which is why we often feel compelled to read them), even though they do not offer adequately tested *solutions* to these problems (which is why we shouldn't read them, at least when our purpose is keeping up to date with advances in clinical management; somewhat different tactics are needed for solving specific patient problems, as we discussed in Chapter 11).

The spectrum of biomedical publication resembles the spectrum of research that we discussed in the introduction to the book. For the scientist, this is exactly what one would want and warrants the high status that journals are accorded in science and academic promotion. *Clinical* journals usually focus on the more applied end of this spectrum by reducing the number of laboratory studies they select for publication or omitting them entirely. However, even in clinical journals, the vast majority of the investigations are from the laboratory or from preliminary studies among humans. When tested more rigorously, most innovations fail to pass. *In other words, many of the studies that are reported in clinical journals provide information that will be discredited or substantially revised on more advanced testing (think about it!).*

One unfortunate consequence of the high concentration of preliminary studies appearing in clinical journals is the premature adoption of innovations. Let's "pick on" case reports and series for a moment to illustrate this point. Where do you think case reports and case series fit in the spectrum of research reports? They are preliminary observations and highly subject to subsequent refutation. As an example, there were hundreds of case reports and case series extolling the virtues of extracranial-intracranial arterial anastomosis for preventing stroke recurrence, until a large randomized trial demonstrated that this technically elegant procedure was ineffective [7] and harmful [2]. It is true that case reports may precede the validation of effective maneuvers, and they are frequently accurate in announcing adverse effects of drugs [11]. Unfortunately, they also introduce what often prove to be useless or harmful treatments, because their methods do not permit discrimination of the valid from the interesting but erroneous. Thus, they cannot provide, by themselves, a sound basis for clinical action [1].

As practitioners, the studies that we must pay attention to are the most definitive investigations, the ones that meet the criteria for critical appraisal of medical evidence that appear in previous chapters of this book, summarized in Figure 12-1 and 12-2. We certainly don't need to feel guilty about skipping the others in our regular attempts to keep up.* Unfortunately, the counterpart of the high proportion of preliminary studies in clinical journals is the low concentration of rigorous clinical studies. This low concentration results in detection problems. Important advances are delayed in implementation in part because clinicians simply are unaware of them (the slippery slope!). Thus, errors of omission (failure to recognize genuine advances) are added to those of commission (premature adoption).

To overcome these problems, we can wait for others to tell us what to do, in which case we will always be behind the times. In doing so, we also will be abrogating critical appraisal of health care advances to others, who may not do it well. Or we can take on the task ourselves. The strategies that we are about to describe are designed to make this task doable, at least for the clinical problems that we see relatively frequently in our practices.

The Medical Library and the Medical Literature

In the first edition of this book, many of the elements of this section appeared in the chapter entitled "How to Use the Library." Any of you who are regular library-users will be well aware of their enormous value as information centers with highly skilled information professionals, large print resources, compendia, and an increasing arsenal of electronic information facilities. No doubt you will keep on using these (heavily subsidized!) facilities. But most of us don't take the time to visit the library regularly (or at all) once we graduate.

This new version of the "library" chapter begins with the premise that the trip to the library takes more time than most of us are willing to spend on a regular basis (even if it is only steps away from where we work). However, thanks to some new information services and technology, this trip is seldom necessary for ordinary information tasks.† In fact, most of what we need to do can be done at home or in the office in less than the 3 hours per week that physicians report they spend in reading journals [9]. (We say "less than 3 hours" here because we tried to convince you in Chapter 11 that part of your weekly reading time should

*As we will see in the next chapter, preliminary studies are better than no studies at all and may be all that are available for solving patient problems. For regular maintenance of one's knowledge, however, most preliminary (and a lot of the more advanced) studies can safely be ignored.

†Please don't take this as an indication that we think that libraries or librarians are obsolete. Quite the contrary. Librarians taught us most of the useful things that appear in this chapter and know far more about information services and management than we ever will. Their work should be consulted for more advanced discussions of the services that are presented in this book.

be devoted to tracking down the answers to specific problems that have arisen in the course of caring for your patients.)

ORGANIZING READING TO MAINTAIN COMPETENCE

Because new information of pertinence to medical practice usually appears first in the peer-reviewed medical literature, it makes sense to devote part of one's time to perusing this literature. Depending on your clinical field, there are many specialized "update" services as well, but these derivative services can appear only after the original journal publication and often are based on unstated (and sometimes expedient) selection policies.

Clearly you will need an aggressive strategy to tame the unruly literature. It is comprised of three basic tactics [4, 10]. Alas, there are no randomized trials of personal strategies that can provide us with guidance for keeping up to date with newly published literature. Bearing this caveat in mind, we offer the following suggestions based on what we do and feel makes sense. First, restrict your regular journal reading mainly to peer-reviewed journals that provide the best yield of articles for your own areas of clinical interest. Second, in browsing through these journals, read *only* those original articles (reports of planned clinical investigations) and systematic reviews (reviews with Methods sections) that, if valid, would be of direct importance to your own clinical practice. Third, scan the methods and results of these articles to determine whether they are likely to be true before reading them in detail. Most journals and articles in journals fail basic standards of methodology. For example, in our own survey of the literature, only 7% of articles in high-circulation general medical journals met minimal criteria for relevance and scientific rigor for general internal medicine [5].* In the rest of this chapter, we will describe the details of how to apply these strategies effectively and efficiently.

Which Journals Should You Read?

Table 12-1 provides a list of steps that can help you to select journals and articles for regular reading. We will take these step by step.

DETERMINE THE YIELD—FOR YOU—FROM GENERAL, HIGH CIRCULATION JOURNALS

To determine which journals you should read on a regular basis, we will assign you some homework. We would like you to conduct a brief survey of the general and specialty journals pertinent to your clinical turf. It is important for you to do your own survey of journals. We can't do this for you, for at least three good reasons. First, our clinical interests are unlikely to match yours. Second, if you are trying to keep up to date you will need to develop and practice the skills to

*This should not be considered as a challenge to the quality of these journals. General medical journals have broad audiences and act as communication channels for scientists as well as clinicians. Once this is understood, it doesn't seem so sacrilegious to extract the few morsels that are nourishing for one's personal clinical competence while leaving the rest.

Table 12-1. Ways to expand personal surveillance of biomedical literature*

1. Determine the yield—for you—from general, high circulation journals
2. Determine the yield from specialty journals of potential relevance to your practice
3. Delete low-yield journals from your regular reading
4. Add as many high-yield journals to your regular reading as you can afford, in terms of both time and cost
5. Collaborate with colleagues by developing and circulating a complementary set of subscriptions
6. Develop a "reading habit": review high-yield journals on a regular basis
7. Review *Current Contents,* or *Reference Update,* or their equivalents regularly
8. Subscribe to the SDI (Selective Dissemination of Information) service
9. Create your own SDI service on a personal computer

*Adapted from Haynes, R. B., McKibbon, K. A., Fitzgerald, D., et al. How to keep up with the medical literature: II. Deciding which journals to read regularly. *Ann. Intern. Med.* 105: 149, 1986.

do so yourself. Third, developing the skills by the route outlined above is not merely an exercise: you can practice on journal issues that you haven't read yet. In doing so, you will not only pick up the articles that are worth your time to read but can also determine the journals that you want to continue surveying on a regular basis.

We will start with the big general medical journals such as the *New England Journal of Medicine,* the *Lancet,* and the *British Medical Journal.** If you already have stacks of different general medical journals at your office or in your home, select about five or six consecutive issues of each and set aside a period of about 2 to 3 hours when you can be free of disturbances.† If you lack medical journals or solitude in your usual habitat or work environment, this sort of personal survey is perhaps better done in a medical library where you can assemble the necessary "subjects" in the same place at the same time.

Whenever and wherever you are ready to go, write down your rules for acceptance of an article as worthy, and create a tally sheet before you start reading. How high you set your criteria for reading an article in detail, and the order in which you apply the criteria, is up to you. As a guide, we have summarized our approach in Figure 12-1.

First, look at the table of contents for a given issue, review the titles of the articles and, based on the titles, count and record the number of *original studies* and *review articles* reported. Then count as a rejection any article with a title

*These general journals often publish the major advances in medicine, *regardless of the field of study,* because the authors of articles on important studies naturally seek the excellent reputation, rapid review, and large audiences these journals provide. Even highly specialized clinicians may need to review these journals regularly.

†The exact number of issues to review depends on the number of articles per issue and the yield. As a guide, you can get a fairly precise estimate by reviewing about 100 to 150 articles per journal. At about 20 seconds per article (with wide variance) this will take you about 30 to 45 minutes per journal, not a bad investment given the high price of journal subscriptions and high value you place on your own time.

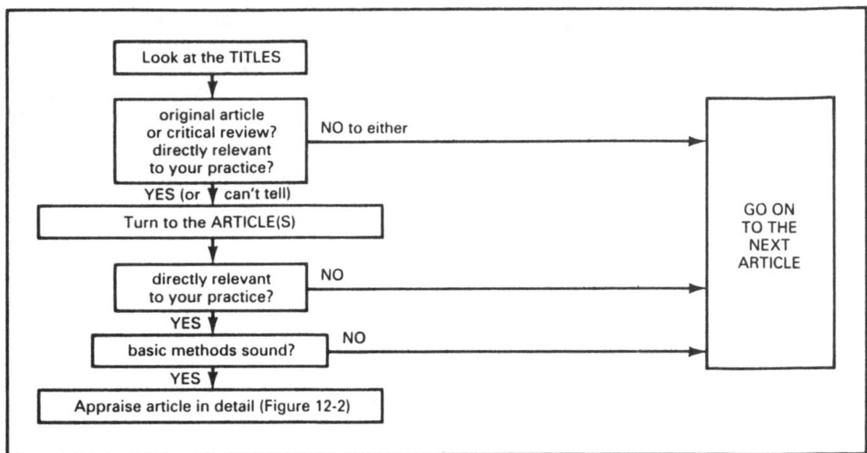

Figure 12-1. Reviewing journals

that appears to lack direct applicability to the patients that you see. Next, turn to the articles whose titles survived this first level of scrutiny. Assess these articles further for clinical relevance to your own patients and for methodologic adequacy. The criteria for the latter are summarized in Figure 12-2. You don't need to read an article any further than is necessary to determine that it has failed to pass one of your criteria. It is probably adequate for the purposes of this comparison of journals to apply only the main methodologic criterion for each type of study. For example, if the article reports the evaluation of a treatment, then it should be a randomized, controlled trial. It takes only a few seconds to run this sort of check and you can therefore review a larger number of issues of each journal (to give a more precise estimate of its likely yield over time) and a larger number of different journals.

Do not be disappointed if your favorite medical journal rates poorly. (If you feel that it is really better than your survey indicates, you can increase the number of issues surveyed—but don't throw out any of the data you have already collected on it.) And don't be surprised if only a small fraction of articles makes the grade. In our application of this approach, only about one or two articles per issue of the highest yield journals pass this screening procedure.

Is this low yield rather discouraging? It certainly does make one conscious of the limitations of reading journals as a means of finding important communications from medical researchers to clinical practitioners. However, if you have been following the logic of the approach we have described, this low yield is actually cause for celebration: The number of well validated advances in medicine that are relevant to each of our individual clinical practices is quite small and, with some fairly simple tactics, these can be winnowed from articles that serve other purposes. It is only because of this low yield that keeping up with important and relevant advances is possible.

What about editorials? You can't critically appraise editorials and, as articles written or invited by editors, they often are not even subject to the same peer-review standards as submitted articles. Nevertheless, they serve at least two useful purposes. First, editorials commenting on original articles you have selected for clinical relevance and validity can provide a useful context and further critique. Second, editorials that refer to articles in *other* journals are signposts to original publications that may merit your direct attention. Two other "early warning systems" for important studies that appear in journals that you don't review regularly are *Current Contents* and SDILINE. These are described in the last three steps on pages 370 to 374.

DETERMINE THE YIELD FROM SPECIALTY JOURNALS OF POTENTIAL RELEVANCE TO YOUR PRACTICE

Depending on the nature of your clinical practice, there may be a small or large number of specialty and subspecialty journals competing for your attention. Although a larger proportion of these journals' articles are about the diseases you treat, this does not ensure that the reports are both relevant to your patients and of high enough scientific quality to warrant your close scrutiny, let alone a change in your practice habits. (Don't be fooled by the frequent claims in the abstracts and discussion sections of these articles that the results have "important implications for clinical practice." This phrase and those of similar ilk are present in so many articles that they should be taken no more seriously than the "Sincerely" appearing at the end of a form letter from a magazine company president, soliciting your subscription to a magazine.)

As with general medical journals, the best way to determine the value of a specialty journal for your needs is to measure its actual yield. To wit, another survey of the sort just described for general medical journals is needed. Put any specialty or subspecialty journals to which you subscribe through this process, along with any other journals that you don't read regularly, but that you feel may harbor advances of importance to your own practice.

Delete Low-Yield Journals from Your Regular Reading

One of the dividends from the foregoing surveys is the identification of journals that aren't giving you enough value for your money or time. You can now rank them in the order of highest to lowest yield and determine how many of them you can really afford the time to read regularly (don't worry about cost for the moment). If you can afford the time to read all of them, you should consider expanding the number of journals that you read. If you currently try to read more journals than you have time for, then drop as many of the journals *from the bottom of your list* as you lack time to read. If you subscribe to any of these low-yield journals, drop the subscription or donate it to your local library. If you are on a circulation list for these journals, take your name off the list.

Some journal subscriptions cannot be canceled easily because they come automatically with membership in a professional organization. This is fine if the journal is of adequate quality, or if the organization news is of interest or importance to you. But if neither of these is the case, arrange to have these journals diverted somewhere before you see them. (The same goes for ALL non-peer-reviewed journals that you receive free in the mail. These contain articles that

Figure 12-2. Critical appraisal of journal articles

Following from Fig. 12-1, is the article a report of an original study or a critical review that is directly relevent to your own clinical practice? NO → GO ON TO NEXT ARTICLE

YES → Purpose of study?

Therapy	Diagnosis	Screening	Prognosis	Causation	Quality of Care	Economics Analysis	Review
Was the assignment of patients to treatments really randomized?	Was the test compared blindly with a gold standard?	Was the study a randomized trial? If YES, see Therapy If NO:	Was an inception cohort assembled?	Was the type of study strong? (RCT > cohort> case control >survey)	Did the study focus on what clinicians actually do?	Did the economic question include alternatives to be compared and viewpoint?	Were the questions clearly stated?
Were clinically important outcomes assessed objectively?	Was there an adequate spectrum of disease among patients tested?	Are there efficacious treatments for the disorder?	Were baseline features measured reproducibly?	Was the assessment of exposure and outcome free of bias? (e.g., blinded assessors)	Have the clinical acts under study been shown to do more good than harm? If not, did the study compare process to outcome?	Were the alternative programs adequately described?	Were the criteria for selecting articles for review explicit?

Was the treatment feasible to use in your practice?	Was the referral pattern described?	Does the current burden of suffering warrant screening?	Were the outcome criteria clinically important and reproducibly measured?	Was the association both significant and clinically important? If not, was power considered?	Were the clinical processes or acts measured in a clinically sensible and valid way?	Have the programs' effectiveness been described?	Was the validity of the primary studies assessed?
Was there at least 80% follow-up of subjects?	Was the description of the test clear enough to reproduce it?	Does the screening test have high sensitivity and specificity?	Was follow-up at least 80%?	Was the association consistent across studies?	Were both clinical and statistical significance considered?	Were all relevant costs and effects identified?	Was the assessment of primary studies reproducible?
Were both statistical and clinical significance considered?	Was the test reproducible (observer variation)?	Can the health system cope with the screening program?	Was there adjustment for extraneous prognostic factors?	Was the "cause" shown to precede the "effect"?		Were the measurements credible?	Was variability in the results of studies analyzed?
If the study was negative, was power assessed?	Was the contribution of the test to the overall diagnosis assessed?	Will positive screenees comply with further assessment and intervention?		Was there a dose-response relationship?		Was a sensitivity analysis performed to assess the effect of assumptions?	Were the findings of the primary studies combined appropriately?

advertisers have paid for you to see. "Throw-away journals" should be thrown away *before* they are read.) If you do not have someone to screen your mail, it is easier to avoid wasting your time on these journals if you toss them before you even glance at their often—and intentionally—seductive covers.

ADD AS MANY HIGH-YIELD JOURNALS TO YOUR REGULAR READING AS YOU CAN AFFORD, IN TERMS OF BOTH TIME AND COST

If you performed the exercises in the first three steps, you will now have "performance rated" several journals of relevance to your clinical practice. Congratulations—you will have come a long way toward organizing your reading. But there is an additional problem to deal with: the dispersion of articles on a given topic in many diverse journals. This problem is referred to by Ed Huth, the former editor of *Annals of Internal Medicine,* as scatter [8]. We will illustrate this with a modern information parable.

Weiner and his colleagues, a group of OBGYN clinicians, became upset that they couldn't find much in their journals about the risk of breast cancer from oral contraceptives. They set out on an odyssey to track down this elusive literature and identify its usual habitats. This turned out to be quite a quest. They managed to locate 741 articles published during the period 1977 to 1980, but only 27 (3.6%) contained original data and only four were published in journals of obstetrics and gynecology [10]. Weiner decried this as a form of censorship, because the result of this dispersal of relevant articles among so many journals was to deny obstetricians access to the literature required for the care of their patients. The literature has not responded to this challenge, and articles on just about any clinical topic continue to be scattered across a large number of journals. There are many factors contributing to scatter, including the large number of journals and specialization of these journals. Authors of articles on oral contraceptives and risk and cancer can send them to journals of obstetrics and gynecology, or to those on endocrinology, epidemiology, cancer, general medicine, family medicine, family planning, human sexuality, and so on. The moral of this parable is that keeping up requires surveying as broad an array of literature as you can afford (in time and expense).

An advantage of surveying a wide range of general and specialty journals is that you will probably identify some high-yield journals that you don't currently read regularly. In order of yield, these journals should replace the low-yield journals that you have identified.

If you can afford it, obtain personal subscriptions to the best of these journals. This is the easiest (albeit the most expensive) way to obtain all issues of a journal in a timely and convenient fashion and permits you to remove specific articles for your reprint file (or to keep the entire issue of the journal, if you prefer to assist gravity in keeping your bookcases and desk firmly on the floor).

COLLABORATE WITH COLLEAGUES BY DEVELOPING AND CIRCULATING A COMPLEMENTARY SET OF SUBSCRIPTIONS

Avoid bankruptcy! A money-saving way to expand the number of relevant journals for your regular review is to use your survey results to convince your colleagues to chip in and develop a set of complementary subscriptions for circulation to all of you. Each member of the "circulation club" could agree to subscribe to a proportion of the journals on your combined high-yield list, and the issues of each journal could be circulated through the members of the group as they arrive in the mail. The order of circulation isn't particularly important, but there should be a record of who has seen the journal and who hasn't. This is easily accomplished by attaching a check-off list of readers to the cover of each issue.

Of course, journals that have high yield for you may not be so useful to other clinicians in your consortium because of differences in your practices or differences in your standards of what constitutes worthwhile reading. Thus, you may need to negotiate and compromise in establishing the journal subscriptions. Obviously, the closer the clinical interests of all group members, the easier the process. However, in view of the tendency of major advances to be published in general medical journals, these can be the common denominator, even if the collaborators are diversely specialized and subscribe to some journals outside the common pool.

There are some other disadvantages to circulating journals, some of which are easier to avoid than others, and it is certainly worthwhile to look into these if you are or will be circulating journals [36]. Fortunately, it is possible to prevent most of the problems by keeping the number of participants small, subscribing personally to the most important journals for your own practice, and setting up guidelines for "circulation etiquette" to speed the rate of passage of journals around the group.

DEVELOP A "LIBRARY HABIT": REVIEW HIGH-YIELD JOURNALS ON A REGULAR BASIS AT THE LOCAL MEDICAL LIBRARY

A low-cost alternative or supplement to personal or group journal subscription is to set aside time each week to visit the nearest or best medical library. This may be at your hospital, your local medical society, or a medical school. Any travel time will obviously be at the expense of reading time, so there is certainly a price to be paid if you have to go far out of your way to get to the library. On the other hand, this habit will take you away from your office and the other places where work and interruptions expand to fill all your time. Furthermore, libraries subscribe to a much wider range of journals than any individual.

Of course, this large number of journals can be a handicap if you aren't selective in your reading. If you define the set of journals carefully on the basis of average yield and are rigorous about sticking to the list, then you can avoid wasting your precious reading time.

Medical libraries usually keep their latest issues separate from earlier, bound volumes, making it easy to review the most recent issues. However, the library is a shared resource, and if someone else is looking at an issue when you would like to, you'll miss it. Furthermore, unless you have a photographic memory, you are very unlikely to remember at one visit which issues you reviewed at the previous visit. This is especially true if you use the rapid review techniques advocated in this chapter. Maintaining a log of the issues you have scanned will protect you from duplicating your reading and remind you, on subsequent visits, of what you haven't read.

The frequency of your library visits will depend on how many journals you wish to review, how frequently new issues of these journals arrive at the library, how much time you set aside for each visit, how quickly you are able to separate the wheat from the chaff, and how much competition there is for the journals you are interested in. Although you will need to judge these things for yourself, 2 hours per week (at one stretch, and at a nonpeak time for the library) will likely keep your medical knowledge in fine fettle. If your clinical schedule permits it, midmorning is a good time in many libraries, because they are relatively quiet then and, more importantly, the journal shelves are likely to be in the best order of the day.

One final word on using libraries. Most librarians are partial to regular customers and often will go out of their way to help you meet your objectives efficiently. More important, as we discussed in Chapter 11, the librarian can also be the key person in helping you to acquire the best information available on specific patient management problems. Get to know your librarian!

REVIEW CURRENT CONTENTS, REFERENCE UPDATE, OR THEIR EQUIVALENTS REGULARLY

Given the scatter of articles on the same topic among many journals, it is not feasible to encounter all the relevant articles by surveying a reasonable number of journals. Fortunately, there are a number of literature services that can direct you to articles published in journals that you don't regularly read. Particularly if you are a subspecialist with the time and inclination to attempt to keep up with all advances in your field, these services can reduce the number of journals you need to review first hand.

The Institute for Scientific Information publishes a weekly compendium of the table of contents of current issues of a wide range of journals. Indeed, some subscribers receive their issue of *Current Contents* even before they receive the journals it covers. *Current Contents* groups journals by general subject to facilitate their review; thus, *Clinical Medicine* is published as a separate version of *Current Contents*. Unfortunately, the term "clinical medicine" is rather broad and one of the major problems of using *Current Contents* is the tedium of perusing page after page of journal titles, looking for those of particular interest. This problem is partly overcome by an index at the back of each issue that lists articles according to the words that appear in their titles. It is also tedious to flip back and forth between index and title pages to see if the title word of potential interest is derived from a title of equal interest.

You can reduce the amount of time it takes to get through *Current Contents* by reading only the titles of articles in journals that have passed your test for high yield. This takes orbicular self-discipline to keep your eyeballs from straying onto the esoterica (for your purposes, at least) that surround the journal title pages of primary interest to you.

Current Contents also includes an index of the addresses of the authors of articles so you can request reprints. If you like to obtain articles by the reprint route, this is certainly a convenience, although it does present some problems. First, the old adage that it isn't fair to judge a book by its cover applies in kind to judging articles by their titles. Many titles imply more promise than the article provides and others are unduly modest; consequently, requesting reprints of articles from their titles can be misleading. Second, many authors don't answer reprint requests, thus, although the cost of mailing a reprint request may be less than the cost of photocopying the article from the journal in your local library, the low yield on mailed reprint requests makes this approach both unattractive and expensive. Third, one waits for the mail. By the time you receive the article (if you get it!), you may have missed opportunities to apply the information.

To avoid the problems of reprints, you may want to use *Current Contents* in conjunction with your own visits to the library, or send someone to the library to track down the articles you are interested in. If you go yourself you will be able to inspect the articles that have caught your eye before you copy them. If you do this, it is important to delay your visit for a few weeks after the arrival of *Current Contents* in order to avoid chasing articles in journal issues that have not yet arrived in the library. Reprints can also be requested through the on-line services, BRS Colleague and Dialog (see the appendix of this chapter) with document delivery by regular mail, courier, or fax, beginning at U.S. $8.95* per article (up to 10 pages) for first-class mail and higher rates for faster service (e.g., U.S. $1 extra for ordering by phone and U.S. $20 per article [up to 10 pages] for fax delivery).

You or your circulation group can subscribe to *Current Contents.* However, you may want to use your library's copy for awhile before you commit your journal subscription funds, as a yearly subscription is expensive (U.S. $400).

Current Contents can also be searched on line, through BRS Colleague and Dialog. These services include a large number of electronic literature databases that you can access from a microcomputer with a modem (see Chapter 11 for details). *Current Contents* is updated weekly in two versions, *Clinical Medicine* and *Life Sciences.* These files can be searched by title words, key words, and authors as well as through requesting printouts of the title pages of specific journals. As we will outline in the section on SDI (page 372), a combination of title pages and topic searches may be the optimal way to review current titles. The charges for these services are a bit dear. As of late 1989, the connect-time charge for *Current Contents* on Colleague was U.S. $81 per hour for prime time and $71 for nonprime time, plus $.99 for printing out a title page or $.23 for displaying an article title. The connect time can be minimized by stacking the commands off line, including the specific journals and subjects you want (most communications software will allow you to store such commands). Reprint delivery is provided for an additional charge, about $10 per document.

Current Contents on Diskette™ is now also available for microcomputer (both IBM and Macintosh), for both *Life Sciences* and *Clinical Medicine.* The programming for this version is very slick. You can browse recent issues by journal,

*The prices quoted here were current in late 1990.

discipline, or title words, and generate a customized letter to send to authors for reprints. There is a high price to be paid for current access, however. The subscription is expensive. Subscribing information is at the end of this chapter.

Though it is the pioneer, *Current Contents* is certainly not alone in providing software for microcomputer access to current literature citations. *Reference Update* is a microcomputer competitor from Research Information Systems, Inc. It provides weekly updates for some 400 medical journals in its basic edition, and 700 journals in its deluxe edition. The updates can be obtained on diskette for IBM-PC and Macintosh computers, or by 9600 baud modem. Journals can be searched by journal issue, title words (and some synonyms), and through author-assigned key words for those few journals that provide them, but there is no further indexing. The lack of indexing for *Current Contents* and *Reference Update* is a handicap that can be overcome by using SDI services (see appendix), but not without sacrificing the speed of having the citations available as the articles are published.

In addition to these general services, there is a rapidly increasing number of specialty abstracting and current-awareness services. Three examples are *Hypertension Database of the Current World Literature* (over 250 journals) and *Current Opinion in Cardiology Database* (over 250 journals), both from Current Science, and the *AIDS Bibliography* from the National Library of Medicine. Most of these types of services are comprehensive within their field and leave the sorting to the user. Thus, their main advantage is in rounding up the literature on a specific topic, and their main weakness is not organizing it further, for example, by relevance for clinical practice. They are, therefore, of more value for scientists than for clinicians.

SUBSCRIBE TO SDI (SELECTIVE DISSEMINATION OF INFORMATION)

If you have highly specialized interests, you may find the yield from reading general medical journals so low that it is difficult to justify the time. If articles of potential value for your practice are published in only one or two journals, then the obvious solution is to subscribe to these journals. However, there are few medical disciplines with only one or two journals to honor them, and there are even fewer medical topics for which publications appear in only one or two journals. The Selective Dissemination of Information (SDI) service of the U.S. National Library of Medicine (NLM)) was created to meet just this specialized need.

The SDI file in MEDLINE contains the current month of new citations. An SDI file is an automatic, periodic (usually monthly) literature search on MEDLINE that can be designed to pull citations (and, at your option, abstracts and indexing terms) on the topics you specify from any of the 3000+ journals that are included in the MEDLINE file. In comparison with *Current Contents* or *Reference Update,* the SDI service is much less expensive (unless you specify a very large number of topics), quite a bit slower (months for most journals), but substantially more powerful in terms of retrieval of relevant citations and avoidance of irrelevant citations. SDI services can also be arranged for other literature databases, including EMBASE, from the Netherlands' *Excerpta Medica,* which covers over 4000 journals (with about a 40% overlap with MEDLINE), but the price is substantially higher.

The service works like this. Pick out the topics that you want to keep up to date on and look up the appropriate medical subject headings for these topics (use the *Medical Subject Headings* manual in any medical library or select the terms from GRATEFUL MED, software from the National Library of Medicine for "end user" searching). Then run (or ask your librarian to run) the search on the SDI file in MEDLINE to ensure that the search retrieves relevant citations, in a quantity that you can live with, and without a lot of junk (quaintly called "false drops" in the argot of the librarian). Your search may benefit from adding in text words or buzz words that have not (yet) become indexing terms. Once you are happy with the search results, the search strategy that you have perfected can be sent as an SDI search request to the National Library of Medicine in the United States on a form that you can obtain from any medical library. You will then receive a monthly printout of the citations retrieved by the search, run on the SDI file of MEDLINE. The charge for this service depends on how many citations meet your requirements, plus postage, but the cost is typically only a few dollars a month for a simple search, as the searches are run in off-hours, when the computer runs faster and the meter ticks slower. SDI services for the MEDLINE file are also available at a higher price from the commercial vendors, BRS Colleague and Dialog.

You can order a separate SDI file for each unique topic in which you are interested or you can put two or more topics into the same SDI file. For example, if you were interested in two particular aspects of AIDS, such as AIDS among drug abusers (the MeSH term that covers drug abuse is "SUBSTANCE ABUSE") and among individuals receiving blood transfusions, use the terms AIDS AND [EXPLODE SUBSTANCE ABUSE OR EXPLODE BLOOD TRANSFUSION].* (This yielded 25 citations when we ran it in early 1990.) Of course, you could set up a more general search (using, for example, just the term AUTOIMMUNE DEFICIENCY SYNDROME or its cross-referenced term, AIDS), but then you would retrieve many citations peripheral to your interests. The search would also need to contain a PRINT command. There are many options for this: the command PRINT INCLUDE ADDRESS, ABSTRACT retrieves the citations, including authors, titles, and journal source, plus the author's address and the article's abstract, if the citation includes one. (Always get the abstracts! They will cost you a bit of money for retrieval but will more than pay for themselves by allowing you to be much more selective about the full-text articles you subsequently seek.)

*As you should recall from Chapter 11, the "AND" in this search is a Boolean AND which retrieves articles that are on both AIDS and the combination of substance abuse or blood transfusion, and the "OR" indicates that the search will retrieve citations on either substance abuse or blood transfusion.

If you do your own MEDLINE searching with software such as GRATEFUL MED, you can run this search yourself and save yourself a bit of money. The AIDS search on the November, 1989 SDI file retrieved 34 references and cost $2.46. If you do decide to do your own updates, it is easy to forget to do the search at the same time each month. Here is a way to get around this problem. Using GRATEFUL MED version 5.1 or higher, add the month to the search strategy (put, for example, "NOVEMBER1990" (no spaces) on the next subject line) and store your SDI search *for the MEDLINE* file—if you store it for the SDI file, you will get booted out when you run it, because the SDI file doesn't recognize the date term. The MEDLINE file is updated about the middle of each month. Thus, when you get around to updating your own file, you should do it in the second half of the month. Retrieve the update search you stored, change the date to include all the months since the previous search (for example, DECEMBER1990 OR JANUARY1991), and run the update search on the MEDLINE file (NOT the SDI file). (If you are using software other than GRATEFUL MED, the MEDLINE equivalent of DECEMBER1990 is 9012 [EM], in which EM stands for entry month.)

You can add additional topics to your update search, and these don't need to be related to your initial topic. You also can retrieve the table of contents for specific journals (as many as you want), creating your own "current contents," though this will not be nearly as current as that provided through the lickety split services described in the previous section.* This is an excellent way to scan the contents of journals you don't subscribe to, but which have some relevance to your field.

More details about SDI and MEDLINE searching (including how to do them yourself on a personal computer) appeared in Chapter 11. If you have only one or two topics for which you want an SDI file, or if you cannot organize yourself to do update searches on a regular basis, it makes sense to ask a medical reference librarian for help in working out the details and placing your order.

There are also a large number of compact-disc products that provide MEDLINE, and more specialized literature files. These are relatively expensive for individual subscriptions at present, and they are not quite as current as the on-line MEDLINE file. However, they often are provided free by medical libraries. By our calculations, for clinicians who do regular on-line MEDLINE searching (that is, at least one search a week), the break-even point for a compact-disc subscription is about five users. Thus, if you work in a group practice, and enough of your colleagues do their own literature database searching and don't mind the inconvenience of using a single workstation,† it may be more economical to subscribe to a compact-disc service. For very large groups, some com-

*Articles from the journals that NLM regards most highly (those with the largest circulation and most frequent citations) are "posted" (i.e., indexed and entered into the NLM computer database, MEDLARS) as early as two weeks after publication. The posting of other journals can take months. Thus, although there is some delay, it usually is not great for the most important clinical articles.

†There are network versions of some of the compact-disc services now, but the capital outlay may be higher than all but the largest group practices could justify.

pact-disc vendors are now offering network versions of their products that can be accessed by modem or cable.

Power Reading

The purpose of the chapter to this point has been to show you how to enrich the literature you peruse on a regular basis. If you apply these tactics, you will focus on those journals that have a higher percentage of articles that meet the criteria of soundness and direct relevance to your clinical practice. Furthermore, if you apply the strategies summarized in Figures 12-1 and 12-2 to each of the issues on your regular reading list, the articles you actually need to read in detail will be few.

Just how vigorously you apply the criteria in Figure 12-2* may vary somewhat from subject to subject, and these criteria should be adjusted to match your time, knowledge of the subject, and purpose. For example, for clinical reading to keep up with important advances, you should continue reading only if the article is *directly* relevant to your patients, and meets *at least* the key methodologic criteria, including the major design criterion (for example, an inception cohort for a study of prognosis), plus a major performance variable (such as following up at least 80% of the inception cohort). We will call this the "preemptive strike mode." On the other hand, if you are highly knowledgeable about the field and know the current state of the art, you might only invest additional time in an article if its methodology is stronger than that of previous studies (whether they were strong or weak) or if it provides important confirmatory evidence.

As we'll discuss in Chapter 13, review articles are most useful if you are unfamiliar with a topic, haven't reviewed the literature on it for some time, or an unresolved controversy about the management of the clinical problem renders individual articles an insufficient basis for action. Reviews also can summarize information on differential diagnosis and underlying mechanisms; original articles are usually too focused to perform these tasks. The methodologic standards for performing overviews of the literature have been improving during the last few years. Some readers' guides for appraising them are summarized in Figure 12-2 and described in detail in Chapter 13. Unfortunately, most reviews still lack a systematic approach to the collection, selection, and analysis of original articles. If a review is directly relevant to your practice and meets high standards, take a peek at its conclusions. If they differ from what you currently believe, look through the article in detail: you will need to consider a change in your practice. If the review methods are not strong, or the recommendations from the review are similar to what you already do, move along to the next article.

If you decide that an article is worth additional attention, you will need to decide how you will remember its findings. If it addresses a clinical problem that you deal with often, rip out the article (if it's your journal!) or copy it, and put it in your clinic coat pocket or reprint file (if you have a file that works) to

*The criteria are crammed onto one page in case you want to photocopy it and have it with you when you browse.

use on the first opportunity that arises. If your pocket is too full or your file might as well be a circular one, inscribe the article's key details on a 3 in. × 5 in. card and stick that in your pocket until you have committed the new knowledge to memory. (This may seem like a lot of work, but this is very close to pay-off time, with the slippery slope we discussed at the beginning of this chapter just about to be sanded.)

If the article is about a problem that you don't deal with often, but find interesting—forget it. There isn't enough space in your brain for the things you really need to know, let alone this interesting but peripheral information. Your energies are better directed to looking up the topic the next time the related clinical problem arises (see Chapter 11) than trying to keep track of potentially useful information until the problem does arise.

When you have finished with an article, *do not go on to the next article*. Head back to the table of contents and scan the titles until you come to another one that appears relevant to your practice (skipping all but the original articles and systematic reviews), then open the journal again at that point.

The Key to Success

It takes considerable self-discipline in applying the simple skills described in this chapter to quickly set aside all but the most clinically pertinent and scientifically sound articles. Clearly, simply collecting articles that make it through this initial screening isn't enough. It takes further self-discipline to review these high quality articles in sufficient detail to determine their true worth to your patients and to learn enough from them to accurately apply their findings in your own practices. In other words, good reading habits don't come easily.

Nevertheless, it is immensely satisfying to be on top of the latest developments in patient care and, with practice, this can generally be done within the amount of time that most practitioners already allot to attempting to keep up to date. It is important, however, to bear in mind that a good part of your "update" time is most profitably spent in finding the answers to specific clinical problems, rather than regular review of journals as they find you.

Appendix. An Annotated List of Medical Information Products Described in the Chapter

The product information included here is for the convenience of readers and does not imply endorsement of the products, except as indicated in the text of this and other chapters. The prices mentioned were accurate as of early 1990. The list is not comprehensive: There are many other products, good and bad, available.

AIDS Bibliography is a monthly printed bibliography from the National Library of Medicine, containing citations to the journal literature (from AIDSLINE), monographs (from

CATLINE), and audiovisual materials (from AVLINE). It is available from the U.S. Government Printing Office, Superintendent of Documents, Washington, DC 20402 (202-783-3238) for $48 per year ($60, foreign), as of late 1989.

Current Contents, in its print and microcomputer forms, is available from the Institute for Scientific Information, 3501 Market Street, Philadelphia, PA 19104 (800-336-4474). As of late 1989, the diskette version was available, at an annual subscription fee of $495 (weekly updates available for both IBM-PC and Macintosh computers). The on-line version of *Current Contents* is available through Dialog and BRS Colleague.

GRATEFUL MED is software (for both IBM-PC and Macintosh computers) intended for easy use by clinical end users of the MEDLARS on-line databases, including MEDLINE. It is available for $29.95 plus $3.00 shipping and handling from the National Technical Information Service, 5285 Port Royal Road, Springfield VA 22161.

Hypertension Database of the Current World Literature and *Current Opinion in Cardiology Database* are products of Current Science, available for IBM-PC. Personal annual subscriptions are $470 for the former and $550 for the latter, and include recommendations and annotations from experts, with bimonthly updates. United States and Canada: Current Science, Subs., 1201 Locust Street, Philadelphia, PA 19107 (800-552-5866 or 215-790-2279). Outside United States and Canada: Current Science, Subs., 34–42 Cleveland Street, London W1P 5FB, UK.

Reference Update is a product of Research Information Systems, Inc., Camino Corporate Center, 2355 Camino Vida Roble, Carlsbad, CA 92009 (Tel.: 800-722-1227 within the United States, (excluding California), or 619-438-5547, elsewhere; fax: 619-438-5573). It is available for both IBM-PC and Macintosh computers in both Basic (400+ journals, $298) and Deluxe (700+ journals, $375) versions. Also available by 9600 Baud modem at slightly lower prices, not including long-distance charges.

ON-LINE SERVICES

BRS Colleague (and BRS After Dark, an off-hours, reduced-rate, more limited service). BRS Saunders, 8000 Westpark Drive, McLean, VA 22102 (Tel.: 800-345-4277; 703-442-0900; fax 703-893-4632).

Dialog (and also Knowledge Index, an off-hours, reduced-rate, more limited service). United States: 3460 Hillview Avenue, Palo Alto, CA, 94304 (415-858-3785); Canada: Micromedia Ltd., 158 Pearl Street, Toronto, Ontario M5H 1L3 (800-387-2689; 416-593-5211).

NLM Direct. United States: National Library of Medicine, MEDLARS Management Section, 8600 Rockville Pike, Bethesda, MD 20209 (301-496-6193); for Canada, consult Health Sciences Research Centre, Canada Institute for Scientific and Technical Information (CISTI), National Research Council, Montreal Road, Ottawa, Ontario, K1A 0S2 (613-993-1604).

References

1. Chalmers, T. C., Matta, R. J., Smith, H., Jr., and Kunzler, A. M. Evidence favoring the use of anticoagulants in the hospital phase of acute myocardial infarction. *N. Engl. J. Med.* 297: 1091, 1977.
2. The EC/IC Bypass Study Group. Failure of extracranial-intracranial arterial bypass to reduce the risk of ischemic stroke: Results of an international randomized trial. *N. Engl. J. Med.* 313: 1191, 1985.
3. Haynes, R. B. Loose connections between peer reviewed clinical journals and clinical practice. *Ann. Intern. Med.* 113: 724, 1990.
4. Haynes, R. B, McKibbon, K. A., Fitzgerald, D., et al. How to keep up with the medical literature: I. Why try to keep up and how to get started. *Ann. Intern. Med.* 105: 149, 1986.
5. Haynes, R. B., McKibbon, K. A., Fitzgerald, D., et al. How to keep up with the medical literature: II. Deciding which journals to read regularly. *Ann. Intern. Med.* 105: 309, 1986.
6. Haynes, R. B., McKibbon, K. A., Fitzgerald, D., et al. How to keep up with the medical literature: III. Expanding the volume of literature that you read regularly. *Ann. Intern. Med.* 105: 474, 1986.
7. Haynes, R. B., Mukherjee, J., Sackett, D. L., et al. Functional status changes following medical or surgical treatment for cerebral ischemia: Results in the EC/IC Bypass Study. *J.A.M.A.* 257: 2043, 1987.
8. Huth, E. J. The underused medical literature (editorial). *Ann. Intern. Med.* 110: 99, 1989.
9. Stinson, E. R., and Mueller, D. A. Survey of health professionals' information needs and habits. *J.A.M.A.* 243: 140, 1980.
10. Weiner, J. M., Shirley, S., Gilman, N. J., et al. Access to data and the information explosion: Oral contraceptives and the risk of cancer. *Contraception* 24: 301, 1981.
11. Venning, G. R. Validity of anecdotal reports of suspected adverse drug reactions: The problem of false alarms. *B.M.J.* 284: 249, 1982.

13

How to Read Reviews and Economic Analyses

The chapters of this book devoted to diagnosis, prognosis, and therapy presented tailor-made strategies for assessing evidence on these clinical acts. These guides, while sharing common threads addressing validity and clinical usefulness, have been specific to the clinical task at hand and have little else in common.

However, two sorts of clinical articles, namely reviews and economic analyses, regularly address issues across the spectrum of the preservation and enhancement of health and the prevention, detection, diagnosis, prognosis, treatment, and rehabilitation of disease. Although they can't be pigeonholed (and therefore have not received much attention in previous chapters), they constitute important sources of information for clinicians trying to make decisions, not only about individual patients but about their practices, hospitals, and health care systems. Moreover, we think that the assessment of these reviews and economic analyses can benefit from the same combination of science and common sense that produced the guides you've encountered in previous chapters. Accordingly, we present them here in their own chapter.

Guides for Assessing Reviews, Overviews, and Meta-Analyses

As we discovered in the preceding chapters, clinicians attempting to keep abreast of current developments must find ways of dealing with the exponentially expanding literature. Efficient strategies for finding and storing relevant articles and for discarding studies which are not valid or applicable are presented throughout this book. However, interrogating the literature about a clinical question remains time-consuming, and when there are dozens of equally relevant and sound articles on the same question it is simply not feasible for clinicians to read all of them.

One solution to this problem is to track down and appraise a review* article. If a rigorous scientific overview has been conducted on the clinical question you are attempting to answer, your time is better spent studying it rather than a grab (and perhaps distorted) sample of its citations. Thus, you may want to seek out review articles right at the beginning of your search (by requesting a "REVIEW" when setting up a GRATEFUL MED search, or by using the MeSH term "META-ANALYSIS"), and that's why we described how to do this in Chapter 11 on tracking down the evidence.

*Three terms are in use to describe such articles, and we use them as follows: when a *review* (the general term for all attempts to synthesize the results and conclusions of two or more publications on a given topic) strives to comprehensively identify and track down all the literature on a topic, we call it an *overview*. When an overview incorporates a specific statistical strategy for assembling the results of several studies into a single estimate, we call this assembly a *meta-analysis*.

Table 13-1. Guides for reading reviews, overviews, and meta-analyses

1. Were the question(s) and methods clearly stated?
2. Were the search methods used to locate relevant studies comprehensive?
3. Were explicit methods used to determine which articles to include in the review?
4. Was the methodologic quality of the primary studies assessed?
5. Were the selection and assessment of the primary studies reproducible and free from bias?
6. Were differences in individual study results adequately explained?
7. Were the results of the primary studies combined appropriately?
8. Were the reviewers' conclusions supported by the data cited?

However, regardless of what we call them, reviews, just like primary articles, must be read selectively and critically. Just as the use of flawed methods in conducting a study of diagnosis or therapy may invalidate its results, their employment in generating a review also may generate incorrect conclusions and useless or even harmful clinical recommendations.

We'd suggest that almost all the reviews published until very recently, and even most of those published today, suffer from these flaws. We think that the reason for this deficiency in reviews lies in the tradition of calling upon content-area experts to produce them. By the very virtue of their expertise, these authors begin their task with a conclusion, backed up especially by their own work, and invested with not a little of their personal reputations.* Little wonder, then, that the results may be skewed in content and citation as well as conclusion.

As a result, the busy clinical reader may find two reviews of the same, important clinical question that come to opposing conclusions and recommendations [1, 4]; how is the reader to decide which one to believe? The solution lies in recognizing the review as a study in itself, in which the reviewer poses a clinical question, gathers data on it (in the form of previous articles), analyzes them, and draws a conclusion. The fundamental difference between a review and a primary study is the unit of analysis—not the scientific principles that apply. Accordingly, just as for articles of other sorts, we can generate strategies for assessing reviews [6], and they are summarized in the eight questions that appear in Table 13-1. They, and much of the following discussion, are based on the work of one of our McMaster colleagues, Andrew Oxman. Before discussing them individually, however, two more comments are warranted. First, these guides apply to reviews addressing pragmatic clinical questions about etiology, diagnosis, prognosis, or management (rather than reviews of fundamental mechanisms of disease or pathophysiology). Second, the term "primary studies" will refer to the research reports (each containing original data) from which the review was generated.

*One of us has described this and other perils of being an expert in an essay calling for their compulsory retirement! (Sackett, D. L. Proposals for the health sciences: I. Compulsory retirement for experts. *J. Chron. Dis.* 36: 545, 1983.)

WERE THE QUESTION(S) AND THE METHODS CLEARLY STATED?

The first task is to decide whether the review is relevant to the reader's clinical practice or interests. This requires a clear statement of each of the three elements of the question(s) being addressed by the review: what is being reviewed (what exposure, diagnostic test, prognostic feature, treatment, and the like); in whom (the clinical population of interest); and for what consequences (which clinical outcomes). When all three elements are clearly specified, the reader can quickly decide if the review is both relevant and clinically sensible.

In addition to a well-defined problem statement, an explicit statement of the methods that were used for the research review is necessary if the reader is to make an informed assessment of the scientific rigor of the review, and the strength of the support for the review's inferences. The middle six guides of Table 13-1 will help the busy reader make a detailed assessment of this issue. However, an early screening of a review article often will reveal that it contains neither a Methods section nor any explicit statement of how it was conducted. Faced with this deficiency, the busy reader can save time by discarding that review article and looking elsewhere.

WERE THE SEARCH METHODS USED TO LOCATE RELEVANT STUDIES COMPREHENSIVE?

Because it is surprisingly difficult to locate all the published (to say nothing of the unpublished) research on even a narrowly defined clinical question (such as all randomized control trials of a given therapy for a given disease), readers require assurance that all articles that could have an important impact on the review's conclusions have been included. The more comprehensive the searching strategy, the more likely all important articles have been found, and readers should be provided an explicit statement of the search strategies used. Ideally, readers would discover that the reviewer used: (a) one or more bibliographic data bases (including a statement of which key words were used, and how); (b) a resource for tracking the earlier landmark articles forward in time such as the Science Citation Index; (c) a search of the references of all relevant papers for citations of other relevant papers; and (d) personal communication with investigators or organizations in the area being reviewed (in order to ensure that important published papers have not been missed, and especially to identify important unpublished reports). The more of these strategies employed in the review, the more confident the reader can be that all relevant reports have been included.

WERE EXPLICIT METHODS USED TO DETERMINE WHICH ARTICLES TO INCLUDE IN THE REVIEW?

A comprehensive literature search will yield both pertinent and irrelevant articles, and readers should be told how they were winnowed to produce the subset that generated the review's conclusions. When this process is unsystematic, opportunities for bias abound, and the all-too-frequent "selective" reviews of just those subsets of papers that confirm reviewers' preconceptions have tarnished the reputation of the review article. Even when explicit, preestablished criteria are employed, however, reviews of the same issue that use different selection criteria can generate different conclusions. For example, two methodologically sophisticated and carefully conducted reviews of whether steroid therapy increases the risk of peptic ulcer employed different inclusion criteria and reached diametrically opposite conclusions [1, 4].

Ideally, the review will report this selection in terms of precise sorts of patients, specific clinical outcomes, and particular maneuvers, tests, exposures, or prognostic factors, plus key elements of study design that identify "quality filters" on the admissibility of evidence; for example, most modern reviews of treatment restrict admission to randomized trials [8].

WAS THE METHODOLOGIC QUALITY OF THE PRIMARY STUDIES ASSESSED?

Reviewers will come to correct conclusions only in so far as they make accurate assessments of the methodologic quality of the primary studies which comprise their reviews. If all the studies addressing a clinical question are methodologically flawed, their conclusions not only may be unsound but, if flawed in the same direction, may display a superficially impressive but spurious consistency. For example, a number of case-series and cohort studies suggested that extracranial-intracranial bypass surgery reduced the risk of stroke, and served as justification for the large randomized trial that showed that the operation was not effective. However, a review that failed to consider the methodologic quality of the former, sub-experimental reports might incorrectly conclude that the operation was a success.

Methodologic standards, in the form of readers' guides, are presented throughout this book and summarized in Table 11-2, and can be compared with those employed by a review if the latter are reported in sufficient detail. Readers can then make their own judgments about the methodologic quality of the primary studies and the appropriateness of their inclusion in the review. This assessment of methodologic quality can be applied in two ways. First, did the individual studies meet minimal scientific criteria which would allow a strong inference to be drawn from their results? Second, can important differences in study conclusions be explained by differences in their methodologic quality? If so, the truth most likely lies in the conclusions drawn from the studies of higher methodologic quality.

WERE THE SELECTION AND ASSESSMENT OF THE PRIMARY STUDIES REPRODUCIBLE AND FREE FROM BIAS?

When two or more experts are asked to select and assess primary articles on the same topic, their disagreement about which articles ought to be included in a review can be both extraordinary and distressing, as we already found in reviews on steroids and peptic ulcer. Of perhaps even greater concern is the finding that, even when independent experts agree that an article should be included in a review, they may disagree about its conclusions! For example, when Thomas Miller examined five reviews that addressed whether the addition of psychotherapy to pharmacotherapy improved outcomes for psychiatric patients, he discovered that 11 studies had been included in two or more reviews [5]. On closer examination, however, six of these 11 studies had been interpreted as "positive" in at least one review and "negative" in at least one other!

So problems with reproducibility and bias can affect three stages of the review process: making the decision about which papers to include, deciding on their quality, and interpreting their results. These problems can be minimized when reviewers apply explicit criteria for the inclusion and assessment of primary articles, and readers should examine the review article for descriptions of what these criteria were and how they were applied. Ideally, each potential primary study should have been assessed for inclusion and if included, for methodologic quality and results by at least two reviewers, blind* to each other's decisions, and with the extent of their agreement documented and quantified (you should look for some statistical measure which quantifies their agreement above and beyond chance, such as the intraclass correlation coefficient we introduced in Chapter 3 or the kappa statistic you met in Chapter 2).

WERE DIFFERENCES IN INDIVIDUAL STUDY RESULTS ADEQUATELY EXPLAINED?

Since reviews often are undertaken in order to settle a controversy, it comes as no surprise that the individual studies they review will have differing, and frequently opposing, results. Moreover, even when individual articles agree that a drug is efficacious, they often disagree about the magnitude of its effect. Good reviews confront these differences and try to explain them.

Differences in study results can usefully be thought of as arising from five sources:

1. Different sorts of patients (with different disease stage or severity, comorbidity, prognosis, or responsiveness to treatment)
2. Different exposures, ways of performing diagnostic tests, or applying treatments (including doses, durations, combinations, and compliance)
3. Different outcomes (defined and measured in different ways and with different degrees of completeness)
4. Different study methods (with different rigor and power)
5. The play of chance

Good reviews often can explain differences between study results in terms of these five sources. For example, back in Chapter 6 you saw how differences in the sorts of patients included in studies of the prognosis of febrile seizures nicely reconciled conflicting results, and in Chapter 7 you learned how randomized trials tend to generate lower estimates of efficacy than more biased, non-experimental methods. Readers of reviews should be alert to whether these five possible explanations of differing study results have been considered, and special

*Indeed, Thomas Chalmers and his colleagues take this one step further in their reviews by what they call "differential photocopying" of the Methods and Results sections of the primary articles. The reviewers who are judging a study's Methods receive only that part of the report, and are blind to the study's results, conclusions, and authors.

caution should attend the interpretation of reviews that attribute differences between study results to just one explanation without adequately considering the other four.

WERE THE RESULTS OF THE PRIMARY STUDIES COMBINED APPROPRIATELY?

Reviews and their readers want a "bottom line." Is serum ferritin helpful in diagnosing iron deficiency and, if so, how helpful? Are patients with ulcerative colitis more likely to develop colon cancer and, if so, by how much? Is tamoxifen good for Stage I breast cancer and, if so, how good? Does treating hypertension reduce the risk of heart attack and, if so, by how much? As you can see, these bottom lines answer two questions: Is there something *really* going on and, if so, *how much*? To answer these questions, reviewers must somehow combine the results of the individual studies they have examined. There are several ways to do this and we want to show you how to recognize them and judge their appropriateness (because some are wrong, and others, though promising, are not universally accepted).

Before scrutinizing how the reviewer combined the results of the individual studies, you should satisfy yourself that it makes sense to combine this particular set of studies. Are the patients, treatments, outcomes, and methods sufficiently similar that it makes clinical and biologic sense to combine them? If not, hope that the overview refrained from trying to combine the results statistically; it nonetheless should state explicitly the basis for any conclusions that it does reach, and still should attempt to provide a unifying explanation for conflicting results. If an overview of dissimilar studies barges ahead and combines their results, be cautious about accepting its conclusions; better still, look for a better overview.

If, on the other hand, it makes sense to combine the results of the studies under review, read on. Consider an overview of randomized trials of the same drug regimen for the same condition (in the same sorts of patients, and for the same outcomes) in which five small trials found "no statistically significant benefit" and concluded the drug was worthless, while two other trials (one small and one big) found "statistically significant benefit" and concluded the drug was efficacious. They certainly are similar enough to warrant being combined somehow. We hope you agree that one wrong way to do this is to compare the numbers of positive and negative studies on an issue and give the nod to the answer with the highest "vote" (in this case, 5-to-2 for the drug to be worthless). Not only should this look wrong on commonsense grounds; if you hark back to the fourth readers' guide for articles on therapy you will want to ask "If the difference is not statistically significant, was the trial big enough to show a clinically important difference if it had occurred?"

It follows that the methods used for combining the results of several studies must take into account the size of each study, and a number of statistical strategies have been developed for this task. They go under the name of "meta-analysis" and are becoming increasingly popular, especially as methods for combining the results of multiple randomized trials. However, their optimal form remains controversial, and clinical readers shouldn't be expected to understand their individual tactics or merits.* Nevertheless, the clinical reader can quickly determine whether whatever meta-analysis was performed generated two important pieces of clinical information. The first is the size of the overall effect, across all the studies reviewed, of the factor under review (the strength of association in an etiologic overview, the likelihood ratio of a diagnostic test, the probability of an outcome in a prognostic overview, the reduction in unfavorable outcomes in a therapeutic overview). The second is some indication of the risk of the false-positive conclusion that something is going on† when, in truth, it is not. As you recall (we hope!) from Chapter 7, this risk typically is expressed as a P value. Meta-analysis is on strongest ground when the methods employed in the primary studies are sufficiently similar that any differences in their results are due to the play of chance.

WERE THE REVIEWERS' CONCLUSIONS SUPPORTED BY THE DATA CITED (OR DID THE REVIEWER SAY, "TRUST ME")?
Whether or not reviewers use meta-analysis, the results of individual primary studies should be reported in sufficient detail that the reader is able to critically assess the basis for the reviewer's conclusions. Tables summarizing crucial aspects of methods and results can be very helpful in quickly deciding whether conclusions really are consistent with data. As with reports on individual studies, both clinical and statistical significance should receive appropriate attention.

While reviews that meet all these criteria are rare, the principles behind these guides have gained wide acceptance. This is happening just in time, for there has been an outbreak of reviews in the medical literature. Readers able to use the foregoing guidelines can look forward to the prospect of being able to choose that subset of valid, useful reviews that can spare busy clinicians the work of searching and summarizing the relevant literature themselves on every issue of importance in their clinical practice.

Guides for Assessing Claims About the Cost-Effectiveness of Clinical and Other Health Care

Whether acting as individual clinicians treating individual patients, as members of a hospital staff, or as health advisers to our towns, voluntary agencies, or governments, we cannot escape making economic decisions. Our need to become at least a bit sophisticated in assessing economic analyses is emphasized quite forcefully when we realize that the *real* cost of every one of our individual

*At the time that this second edition was written, the "Observed-Expected" approach, as developed by Richard Peto and Rory Collins, was widely used and accredited (Peto, R. Why do we need systematic overviews of randomized trials? *Stat. Med.* 6: 233–40, 1987).

†The "something going on" could be a relative odds that appears elevated in an overview about etiology, a likelihood ratio that appears decisive in an overview of a diagnostic test, a relative risk reduction that appears clinically significant in an overview of a treatment, and the like.

Table 13-2. Guides for assessing an economic analysis of clinical and other health care

1. Was the economic question properly posed?
2. Were the alternative programs adequately described?
3. Has the programs' effectiveness been validated?
4. Were all important and relevant costs and effects identified?
5. Were credible measures for these costs and effects selected?
6. Was an appropriate analysis carried out?
7. Were comparisons between programs properly adjusted for time?
8. Were the presence and magnitude of bias identified?

or collective clinical acts is our inability to use that time, those people (including ourselves!), or that budget doing anything else.* Even when we are doing something of great benefit to our patients, by doing it we cannot do something else.

Although there is an understandable reluctance to pay greater attention to economic issues in the management of individual patients (after all, if we're not striving to obtain the best treatment for our patient and hang the costs, who is?), all sides agree about those other occasions when we are acting as a member of a clinic or hospital staff or as an advisor to a health agency or a government, where we regularly face economic decisions about which programs to launch or expand and which ones to abandon. Increasingly persuaded that the supply of doctors, nurses, other professionals, hospitals, and other facilities and technology cannot meet the wants or even the needs of all our patients, those who plan, provide or pay for these health services must ask the question: How can we apply our limited resources where they will do the most good? Because this question involves both costs and consequences, and because it implies a choice between alternative courses of action, it is said to constitute an economic analysis. In such a comparative analysis, money is usually (but, as we shall see, not always) the unit of measurement. The "real" cost of any health program, however, is the sum of effects or benefits forgone by committing resources to this program rather than to another one.

The strategies for evaluating economic claims will be described within the context of eight "guides" for the reader of such reports, and we acknowledge our debt to Greg Stoddart, Mike Drummond, and George Torrance for teaching us about them [2, 3]. Before presenting these guides, however, it should be stressed that in economic evaluations (as with the evaluation of the quality of care) the effectiveness of the maneuver being "optimized" must be established beforehand; the strategies of economic evaluation assume effectiveness at the outset.

The eight guides for readers of efficiency reports appear in Table 13-2 and can be posed as questions.

*Often you will encounter this *real* cost referred to as the "opportunity" cost, denoting the opportunities (for doing other things) that we lose when we commit our time and effort, and somebody's resources, to a given action.

WAS THE ECONOMIC QUESTION PROPERLY POSED?

Consider the question "How much does it cost us to run the immunization program in this town?" Although this may appear to be a question of efficiency, it lacks two essential elements of an economic analysis. First, it fails to specify the alternative *choices* (How much does it cost compared to other ways we could spend these resources?). Second, it fails to specify the *viewpoint* from which costs and benefits are to be considered. Is it concerned with the out-of-pocket expenses to the patient; the costs of rent, staff, and supplies to the clinician; the budget line of the Ministry of Health; or is the viewpoint that of society: "all costs and benefits to whomsoever they accrue"?

Now consider the following questions: "Should our county provide free immunizations through the Public Health Department or should they be provided on a fee-for-service basis through private doctors' offices?"; "Would it be cheaper and better for our hospital to treat varicose veins by outpatient injection rather than by inpatient stripping?"; "Should our province 'automate' breast cancer screening for women over fifty as opposed to the present 'hit-or-miss' system?" All three of these latter questions present specific choices and identify the viewpoint for costs and effects; accordingly, they are properly posed economic questions about the efficiency of clinical and other health services.

WERE THE ALTERNATIVE PROGRAMS ADEQUATELY DESCRIBED?

Readers of economic analyses should be able to replicate the preferred programs in their own setting. Therefore, the reports must describe both the costs (who does what to whom, where, and how often) and effects (with what health results) of the programs being compared.

HAS THE PROGRAMS' EFFECTIVENESS BEEN VALIDATED?

There are efficient ways of providing services for blood-letting, but they should be applied to blood donors, not patients with g-i hemorrhage. As emphasized earlier, effectiveness is assumed rather than established in efficiency studies, and we must insist here, as elsewhere, on hard evidence from randomized trials.

WERE ALL IMPORTANT AND RELEVANT COSTS AND EFFECTS IDENTIFIED?

Readers should satisfy themselves that all factors both pertinent to the question posed and contributing significantly to the cost or effect of the programs under scrutiny have been included. In general, both the costs and the effects can be of three sorts. On the cost side, you need to decide whether the report need only consider the actual costs of organizing and operating the program, or whether it should include any additional costs borne by patients and their families, or even the costs that arise from changes in the use of resources outside the health sector. On the effects side, you need to decide whether the report need only consider the "hard" clinical outcomes of mortality, morbidity, and function, or whether it should include the important area of the quality of life (or utility) that we discussed in some detail in Chapter 7. Finally, you may even want the report to have considered the program's effects on the availability and use of future resources (treating hypertension frees up resources for treating stroke now, but increases the need for resources to treat the longer-lived hypertensives later). It is unrealistic to expect all relevant costs and effects to have been measured and valued in an economic analysis (especially if they have only small impacts), but you should be sure that key bases are covered.

WERE CREDIBLE MEASURES FOR THESE COSTS AND EFFECTS SELECTED?

Most costs can be translated into units of local currency on the basis of their "prices" in the local setting, and the readers should satisfy themselves that these prices are appropriate.

Effects tend to be measured in one of three ways: first, they can be measured in a common unit of health (lives or years of life saved, levels of function, proportion of hypertensives at goal blood pressure, etc.); as we shall discover shortly, such measures lend themselves to "cost-effectiveness" analysis. Second, effects could be measured in several different units of health and then all converted into a common unit of currency. Although this method presents major conceptual difficulties (What is the money value of a life?; How much is good physical function worth in comparison to good emotional function?) it is in common use in the form of "cost-benefit" analysis. The third method of measuring effects addresses not the outcomes themselves but the relative social value (or "utility") of these outcomes compared to those achieved through other programs. One advantage of this third approach is that it can incorporate the "utilities" of the actual consumers of health services rather than the providers [9] and can be incorporated into "cost-utility" analyses.

WAS AN APPROPRIATE ANALYSIS CARRIED OUT?

The analysis must be appropriate to the nature of the effects produced by the alternative programs. If the effects are equal, they can be ignored and a simple comparison of costs will identify the preferred program; this is usually called "cost-minimization" analysis, and is illustrated in Table 13-3 for the varicose

Table 13-3. A cost-minimization analysis of outpatient injection versus inpatient stripping of varicose veins

	Effects among patients			
	Cost to the hospital per patient	No further treatment required	Prescribed support stockings	Further treatment required
Outpatient injection	9.77	78%	9%	13%
Inpatient injection	44.22	86%	11%	3%

Table 13-4. The costs and effects of breast cancer screening versus the current practice

	Effects		
	Costs	Well years	Years of life
Screening	Higher	Fewer	More
Current practice	Lower	More	Fewer

vein example. These data arose from a randomized trial of injection versus stripping and the author concluded that the results (effects) of the alternative procedures were the same [7]. The hospital costs are so different that even if one hospitalized the injection failures, the outpatient injection would still be the procedure of choice. This trial also determined the number of "disability days" required for treatment and convalescence under the alternative programs, and found that these averaged 6.4 days for those treated by outpatient injection and 31.3 days for those treated by inpatient stripping. Here the effects are unequal but are measured in the same common unit of health (the disability day); the efficiency analysis here is therefore *cost-effectiveness* analysis. Because in this example both the costs and the disability days favor outpatient injection, the conclusion is obvious. But what if injection led to longer disability than stripping? It is here that cost-effectiveness analysis is helpful, for it can tell us how much more we will have to pay (by substituting the more expensive procedure) in order to prevent one additional disability day.

The effects of alternative programs may be both unequal and measured in more than one kind of unit of health. For example, the randomized trial of clinical exam plus mammography for detecting and treating cancer of the breast in its early stages has shown that one in three older women may be spared a premature death in the process [10]. However, both she and her two peers who are not saved through early detection have a reduction in their "well years" by the very act of this early detection and "labeling." When we also take into account the great expense of launching and running such a program, we can develop the efficiency analysis shown in Table 13-4.

How are we to identify the preferred program when the effects of the alternatives are both multiple and conflicting? Two approaches can be used. First, both sets of effects can be converted (easier said than done!) into monetary units and combined; the evaluation of efficiency thereby becomes *cost-benefit* analysis. Alternatively, the common unit for the effects can be the value or *utility* of these outcomes to the women who would experience them; the efficiency evaluation then becomes *cost-utility* analysis.

WERE COMPARISONS BETWEEN PROGRAMS PROPERLY ADJUSTED FOR TIME?

The perceptive reader has already recognized that the two types of effects of the breast cancer screening program ("well years lost" and "years of life gained") sum to a quite different net effect at different times after the program begins; early on, well years lost will predominate and only later will we accumulate the large numbers of women who were saved from premature cancer death and therefore tipped the balance in favor of years of life gained. Similarly, once the initial cost of setting up the screening program has been met, it will become cheaper to operate. Finally, a bird in this year's hand is worth two in next year's bush; the importance of both costs and effects diminishes with distance in time as well as space, and this must be taken into account in the analysis of efficiency. The strategy for doing so is called "discounting" and is analogous to being willing to pay interest tomorrow for a loan of cash today.

WERE THE PRESENCE AND MAGNITUDE OF BIAS IDENTIFIED?

It is clear that these efficiency analyses call for exact statements (or "point-estimates") about costs and effects. But what if these point-estimates are wrong? What if a year of healthy life is worth 40 ounces of gold rather than 36? What if the health utility of the postmastectomy state was 10% higher? What if we have underestimated the cost of a program by one-fifth?

The comprehensive evaluation for efficiency will have tested for the possible effects of these biases by plugging them into the economic analysis to see whether they would materially affect its conclusion. These additional calculations, called "sensitivity analyses," can provide reassurance about the robustness of the conclusions drawn from the evaluation. They can also underscore, however, the aphorism that efficiency analyses are only as good as the data upon which they operate.

We hope that this chapter has rounded out your skills in assessing the sorts of articles and other evidence that you use in making clinical decisions. The next, and final, chapter in this book will focus on strategies and tactics for keeping these skills sharp and for transmitting them to others.

References

1. Conn, H. O., and Blitzer, B. L. Nonassociation of adrenocorticosteroid therapy and peptic ulcer. *N. Engl. J. Med.* 294: 473, 1976.
2. Department of Clinical Epidemiology and Biostatistics. How to read clinical journals: VII. To understand an economic evaluation (Part A).*Can. Med. Assoc. J.* 130: 1428, 1984.
3. Department of Clinical Epidemiology and Biostatistics. How to read clinical journals: VII. To understand an economic evaluation (Part B). *Can. Med. Assoc. J.* 130: 1542, 1984.
4. Messer, J., Reitman, D., Sacks, H. S., et al. Association of adrenocorticosteroid therapy and peptic-ulcer disease. *N. Engl. J. Med.* 309: 21, 1983.
5. Miller, T. I. The effects of drug therapy on psychological disorders. Ph.D. Dissertation, University of Colorado, 1977.
6. Oxman, A. D., and Guyatt, G. H. Guidelines for reading literature reviews. *Can. Med. Assoc. J.* 138: 697, 1988.
7. Piachaud, D., and Weddell, J. M. Cost of treating varicose veins. *Lancet* 2: 1191, 1972.

8. Sackett, D. L. Rules of evidence and clinical recommendations on use of antithrombotic agents. *Chest* 95: 2S, 1989.
9. Sackett, D. L., and Torrance, G. W. The utility of different health states as perceived by the general public. *J. Chronic Dis.* 31: 697, 1978.
10. Shapiro, S. Evidence of screening for breast cancer from a randomized trial. *Cancer* 39 (Suppl.): 2772, 1977.

14

How to Get the Most from and Give the Most to Continuing Medical Education

Here we are at the end of the book. Much of what has gone before has documented the gaps that exist between what we, collectively, know about how to evaluate and manage human illness and what we, individually, do to and for patients with these illnesses. This final chapter will describe some strategies for closing these gaps.

If you have worked your way through the preceding chapters, you have already demonstrated that you are a highly motivated (and tolerant!) learner who is striving to narrow these gaps. But to illustrate "the trouble with gaps," take a crack at the following self-evaluation.* (Brace yourself, the questions are undoubtedly impertinent!)

1. You have a 27-year-old female patient with systemic lupus erythematosus who asks you about her future and particularly the advisability of pregnancy. Name at least five "critical appraisal" principles you could apply in looking into the medical literature for answers to these questions. (If you are *really* game, go ahead and find the best articles available on these subjects.)

2. *Either:* Calculate likelihood ratios for the following table:

		Target Disorder	
		Present	Absent
Test Result	+ + +	100	1
	+ +	50	10
	+	30	30
	0	2	40
	Total	182	81

or: If you had to dichotomize the test results into either "positive" or "negative," and false-positive and false-negative patients were equally harmed by being misdiagnosed, what cutoff point would be the best one for these 263 patients?

3. The nurses on your team at the hospital asked you 2 weeks ago for an update on the precautions they should take in dealing with

*Our answers appear beginning at the bottom of page 421.

AIDS patients, but you have not had time to get to it until the day you promised to report back to them. They want a statement they can post and circulate, and you have 30 minutes to come up with something. Go to your hospital library and actually carry out this search.

4. Since you began reading this book, how many opportunities have you had to apply its principles in your own clinical practice? Of these, on how many occasions did you actually apply the principles?

If you are reading this *after* doing the exercises above, congratulations! If you *have not* done the exercises, you are living proof of the gap between theory and practice: By saving the energy required to cross that gap, you risk joining the others who are "too busy" to keep up to date. Unfortunately, without some form of performance review we may even be unconscious of the gaps. Ironically, when the need arises for the competency or performance we lack, it is not we, but our patients, who suffer the consequences.

We therefore devote the first portion of this final chapter to answering the question "How can I make my own continuing education as effective as possible (and avoid premature clinical senility)?" Among the knowledge, attitudes, and skills that are essential for continued effectiveness as a clinician, we shall focus on three skills: clinical skills, skills in the critical appraisal of clinical evidence, and self-directed learning skills. We will therefore discuss Continuing Medical Education (CME) as it applies to each of these skills, adding the pertinent educational principles along the way.

Our own continuing education about continuing education has benefitted from the efforts of several colleagues, especially Vic Neufeld [25] and Dave Davis (who chaired the CME Committee at McMaster University).

Clinical Skills

Clinical skills include the *precise and accurate collection of clinical* (symptoms and signs) *and paraclinical* (laboratory and other diagnostic tests) *data*. We have provided several examples of faulty clinical skills in previous chapters, plus evidence that these skills can be improved by supervised training, by comparing your findings with those of colleagues and mentors, and by comparing your findings against more definitive tests. As we showed you in Chapter 10, clinicians who keep track of their success rates for key clinical observations have a performance review and feedback system that is invaluable for brushing up their clinical skills when they are deficient or become rusty. However, inertia prevents most of us from even adopting a performance review and feedback system, let alone responding to it (have you tried the system described in Table 10-1?). If you have not yet tried keeping a scorecard on yourself, why not copy the headings from Table 14-1 on a card, stick it in your pocket, and try it on your next 10 patients.

Unfortunately, as has been demonstrated for patient compliance, feedback alone is not sufficient to modify behavior [2]. In order to improve a skill or maintain it at an optimum level, there must be some reward for doing it. After all, if virtue were its own reward, we would not have needed to write this book. In view of all this, why don't you make the same sort of deal (contingency contract) with yourself that has been successful in improving patient compliance [30] (Fig. 14-1)?

Then, if you complete the task successfully, you simply give yourself the agreed-upon reward! Alas, there is a penalty in applying this tactic to oneself, as the joy of winning the reward is tempered by the sorrow of having to pay for it—i.e., it is difficult to reward oneself. We do not know of a tested solution to this problem but suggest that you try a tactic employed by psychologists when they deal with very difficult behaviors such as overeating, smoking, alcohol abuse and the like (after all, we *are* talking about bad habits!). Their approach is to have patients pay an up-front entry fee for the program and make its return contingent upon achieving negotiated goals. Why not finance your continuing education in clinical skills by putting enough money in a safe place to permit you to buy some luxury item you wouldn't ordinarily buy yourself (a wide-angle camera lens, an expensive book, a stereo component, etc.), and retrieving appropriate amounts of it as you achieve the goals you have set down in advance? That way you will turn what can be an expensive proposition these days (faulty skills are one cause for malpractice suits, and formal CME costs plenty) into at least a break-even proposition.

At this point you no doubt are questioning our sanity (or, at least, our perverted sense of humor). The truth is, we are deadly serious about the difficulty that physicians have in acquiring and maintaining their clinical skills. And we are convinced by randomized trials of compliance-improving strategies that these interventions are worth applying to our own patients. What we do not know is whether clinicians can apply these techniques *to themselves*. Thus, we are cautious in proposing them to you now. If they work for you, by all means use them (no clinical trial needed!); otherwise, caveat emptor—it may be a waste of your time.

Figure 14-1.

I agree to:

Check my accuracy for at least
one clinical observation on my next 10 patients

In return for:

Treating myself to a ticket
to the next baseball game in town

The alternatives, of course, are to do nothing or to engage in formal, skills-training programs. If you are a medical student or house officer, you are already in such a program, but may need to work hard to get your money's worth. The tactics outlined in Chapter 2 should be useful for this.

If you have completed your formal training, the opportunities to improve your clinical skills are fewer and more expensive. Many formal CME activities pay little attention either to relevance to the practicing clinician or to adherence to basic educational principles; as a result, many CME programs merely go through the motions. Thus, the question arises of how one can select a CME course or program that will, for a reasonable investment of time, money, and effort, have a positive impact on one's practice and patients.

Starting with common sense, some guidelines for this selection are fairly obvious. First, you should concentrate on courses that focus on skills that are really important to your clinical practice. If you are an emergency-room physician or a member of a cardiac-arrest team, you will certainly want to take advantage of some of the advanced cardiac life support programs (ACLS) [3]. However, if you have no opportunity to employ such skills, you should hone your basic life support skills and leave it at that—even if an excellent ACLS program is offered for free in your vicinity and the emergency-room physicians in your hospital claim that everyone should have the skills. This is because such skills deteriorate rapidly if not used [32] and you are better off seeking enhancement of "every-day" skills.

The second commonsense guideline (that we will verify empirically in a moment) is that skills are best learned by a "hands-on" supervised experience, complete with feedback and comparison with an acceptable "gold standard" of performance. If you can't learn to swim by reading a book about swimming, why should you expect to learn how to do expert ophthalmoscopy by attending a lecture on it?

Beyond these two bits of commonsense, there actually is evidence from controlled trials that will help you select an appropriate format. One of us collaborated in a study [29] in which physicians were provided with a list of topics that were available for home study and asked to rank them in terms of preference. They were then allocated randomly to receive or not receive the continuing-education materials related to their two most preferred topics plus two of their least preferred topics. When the actual clinical performance of these physicians was reviewed, it was discovered that they improved their performance in the topic areas in which they were most interested, *regardless of whether or not they received the continuing medical education materials!* On the other hand, for least preferred topics, only physicians who were allocated to receive instruction showed improvements in their performance. We draw two conclusions from this study. First, you can probably improve, by yourself, those skills that you are clinically interested in perfecting. Second, however, you ought to force yourself to attend formal CME events for those clinical topics you enjoy least, but must be good at to do your job properly.

Trials that have assessed the impact of continuing medical education on *patient* outcomes are few and far between—but it is exactly these studies that ought to form the basis for our recommendations as to what sort of CME is worth your while. When we and other colleagues reviewed 248 CME studies, we found only 30 were randomized control trials, only seven of these RCTs were rigorously executed, and only three evaluated patient outcomes [12].

The only study of the lot to show an improvement in patient outcomes [17] took on 20 hospitals that did not have formal "burn programs." These hospitals were randomly allocated to receive or not receive a CME program on burns, and then were compared on the subsequent outcomes of burn patients who presented to their emergency rooms. The continuing medical education program was multifaceted, including seminars, a manual of protocols for patient management, performance reviews, feedback on individual cases, and a telephone hotline for expert consultation.

Several outcomes were correlated with the process of care, and two of these were significantly influenced by the experimental interventions: Compliance with therapy rose among discharged patients and early complications fell among patients who were admitted to the hospital. The hotline was never used, however, and it was not clear which of the other elements of this program were important to the beneficial results that were observed; the investigators singled out rapid feedback on deviations from the burn protocols as likely being of particular value. As feedback and supervision are key ingredients in improving patient compliance, it makes sense to join CME programs that offer this performance review and feedback in areas that are pertinent to your clinical practice.

Such continuing medical education programs are currently scarce. However, the wave of the future may be signaled by a randomized control trial of computer reminders reported by McDonald and his coworkers [22]. This trial computerized the records of general medical patients, added 410 management rules concerning the ordering of diagnostic tests and the management of medications, and sent appropriate automatic reminders to the house officers and nurse practitioners who were looking after a random half of the patients. This maneuver resulted in a significant increase in "appropriate" responses by the clinicians (in terms of test orders and treatment changes) to the clinical situations detected and reported by the computer. However, most of these responses concerned management, not clinical skills, and patient outcomes were not assessed in this brief study, so we don't know if these patients actually benefited from the changes produced.

Looking for common themes in the seven soundest studies in our CME review, the most useful tactic for improving practitioner performance is to provide individual clinicians with both an audit of their own performance and a comparison between it and some standard of care. This individualized audit and feedback was present in each of the studies we described earlier [17, 22, 29] as well as in others [28]. It is important to realize that "group feedback" of the sort that often occurs in hospital-based quality assurance efforts was not effective in changing individual performance in, for example, the use of caesarian sections [20].

To sum up, to enhance clinical skills that you are keen on improving or maintaining, pay attention to the strategies outlined in the first part of Chapter 2, and keep tabs on your track record through the self-monitoring tactics described in Chapter 10. If you cannot or will not do this without incentives, create your own incentive system. For those clinical skills that you need but lack completely, or have but tend to neglect, look for educational opportunities that provide a supervised, hands-on experience with rapid individualized feedback. These often take the form of spending some time seeing patients together with an acknowledged clinical expert who can show you how to do it and give you feedback on whether you do it correctly. To maintain your skills, you also should arrange for periodic review. Finally, in the future, you should be on the lookout for articles describing more sophisticated information systems that will take the drudgery out of the meticulous bookkeeping that is required to keep most of us up to scratch.

Critical Appraisal Skills

Whereas we defined clinical skills (somewhat narrowly) as the precise and accurate collection of clinical and paraclinical data, we define the critical appraisal of clinical evidence as the *application of certain rules of evidence to clinical* (symptoms and signs), *paraclinical* (laboratory and other diagnostic tests), *and published data* (advocating specific treatment maneuvers or purporting to establish the etiology or prognosis of disease) *in order to determine their validity* (closeness to the truth) *and applicability* (usefulness in one's own clinical practice).* For our purposes at least, clinical skills have to do with the *acquisition* of clinical data, while critical appraisal has to do with the *interpretation* of these data.

To understand and improve on our mastery of critical appraisal skills, we will need to explore the three dimensions that comprise the clinical learning experience. These three dimensions are the clinical problem to be solved, the clinical evidence upon which the solution hinges, and the critical appraisal skills with which we assess the data for their validity and applicability.

THE CLINICAL PROBLEM TO BE SOLVED

This dimension spells out the motivation for learning and is shown along a vertical axis in Figure 14-2.

At the highest level, an actual patient under the learner's care serves as the motivation for learning, and this is acknowledged to be the most powerful stimulus for effective learning and retention. Thus, we hope that the reason you are reading this book is your conviction that specific patients of yours will be better off if you became adept at critical appraisal. At a lower level, teachers may provide descriptions of real or imagined patients in the form of case-presentations, a printed scenario such as the biomedical problem (BMP), or a simulated patient. Thus, we have incorporated many such descriptions in this text, and both BMPs and simulated patients are standard stimuli at our medical school. If we have described patients that you often encounter, so much the better. But

*Around our town, the incorporation of critical appraisal into clinical practice often is called "evidence-based medicine."

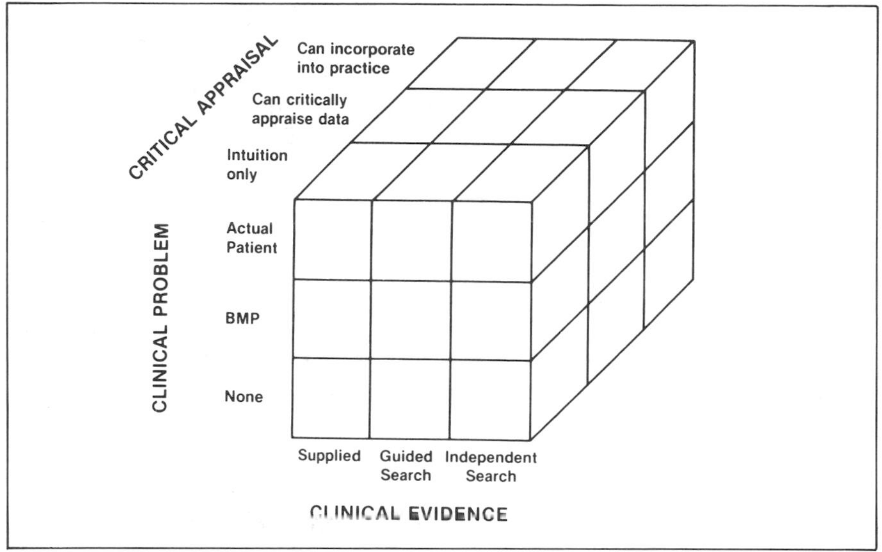

Figure 14-2. Clinical learning.

there are obvious limits to the stimulus that any book can provide, and it cannot compete with the stimulus to learning provided by your own patients. Finally, at the bottom of this dimension there may be no clinical problem at all, only the admonition (with or without coercion) by the teacher that what is being taught had better be learnt. We have avoided (successfully, we hope) any such admonitions in this book, and trust that no one who has persisted to this point has done so simply because some prof cajoled or threatened.

THE CLINICAL EVIDENCE TO BE ASSESSED

This dimension spells out the responsibility for tracking down the clinical data (signs and symptoms), paraclinical data (laboratory and other diagnostic tests) and published evidence (advocating specific diagnostic and treatment maneuvers or purporting to establish the etiology or prognosis of disease) required to solve the clinical problem, and is shown along the horizontal axis in Figure 14-2.

At its highest level of development (to the extreme right) the clinical evidence is tracked down by the learner, using either clinical skills or various tactics for searching the biomedical literature. If you took us up on the exercises at the beginning of this chapter, or have applied some of the strategies we described in Chapters 2 and 11 to obtaining evidence from your patients or the medical literature, you were operating at this level. At a lesser level, the teacher guides the search for clinical and paraclinical data and published evidence, showing the learner how to do it. Again, much of this book was written at this level; such are the limitations of textbooks. At the lowest level, all of the clinical evidence is supplied by the teacher, and the learner is passive in this dimension.

THE CRITICAL APPRAISAL SKILL

This dimension describes the degree of sophistication and independence with which the learner determines the validity of the evidence and its applicability to solving the clinical problem, and is shown along a diagonal axis in Figure 14-2.

In its most highly developed form (in the "northeast" corner of Figure 14-2), learners are not only able to critically appraise the clinical evidence they gathered but also can incorporate conclusions about the validity and applicability of this clinical evidence into their evaluation and management of patients. As with learning to play hockey, this level can only be achieved with practice and experience. At a lesser level, learners have mastered the critical appraisal of clinical and paraclinical data and published evidence, but remain unskilled at incorporation of their conclusions into clinical practice. At the lowest level, learners must fall back on their intuition and cunning to keep themselves from being misled by invalid or inapplicable clinical evidence; many of the examples cited in this book attest to the frailty of this approach.

These three dimensions, each with three levels of development, can now be joined to generate the 27 different learning situations depicted in Figure 14-2. They can be used both to describe and understand continuing medical education events and to identify ways of making them more effective.

Continuing Medical Educational Events

THE "CORE-KNOWLEDGE" APPROACH (or the "this is what everybody needs to know" approach)

In its extreme form, this runs the risk illustrated in Figure 14-3, and is familiar

Figure 14-3. The "core-knowledge" approach in its extreme form.

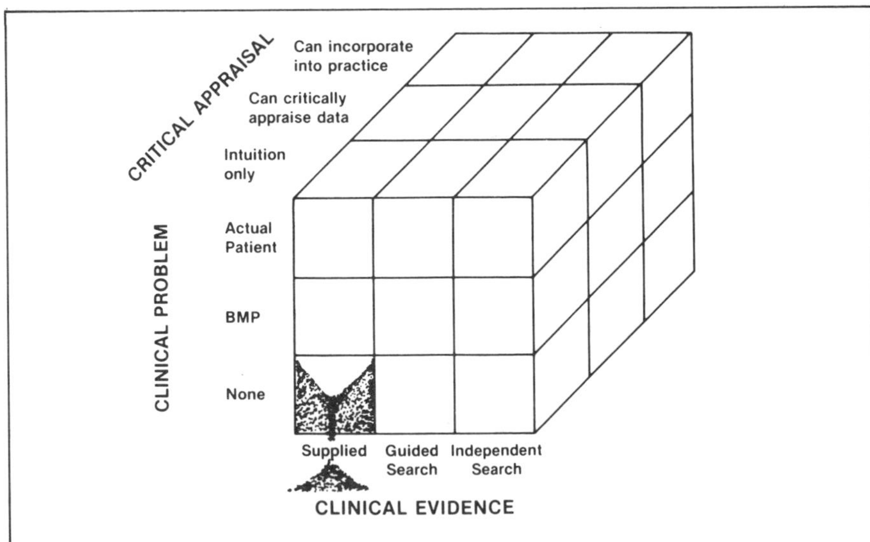

to just about everybody who has been to any educational event of any sort, any time.

If you are subjected (by others or yourself) to this approach, you will learn *what*, not *how* or *why*. There is no critical appraisal, only the mastery of current "facts." Learning is virtually one-dimensional, since what is to be learned is decided by curriculum committees or textbooks (rather than provoked by the clinical problems you face) and there need not be any attention paid to the methods whereby the body of facts was generated. Success is measured by computer (e.g., most medical licensing exams), or by mere attendance (e.g., CME credits for showing up).

Stuff learned this way is rarely remembered. Indeed, this time-honored approach to undergraduate, postgraduate, and continuing medical education has been documented to produce clinical clerks who fail the same anatomy exams they passed two years earlier (although they didn't flunk nearly as badly as senior staff surgeons) [23], and practicing physicians whose knowledge and application of the basic elements of the up-to-date work-up and management of hypertension are *inversely* proportional to the time elapsed since they left medical school [11, 19].

If, however, learners and teachers shift the emphasis from core-*knowledge* (to be memorized) to core *clinical problems* (to be solved), a vast improvement in education can occur [10], as shown in Figure 14-4.

Even if the search for clinical evidence is guided and critical appraisal falls short of incorporation into clinical practice, education can be arranged so that learners confront a proper mix of patients who collectively present the core clinical problems that they must learn to solve. Independence in tracking down and

Figure 14-4. The "core-problem" approach.

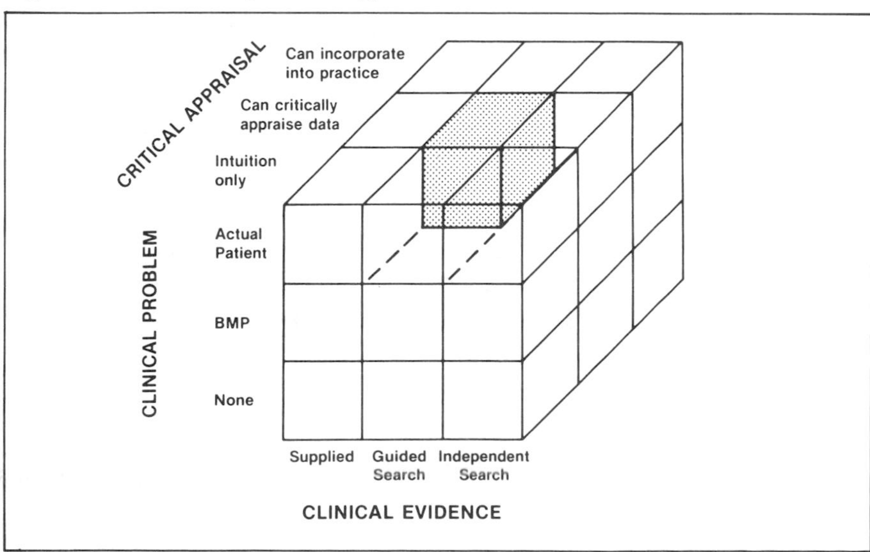

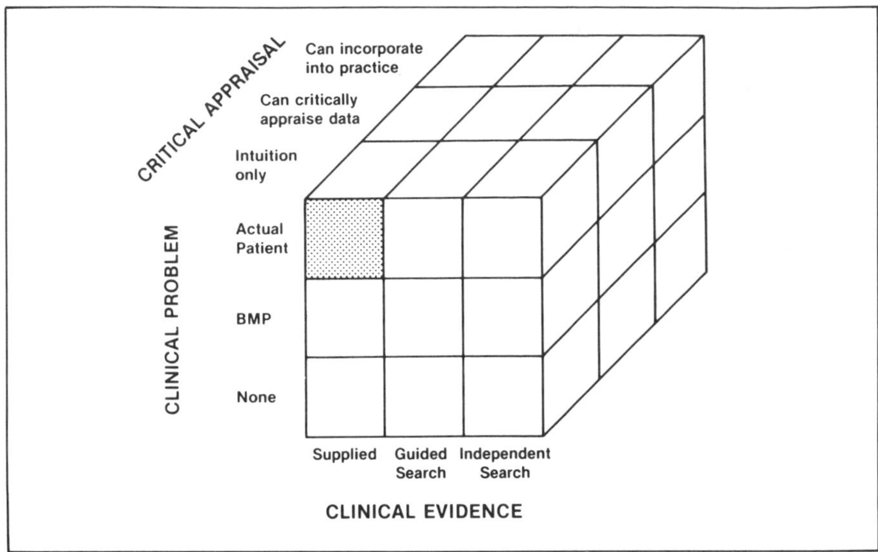

Figure 14-5. The Authoritarian Attending Round.

critically assessing clinical evidence can be encouraged, not squelched, and learners can become competent for the future, not just the present.

THE ATTENDING ROUND

As described earlier, one of the effective strategies for keeping up-to-date is the clinical preceptorship, and this often involves accompanying senior clinicians as they make their attending rounds. The extremes of such attending rounds are shown in Figures 14-5 and 14-6, and this passage is unabashedly directed mainly at teachers, not learners (although the latter may emit catcalls from the side-lines).

At worst, the Authoritarian Attending Round (Fig. 14-5) is a series of monologues of what to do, triggered by case-presentations from cowed learners who are there to absorb, not appraise. Once again, such events are virtually one-dimensional and names have been omitted to protect the guilty and, especially, the repentant. (We suspect that each of you already has a name for this sort of round; at one of our schools, they were labeled "Shifting Dullness").

At best, (Fig. 14-6) attending rounds can be two-stage affairs which begin with the identification of the key elements of the diagnosis and management of a given patient and end with the critical appraisal of the validity and applicability of the evidence tracked down and used by the clerks and house staff to justify each of their diagnostic and management decisions. Sometimes these two stages can be accomplished within the same session, through adequate advance preparation. More often, however, critical appraisal "tasks" are identified at the first of a pair of rounds, "worked up" over the intervening days, and then presented at the beginning of the next round. Such rounds are not only three-dimensional but utilize higher levels of each of the three dimensions of clinical learning (the

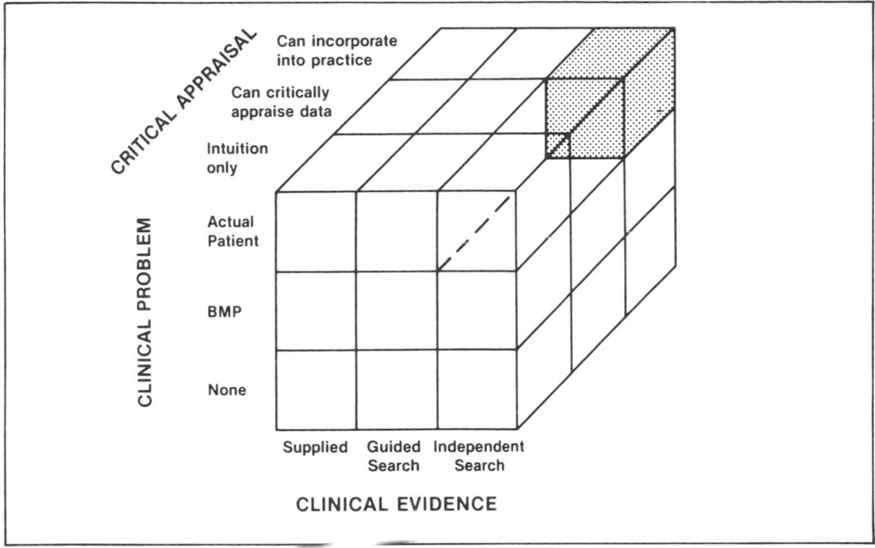

Figure 14-6. The Hirsh Round.

problems are those of the learners' own patients, they can independently track down the clinical evidence, and can incorporate their own critical appraisal of this evidence into the actual care of these patients).*

The foregoing passage provides a nice bridge between learning and teaching; the next section of this chapter asks you to shift from "getting the most from" to "giving the most to" continuing education.

Teaching Critical Appraisal at the Bedside

A busy internist, you are asked to see a fat man with high blood pressure so that you can advise his family physician whether he should be on treatment and, if so, with what. Your clinical clerk and resident are with you in the clinic, anxious to learn how an expert handles such a patient.

Because you see dozens of patients like him a year, learned how to work them up from experts during your own residency, and keep up with advances in this field by employing the strategies described in this book, it's easy to sort the patient out and equally easy to give your clinical clerk or resident either the short or the long version of your standard talk on how to do it (including citations for key articles). If they simply copy your clinical behavior, they'll give good care to hypertensives.

*Referred to in our town as the "Hirsh Round" when they were introduced by Jack Hirsh (who was our Chairman of Medicine when the first edition of this book was written); they could as easily have been called the "Goldberg Round" after Bill Goldberg (a master clinician at St. Joseph's Hospital in Hamilton) or the "Laidlaw Round" (one of our former Deans whose clinical clerks presented him with a desk plaque bearing his most common query during ward rounds: "What's your evidence for *that?!*"); it is simply that our first experience in conducting such rounds was in collaboration with Jack Hirsh.

But for how long? Back in Chapter 10 you learned that whether a hypertensive patient was treated had more to do with the clinician's year of medical school graduation than the patient's target organs. If you need fresher examples, a more recent survey of physicians in the United States revealed that over a third were unfamiliar with advances such as the use of hemoglobin A_{1c} in monitoring diabetes or the appropriateness of a "trial of labor" in many patients with prior caesarian section [33].

For those of us who teach, the message is clear. Although we may do a good job of teaching our students and house officers the best medical practice available today, we do a poor job of teaching them how to decide when what they learned from us is no longer good enough and needs to be changed. We do not teach them how to keep up to date. Thus, clinicians continue, therefore, to mimic their teachers even decades after completing training, and tend not to alter their previously learned diagnostic behavior and treatment decisions, even when later evidence dictates that they should.

In order to keep up to date, clinicians must be able to do two things. First, they must be able to tell when their current diagnostic and management practices are no longer good enough. Second, they must be able to identify which of the other, alternative diagnostic and management practices are better, and therefore should be adopted. This first ability was introduced in Chapter 10. The second ability, deciding which diagnostic and management procedures are the best ones, is central to this book, and was summarized in our discussion of "critical appraisal." How can we incorporate this into bedside teaching?

Of course, if you've assimilated much of the spirit and content of this book, you should have read the preceding few paragraphs with increasing skepticism. Where is the evidence that this approach to teaching and learning makes for better clinical decisions and better clinical care? We shared your skepticism, and therefore carried out a trial of teaching critical appraisal to our clinical clerks in the McMaster M.D. program (see Fig. 14-7) [1].

In this trial, clinical tutors at half the Hamilton hospitals were invited to undergo tutor-training in how to incorporate critical appraisal into their tutorials (90% of those invited took part). After reviewing (or learning anew) the rules of evidence for appraising the validity and applicability of articles about diagnostic tests and treatments, each experimental tutor identified specific tests and treatments that were bound to crop up during the discussion of patients on their rotation (in family medicine, internal medicine, surgery, or pediatrics). Relevant clinical articles were tracked down for each test and treatment, and each article was assessed (by the experimental tutors and the tutor-trainers) for validity and applicability, using the relevant rules of evidence.

In this way, each experimental tutor was armed with educational "packages" that could be introduced when the clinical clerks, in the routine course of discussing a real patient under their care, took stands on whether they should (or should not) carry out a certain diagnostic test or initiate a certain therapeutic regimen. When this happened, experimental tutors could distribute the package that contained both the clinical evidence on the specific test or treatment and an

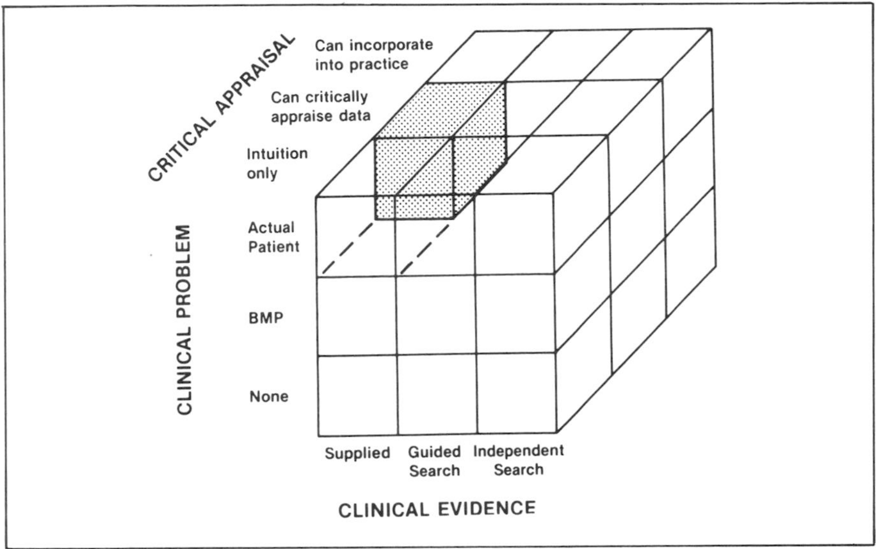

Figure 14-7. The McMaster controlled trial.

essay on how to critically appraise that evidence. The contents of the package then served as the resource for part of the subsequent tutorial meeting.

The results of the trial gave us both encouragement and a sense of urgency. Students who had been in tutorial groups led by experimental tutors, when presented with paper-based patient problems and evidence in the form of articles from current clinical journals, demonstrated clinically and statistically significant increases in their clinical judgment as shown in their ability to take and defend stands on whether specific diagnostic tests and treatments were valid and applicable to these specific patients. That was nice. Moreover, and by extension of the "number needed to be treated" you met in Chapter 7 to the "number needed to be taught," our 8-week trial showed us that we needed to teach four clinical clerks weekly for 8 weeks in order for one of them to sharply improve in the ability to take and defend therapeutic decisions. If these same rates of learning were sustained over longer critical appraisal curricula, we would have succeeded with all our clerks by 32 weeks.

The other result of our trial was the one that gave us a sense of urgency. Students who had been in tutorial groups led by control tutors demonstrated statistically significant *deteriorations* in their critical appraisal skills. These results led our Education Committee to institute tutor training across all disciplines and to incorporate critical appraisal as one of three basic skills (the others are clinical skills and self-directed learning skills) to be mastered during our M.D. program.

Other skeptics have conducted similar trials elsewhere. James Kitchens and Mark Pfeiffer found that residents who had undergone a literature-based curriculum in critical appraisal (35–40 minutes per week for 8 weeks) as part of their ambulatory rotation exhibited much greater improvement in tests of critical appraisal skills than control residents who had not had this brief exposure to it [15]. The number of their residents who "needed to be taught" for one of them to exhibit a large increase in test scores was 6 (and if the effectiveness of their curriculum was sustained, all the residents would have markedly improved by 48 weeks). On the other hand, although Mark Linzer and his colleagues found that interns taught clinical epidemiology were motivated to change their reading habits and showed some improvement in basic biostatistical knowledge, they performed no better than control interns in critically appraising articles [18]. This latter result suggests that putting all one's efforts into the internship year (with all its terrors and other stresses) may not be successful.

The ultimate test of the value of being taught critical appraisal rests in whether its recipients are more up to date 10 and 20 years after they have completed their clinical training.* The short-term "know" results described above, while sufficiently encouraging to cause the rapid and widespread adoption of critical appraisal curricula, cry out for longer term "can" and "do" studies of their impact on clinical performance.

Given that you decide to proceed to teach critical appraisal at the bedside, what are the strategies and tactics for doing so? Our experiences over the last two decades have led us to the following approach: Our basic strategy is to start and finish with the patient and the patient's problem. There are two elements in this strategy. First, critical appraisal is introduced in the same fashion as anatomy, physiology, pharmacology, microbiology, and the other basic sciences of medicine; it is initiated if, and only if, its consideration is relevant to figuring out what the patient has, and how to evaluate or manage it. This approach recognizes and supports the learner's prime objective of trying to become a better clinician, not a better epidemiologist. Second, critical appraisal is introduced naturally, unannounced, and woven into the discussion (turned on and off as required) rather than presented as a separate block or "sermonette." Thus, critical appraisal is presented as a set of skills for approaching the examination, diagnosis, and management of patients that makes the user a better clinician, not a better researcher.

How is this strategy translated into practical tactics? First, how do we show learners that critical appraisal skills will really make them better clinicians? And second, having shown them, how do we get them to do it themselves? Through trial (occasionally by fire) and error (repeatedly), by 1990 two tactics have emerged on the clinical teaching services in our town, the "Instant Resource (Red) Book" and the "Educational Prescription."

TACTIC 1: THE INSTANT RESOURCE BOOK

Our fat hypertensive patient can be used to demonstrate both of the tactics, as well as the overall strategy. The teacher can begin by asking the learner a crucial

*As this edition went to press, a study comparing the "know" dimension of clinical competency between alumni of medical schools with and without critical appraisal curricula suggested that this is, in fact, the case.

clinical (*not* epidemiologic) question: Is the patient hypertensive? The answer inevitably gets into the act of measuring blood pressure, and although most learners know that arm girth has something to do with it, and that the circumstances of measurement can affect the reading, few will know all the major determinants and none will know the magnitudes of their effects. Most teachers will know all the major determinants (but, if asked to list them, would forget to mention some), will be unable to reel off the average magnitude of their individual effects, and will be extremely unlikely to be able to give the correct citation for a useful review on the subject. Enter the *Instant Resource Book,* a collection of summaries (usually a page or less in length) of evidence on the accuracy of the clinical examination (or history, or diagnostic tests, or prognostic markers, or on the efficacy of treatments) and key references.* Figure 14-8 is a replication of the relevant page for this patient, and is an example of the early, "bare bones" format we originally used. Figure 14-9, on the diagnosis of liver metastases, represents the more recently adopted format which has three sections: "Recommendations" (the bottom line on what to do), "Evidence" (a summary of the data used to generate the recommendations), and the *Annotated Bibliography* (with the citations for the studies that generated the data). This more recent format lends itself both to quick use at the bedside and to easier updating when newer, better evidence becomes available.†

The effects of introducing a page of such "pearls" into a bedside discussion are several. First, and most important, learners learn how to become better clinicians on the spot, by doing a better job of examining the patient (blood-pressure measurement) and making a better clinical decision (as to whether the patient is hypertensive). Second, given the proximity of photocopiers to clinical sites, they can go away with their own copy of the relevant resource‡ (indeed, many ask for copies of other items in the *Instant Resource Book,* and occasionally for all of it). Third, unless the service is swamped with other patients to see, the learners raise a series of issues about their own continuing education: They ask how they should keep track of the photocopy, how this particular page came to be generated (permitting the discussion of using patients in one's care as the stimulus for learning), and how the page was prepared (permitting the discussion of how to track down [Chapter 11] and critically appraise useful references and when to get one's own computer§). The availability of the "Critical Appraisal Readers' Guides" on handy wallet cards such as those in the pocket of this book# reinforces this stimulus.

*Anticipating your curiosity over where (on earth!) the *Instant Resource Book* came from, it is the continuously evolving product of carrying out the second tactic, which we'll get to in a moment.

†Indeed, it already has! This entry is now being revised in light of newer, better evidence.

‡Thereby fulfilling the adage: "The photocopy is the wampum of clinical teaching," and complying with the Fourth Law of Sackett's Clinical Team: "The next best thing to knowing is to photocopy."

§Now.

#If yours have been stolen, or if you want extra copies, they are obtainable at cost from the authors.

BLOOD PRESSURE, MEASUREMENT OF (also see HYPERTENSION)

Proper cuff width = 0.4 × arm circumference
12 cm × 23 cm for circumference < 33 cm
15 cm × 33 cm for circumference 33–41 cm
18 cm × 36 cm for circumference ≥ 41 cm

Two arms should read within 20 mm Hg

Diastolic Blood Pressure is RAISED by:

Talking: + 10 mm	Clinic (vs. home): +5 mm (*J. Chron. Dis.* 33: 197–206, 1980)
Strange doctor: +15 mm (*Lancet* 2: 695–97, 1983)	Loose cuff
Unsupported arm: +8 mm	Unsupported back: +8 mm
Too slow release	Arm at xiphoid: +6 mm
Afternoon: +8%	Cold
Pain	Full bladder

Standing: +4 (if normotensive) to
+8 (if hypertensive)
(and pulse rises 7 bpm)

Diastolic Blood Pressure is LOWERED by:

Arm at manubrium: −5 mm	Familiarity: −12 mm (*Primary Care* 7: 637–51, 1980)

Meals: −7 mm supine; −3 mm standing
(Fagan talk in 16 April 1985 *Medical Post*)

Blood Pressure UNAFFECTED by:

4 to 30 times manufacturer's recommended doses of ephedrine nose drops (up to 4 mg at a blast) in normotensives with stuffy noses and hypertensives on beta blockers (Myers. *Can. Med. Assoc. J.* 127: 365–68, 1982)

Figure 14-8. An "old" page from the *Instant Resource Book*.

Although the foregoing tactic is very popular among learners, and graphically illustrates how critical appraisal can make one a better, faster clinician, it can only serve as an introduction. By handing "the answer" to the learners, it fails to help them become independent in any of the three dimensions of self-directed learning (using their own patients to decide what they need to learn, tracking

Figure 14-9. Diagnosis of cancer, metastases to the liver.

A. *RECOMMENDATIONS*

1. If pretest probability is *low* (<20%), start with *Liver Scan* (SnNout): a *completely negative* scan *rules out* liver mets. If the liver scan is positive, go on to CT to sort out false positives.
2. If pretest probability is *high* (≥ 80%), start with *Ultrasound* (SpPin): A *positive* ultrasound *rules in* liver mets. If the ultrasound is negative, go on to CT to sort out false negatives.
3. If pretest probability is *intermediate* (20–80%), go immediately to *CT.*

B. *EVIDENCE*

	SENSITIVITY	SPECIFICITY
1. *Direct examination at surgery:*	[35%]	"High"

Old autopsy studies reported only on specificity. A recent study of sensitivity documented positive palpation in only 6 of 17 cases with liver mets.

	SENSITIVITY	SPECIFICITY	LIKELIHOOD RATIOS: POS.	NEG.
2. *Alkaline phosphotase:*	65%	65%	1.9	0.54
3. *GGT:*	75%	45%	1.4	0.56
4. *CEA* (in colorectal Ca):				
Any result > normal	86%	60%	2.2	0.23
≥ 5 ng/dL	80%	72%	2.9	0.28
≥ 10 ng/dL	70%	87%	5.4	0.34

Blood tests have not been very useful here. Creating more levels of test results has not been very helpful.

	SENSITIVITY	SPECIFICITY	LIKELIHOOD RATIOS: POS.	NEG.
5. *Radionuclide Liver Scan:*				
Any abnormality	90%	70%	3.0	0.14
Focal lesions(s)	80%	90%	8.0	0.22

Technetium-99 has sensitivity of only 30% for lesions 1–2 cm in diameter. The trade-off between sensitivity and specificity is shown nicely. Most useful in SNOUT situations (using the absence of any abnormality as the definition for a negative study).

	SENSITIVITY	SPECIFICITY	LIKELIHOOD RATIOS: POS.	NEG.
6. *Ultrasound:*				
All studies attempted	70%	90%	7.0	0.33
Successful studies only	80%	90%	8.0	0.22

The problems are two: variation in echogenicity of different patients and variations in the skill of different ultrasonographers. Most useful in SPIN situations.

	SENSITIVITY	SPECIFICITY	LIKELIHOOD RATIOS: POS.	NEG.
7. *CT:*	90%	90%	9.0	0.11

The best, but also the most expensive. Should be reserved for intermediate pretest probabilities.

C. ***REFERENCE***

Griner, Panzer, and Greenland. *Clinical Diagnosis and the Laboratory Yearbook,* 1986. Pp. 284–96. Includes 12 references to individual studies.

Figure 14-9 (continued)

down evidence on the matter, and then both critically appraising this evidence for its validity and clinical usefulness and applying it in the clinical situation). For this reason, the *Instant Resource Book* is only a start-up tactic for teaching critical appraisal at the bedside, and a handy record of previous, successful appraisals. Total reliance on it would simply perpetuate the old, discredited system in which learners stop learning when there are no teachers to hand out this year's "right" answers.

TACTIC 2: THE EDUCATIONAL PRESCRIPTION

The next step requires that learners become much more active, and a tactic for accomplishing this that we have used with increasing success over the past several years is the "Educational Prescription." Consider once again the fat hypertensive patient from the start of this discussion. Although the instant resource on blood pressure measurement (Fig. 14-8) can whet learners' appetites for critical appraisal, it cannot teach them how to do it. To accomplish the latter, they must begin to work on their own, and the Educational Prescription helps them do just that.

The discussion of this patient can proceed in several different directions, depending on how much learners already know and what additional things they need to know in order to serve the patient and the referring physician. Thus, on our service the issues that arise when learners care for such patients can go in anatomic, physiologic, pharmacologic, or clinical directions. Although, when beginning work with a new team, it often is less threatening (on both sides!) to orient the first Educational Prescription toward a more traditional issue in pathophysiology, we soon must deal with the patient and consider questions such as: What forms of secondary hypertension are worth seeking in such a patient? (leading, in turn, to questions on the frequency of secondary hypertension and the yield of tests for it); what levels of systolic and/or diastolic pressure ought to be treated in such a patient? (leading to questions of the efficacy and effectiveness of antihypertensive drugs); could this man be treated with weight reduction alone? (leading to questions of the efficacy and effectiveness of nonpharmacologic approaches to controlling high blood pressure); and, how do we get this patient to follow our advice and take his medicine? (leading to questions of strategies for improving compliance with therapeutic regimens). These questions have two important features in common—all are directly relevant to the care of this specific patient (so that their answers will be clinically useful today), and the answers to all of them are constantly changing (so that this year's answer will be wrong at a future date that is inevitable but unpredictable).

An Educational Prescription (Fig. 14-10) is written when learners don't know the answer to a question that is pertinent to the evaluation or management of their patient. Early on, this identification can be made by the teacher. Later, learners who recognize the educational advantages of the approach will begin to request and write their own Prescriptions (by the end of a month on one of our clinical services, about one-third are "self-prescriptions").

At this point many readers must be protesting that they already apply this tactic every teaching day, in the form of verbal assignments to the members of their team. We'd argue (based on our own experience and the confessions of other teachers and learners) that such verbal assignments are incapable of reminding either you or their recipients what the assignment was and what it was for.* Four entries on the Educational Prescription are designed to provide these reminders. First, the specific patient problem that serves as the stimulus for learning is identified, so that the ultimate objective (improving the care of that patient) can be kept in mind. Second, the specific educational task to be performed, and by whom,† is specified, so that the educational target is not forgotten. Similarly, the time and place for reporting the results of the effort are specified at the start. Third, the notation at the bottom of the Prescription reminds learners that their presentation must begin with a description of how they found what they found (so that they can learn how to track down evidence more efficiently) and end with a description of how their critical appraisal of this evidence will change the way that they look after the patient (so that the purpose for the entire exercise remains in focus). This notation also reminds the learner that a critical appraisal, rather than a mere repetition, of the evidence is required. Finally, our Educational Prescriptions are written in duplicate. The original goes to the learner, and the copy is held by the attending or chief resident to monitor completion.

*And we have yet to meet a learner who will volunteer the fact that a verbal prescription hasn't been filled!

†Teachers also should be prepared to be the recipients of Educational Prescriptions when they make unsubstantiated claims about clinical findings, diagnosis, prognosis, or therapy.

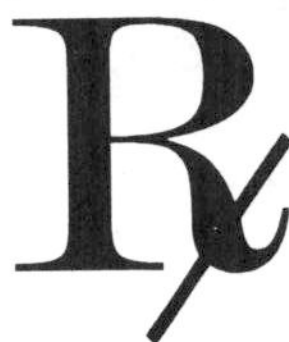

EDUCATIONAL PRESCRIPTION

For The Session on ____________ at ________ Hours at ______.

THE PATIENT PROBLEM: ______________________________

____

____

EDUCATIONAL TASKS TO BE COMPLETED BEFORE THE SESSION:

"Volunteer:"	Task:
____________________	____________________
	____________________
____________________	____________________
	____________________

Presentations will cover:

i. HOW you found what you found.
ii. WHAT you found.
iii. The VALIDITY & APPLICABILITY of what you found.
iv. How what you found would ALTER your MANAGEMENT of the pt.

Figure 14-10. The Educational Prescription.

Each weekday on the typical inpatient service where we work, attending physicians, house staff, and clinical clerks make their individual rounds and then, 3 to 5 days a week, meet as a group for a 2-hour teaching round where we present, jointly examine, and discuss our patients. During the course of these examinations and discussions, questions inevitably arise, the answers to which will determine how a particular patient is evaluated or managed. If the question is judged (usually by consensus) to be an important one, the answer to which would affect not just the specific patient but other, similar patients, an Educational Prescription is written and assigned.

If the patient problem is an urgent one, the prescription may have to be filled and reported upon that same day, often relying on expert consultants as sources of evidence. More often, an interim solution can be implemented while the prescription is being filled, and reporting is done a day, or a few days, later. To ensure the latter, the results of the Educational Prescription are discussed when the patient who generated them is being reviewed; this critical appraisal discussion is thus an integral part of the everyday running of the service, demonstrating its central role in the care of the patient. A sample of the tasks assigned on Educational Prescriptions on our inpatient service appears in Table 14-1.

Table 14-1. A sample of 12 tasks from the first 175 educational prescriptions

If this anemic patient's bone marrow has shut down, what would be the daily changes in her formed elements?

Could this patient's campylobacter jejuni diarrhea have caused his Guillain-Barré syndrome?

Is retinal vein pulsation still a useful sign for intracranial pressure in this woman with a posterior fossa tumor?

What is the accuracy of sigmoidoscopy in ruling out pseudomembranous enterocolitis as the cause for this antibiotic-associated diarrhea?

Could a normal thallium exercise test rule out clinically important coronary heart disease in this man with 6 CCU admissions for atypical chest pain (but never a myocardial infarction)?

Can we generate the first draft of an algorithm for detecting reversible causes of delirium and dementia by studying this confused woman with a fractured hip?

Would the computer program "Internist" help us achieve a diagnosis in this man with multiple unexplained symptoms, signs, and laboratory abnormalities?

Which noninvasive test is best for deciding whether this man's gastric cancer has metastasized to his liver?

Is there a quick way to estimate whether this stroke patient will return to independent living?

Should this vigorous 75-year-old woman with an uncomplicated myocardial infarction receive long-term beta blockers?

Is there a way to help this man with advanced cancer achieve his goal of maintaining excellent pain control on a simpler opiate regimen?

Can we justify (to the hospital administration) the cost of plasmapheresis for this man with Guillain-Barré syndrome?

An analogous approach is used in the office or outpatient clinic. If learners appear weekly, the interval between writing and filling a prescription is a multiple of 7 days. As on the inpatient service, time is set aside for filling Educational Prescriptions (if the clinic is "too busy" to permit this sort of learning, we shouldn't kid the trainees that we are there as teachers).*

One product of an Educational Prescription should be a one- or two-page written summary of the critically appraised evidence, organized either as in Figure 14-8 or, preferably, as in Figure 14-9. This summary of the key evidence and citations serves four purposes. First, it can be copied for each member of the team. Second, it can be used to start the learner's own *Instant Resource Book* (thus contributing to the formation of a pattern of lifelong continuing education). Third, it can be added to the ward's or clinic's *Instant Resource Book* and consulted the next time a similar patient appears. Finally, a subsequent Educational Prescription on a similar patient can use the product of the first prescription as the starting point for an update when a similar patient comes on the service later.

PROBLEMS IN INTRODUCING CRITICAL APPRAISAL AT THE BEDSIDE

As we and our colleagues at other institutions have introduced these tactics on busy clinical services, we have had to solve three problems. The first one arises from the disparity that may exist between the attitudes held by the writers and readers of this book, on the one hand, and the attitudes that prevail in many medical institutions, on the other. Several attitudes are implicit (and explicit!) in the approach to clinical practice advocated in this book. They include skepticism, placing a low value on authority, and tolerating uncertainty. These attitudes are not inculcated in some medical schools, and in others it could be argued that the predominant attitudes are quite the reverse. If you work at one of these latter places, you may be teaching medical students and house staff who believe that the "right" answer always can be found, either in the pages of an authoritative textbook or at the feet of an authoritative attending. Because this latter perspective resolves clinical controversies through appeal to authority (the clinician with the most experience, or the academic with the most prestigious research record), students raised in such a tradition may well be confused or downright hostile when being asked to answer a clinical question by tracking down and critically appraising the primary literature themselves.

How might you respond when the clinical clerks and house staff in your clinic or on your teaching ward display mystification, resistance, or hostility of this sort? The first, and very powerful, strategy is for you to display, right from your first encounter with your learners, the behaviors and attitudes you want them to develop; that is, you can provide a role model of skepticism, tolerance of uncertainty, and the critical appraisal of evidence, regardless of its source. You can start by showing a willingness to say "I don't know." Initially, this admission may be an extraordinarily difficult one to make in public, especially if the implicit message in your medical environment is that uncertainty represents ignorance, inadequacy, and incompetence. Your trainees' expectations may be that

*Of course we learn in busy clinics, but too often at the expense of the patients.

good attendings have all the answers and that attendings who don't have all the answers aren't good. As a result, you are under pressure to answer every question with confidence, even when you are uncertain or unable to cite evidence that supports what you think is correct.

Starting to respond, "I don't know," or "I've been told such-and-such, but I'm not sure of the evidence to support it" will be difficult in such settings, but there are two distinct advantages to doing so. First, because this is exactly what your trainees are saying to themselves almost every time they are asked a question, they will be enormously relieved to discover that they are not hopelessly incompetent and that even attendings have something yet to learn. Second, such responses on your part can be remarkably liberating, for they dramatically decrease the pressure on you to cover up your lack of knowledge or deny your uncertainty. As a result, it now becomes much easier for everyone on the clinical team to admit their ignorance and uncertainty, and teaching rounds can be converted from contests in which everyone is, at least part of the time, bluffing one another about what they know into real opportunities for defining what members of the team don't know and what they are going to do about it.

To be sure, clerks and house staff who are not used to hearing staff members acknowledge ignorance or uncertainty may be taken aback, and their loss of fear may be accompanied by some initial loss of respect. The latter is blunted by their recognition of your expertise in other areas (such as the clinical examination, or the current literature in an area you've recently examined), and is followed by even greater respect when they see how quickly you can track down, critically appraise, and integrate the evidence required to correct your ignorance or uncertainty.

For, of course, you can't stop at saying "I don't know." You have to follow this up by modeling the finding and assessment of whatever evidence is available so that you can come back saying "Now, I do know." Ideally, your admission of uncertainty about an issue in a patient's care today is followed by your appearance on the ward tomorrow with a printout citing the 10 best relevant articles (and a notation that the computer search took 8 minutes), plus photocopies of the two most informative papers for each member of your team. The stage is now set for a critical appraisal of the papers and a discussion of how their results should affect your management of the patient.

After you have taken your time to demonstrate this exercise once or twice for your team, you now have the moral authority to ask them to copy it, conducting their own searches on their own uncertainty or ignorance about their own patients and appraising the resulting evidence. Teaching your clerks and house staff by modeling a literature search on your own computer is extremely powerful and exciting, and the ease with which relevant literature can be obtained in this way may provide a lasting stimulus to them to pursue the scientific approach to the practice of medicine. Moreover, you may want to direct the initial Educational Prescriptions toward more traditional topics such as pathophysiology or pharmacodynamics, introducing critical appraisal topics only after learners are comfortable with the educational tactic.

A complementary strategy for winning over clerks and house staff from an authoritative "must know" style of learning is to be alert for, and capitalize on, controversy and disagreement. Members of your team often will voice different opinions about the meaning of a clinical or laboratory finding, a diagnosis or prognosis, or a plan of therapy. Rather than immediately resolving the dispute (and reinforcing appeal to authority as the only route to truth) by providing the "right answer" (even if you know it), you can begin to move your team along by challenging the disputants to substantiate their conflicting opinions. If, in their initial response, each obtains support from an authoritative textbook or senior subspecialist, so much the better: they will have to admit that even respected authorities manifest fundamental disagreement. If, on the other hand, a critical examination of the relevant literature by both disputants leads them to agreement, team members will begin to get a sense of the power of this approach to guiding clinical practice.

The second problem that surfaces when critical appraisal is introduced into a clinical service arises when learners discover that only a portion of the clinical literature they track down can survive their critical appraisal. This leads to complaints about the scarcity of valid, useful evidence. Although this realization is healthy, it is nonetheless frustrating, especially when learners discover that it applies to such fundamental issues as the accuracy of symptoms, signs, and laboratory data. One effective response to this problem is to combine the encouragement of their continuing efforts at independence in tracking down clinical evidence with helping them identify the modern medical texts and computer software that present organized summaries of the sensitivities, specificities, and likelihood ratios for the clinical history, physical and laboratory examination or imaging procedures in a wide range of presenting complaints, and the therapeutic alternatives for managing these problems. A list of the texts and software we were using at the time this second edition was being prepared appears as an appendix to Chapter 11.

The third problem that surfaces when critical appraisal is introduced follows from the fact that different learners have different amounts of time for learning; at most centers, clinical clerks have the most time, and first year postgraduates the least. Although it can be argued that learners who don't have time to fill Educational Prescriptions because of the pressures of patient care are following too many patients, this admonition won't help them find extra time. The short-term solutions are two. First, time-pressured learners can at least sit in on the prescription writing and filling being done by others, and benefit from hearing these discussions as well as the new information. Second, they can take on Educational Prescriptions that are either limited in scope (to minimize the time spent on searching and sifting) or less urgent (so that they will have additional time to fill them).

OTHER SITES FOR CRITICAL APPRAISAL

It's My Turn to Run Grand Rounds. How Can I Incorporate Some Critical Appraisal into the Session?

The potential for incorporating critical appraisal into Grand Rounds is shown in Figure 14-11.

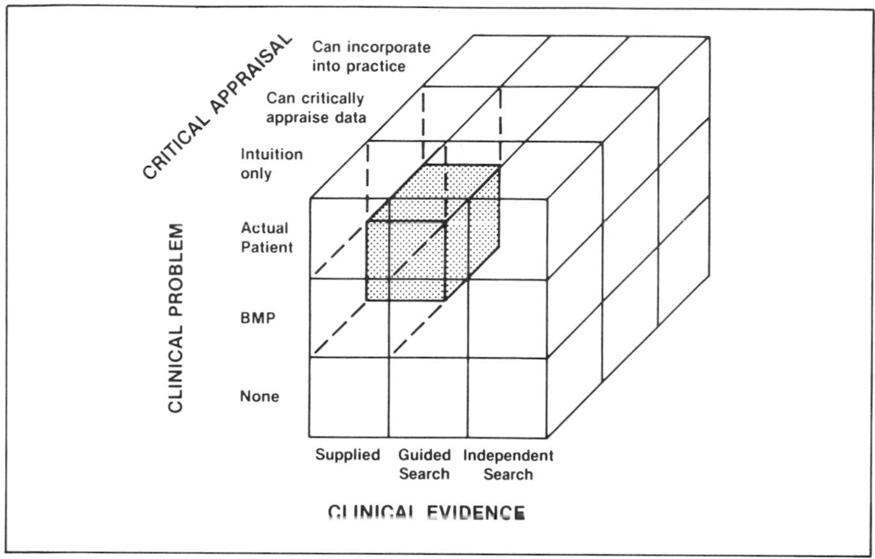

Figure 14-11. Potential for Grand Rounds.

These rounds can become three-dimensional and, with time, shift deeper into the critical appraisal of clinical evidence by coupling the clinical and published evidence together.

After presenting the case and identifying the issue in etiology, diagnosis, prognosis, or therapy raised most prominently by the case, the presenter can synthesize: (a) the actual evidence on the issue (rather than the conclusions drawn from the evidence), and (b) the rules or guides for critically assessing this evidence.

The result is both a conclusion about the case presented at the rounds and an approach to assessing evidence about other cases; the latter is reinforced by citing appropriate critical appraisal essays and by providing throw-aways that specify and explain the critical appraisal guides.

Our Journal Club Is Foundering. How Can We Make It More Exciting and Useful?

Journal clubs often assign individual issues of periodicals to their members, requiring them to review their contents for the other members of the club. Thus, the operation of the journal club replicates a journal subscription, as shown in Figure 14-12.

Journal subscriptions and some journal clubs are in the basement. Clinicians read an article because it arrives in the mail, not because it relates to a patient, and may not realize that most authors discuss only those critical appraisal issues they have solved, not the ones they have failed to solve or have overlooked.

Journal clubs have the option to change. They can elevate themselves toward the far "northeast" by strategies such as:

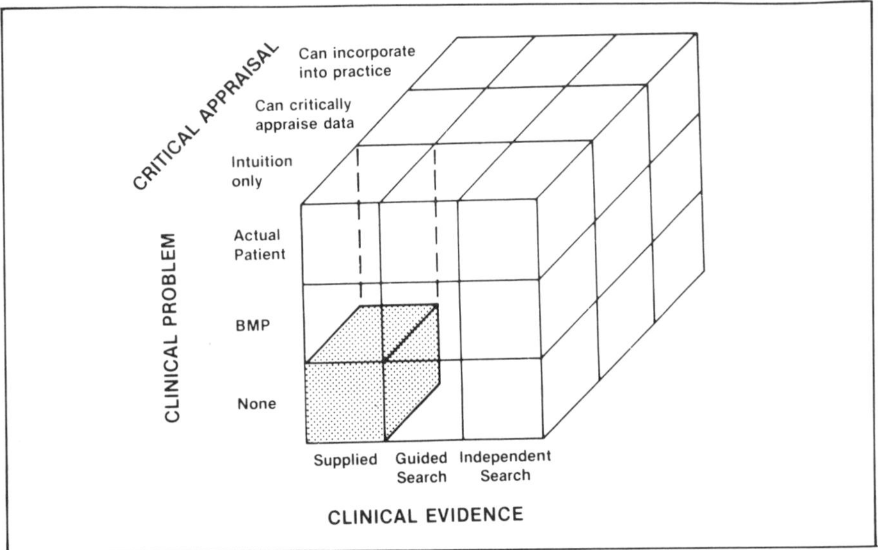

Figure 14-12. A journal subscription and some journal clubs.

a. Providing critical appraisal worksheets (see Fig. 12-2) along with the journal articles, and discussing how the former affect the clinical conclusions drawn from the latter.
b. Going further to using actual patients as the basis for selecting which articles will appraised.
c. Going further still and asking members to identify problem patients in their own practices, find pertinent articles, use them as the focus of discussion, and incorporate the discussion into the care of these patients. The members of this sort of journal club are heading to the "northeast" corner of the learning cube, developing skills in tracking down, as well as critically appraising, those articles that will help them solve their patients' problems.

We've seen some previously moribund journal clubs take on new life by adopting the third strategy. Indeed, one group of our medical students ran their own journal club during their preclinical year, using the paper-based biomedical problems (BMPs) that form the basis for our preclinical curriculum as their starting and ending points [16].

THE FUTURE

As more and better people have become involved in this approach to clinical learning, four things have begun to happen. First, the quality and quantity of *Instant Resource* materials is expanding, so that there are better examples to help learners get started in all the medical specialties, including primary care. Indeed, as this edition was being prepared a group of us banded together to write a very different sort of clinical skills book in which, for inclusion, an item of the medical history or physical examination will have to be both precise (that is, documented to be reproducible within and between clinicians) and accurate (that is, validated against some gold standard of anatomy, physiology, prognosis, or responsiveness to therapy).*

Second, as you learned in Chapter 11, cheaper and more efficient methods (many of which will be computer-based) of tracking down high-quality evidence are becoming available to learners (often through their own computers), making this approach to clinical learning and keeping up to date easier for everyone. When one of us placed microcomputers in the emergency room, intensive care unit, mixed-service ambulatory clinic, and two medical wards of one of our teaching hospitals and gave free access to MEDLINE (through GRATEFUL MED) and BRS/Colleague [13], over 80% of potential users logged in, and although their searching skills left a fair bit to be desired (they missed almost half the relevant articles that reference librarians found on their topics, and about half the articles they did find were irrelevant), their clinical decisions were affected by 47% of the searches.

Third, we think that clinicians increasingly will face up to their need for more up-to-date information about patient management, thereby accelerating the former two trends. For example, and in contrast to their self-reports (of only one such question requiring additional information arising per week, and this additional information usually easily obtained from texts, journals, and drug compendia), direct observation of practicing clinicians has documented two problems arising for every three patients [7]. However, 70% of these questions went unanswered. Moreover, because these clinicians judged their texts to be out of date, their journals too disorganized to permit them to find a particular article, and their time too short for a proper search, most of the 30% of the questions that did get answered were addressed by consulting colleagues. Thus, continuing practice in tracking down, appraising, and applying pertinent information is needed to overcome these flaws in perception and performance that interfere with answering clinical questions as they arise.

Which brings us to the fourth thing that is beginning to happen. As more and brighter clinical epidemiologists tackle the challenges of teaching critical appraisal at the bedside, newer and more effective learning strategies and teaching tactics are being developed and tested. We all look forward to learning about them so that we can apply them in our own clinical teaching and learning.

Self-Directed Learning Skills

The key to continuing effectiveness as a clinician is illustrated in Figure 14-13.

Clinicians judged by their peers to be the most effective practitioners in town exhibit quite vigorous self-directed learning [31]. Despite the pressures of full-time practice, they are stimulated by their patients to track down and critically appraise the latest evidence about the importance and reliability of specific signs and symptoms, the accuracy and power of specific diagnostic tests, the validity of claims about the etiology or prognosis of disease, and the validity and appli-

*To our surprise, the first edition will not be as slim a volume as we initially suspected!

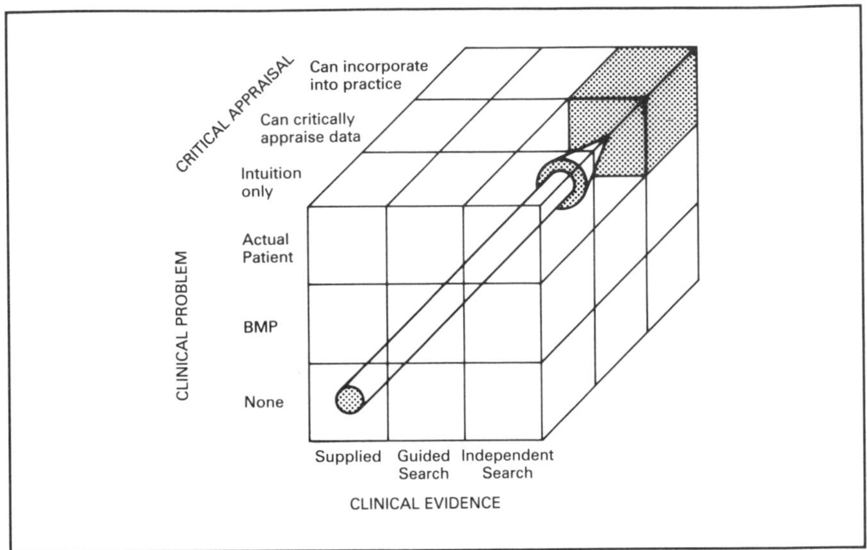

Figure 14-13. Self-directed learning and the effective clinician.

cability of claims that specific preventive, therapeutic, and rehabilitative regimens do more good than harm. They thus are able to tell when the way they have been evaluating and managing patients is no longer good enough and needs to be changed. In short, they keep up to date.

In the preceding portions of this chapter, we have stated the direction in which we think your self-directed learning should take you in developing your clinical and critical appraisal skills. Along the way, we have alluded to several self-directed learning skills. We will end this chapter, and the book, focusing on these skills, because they are a prerequisite for any success in improving and maintaining your clinical competence, especially once you have completed your training. It follows that these skills must be developed to the point of "second nature" by the time you graduate into clinical practice—for they are unlikely to develop de novo thereafter. Table 14-2 provides a list of these skills and we will close with a summary of them.

The importance of formulating clear learning objectives is illustrated in a tale told by Robert Mager [21]. A sea horse set out to find his fortune, supported by a modest amount of cash. As he wandered along his way, he met an eel who convinced him he could wander faster with a pair of expensive flippers. Thus equipped, he speedily met a sponge who relieved him of more of his cash in return for a jet-propelled scooter. Zooming along at five times his former speed, he encountered a shark who offered a shortcut, pointing to his open mouth. Once again, the sea horse accepted the offer of a more rapid transit, and was never seen again. The moral, as Mager puts it, is that "If you're not sure where you're going, you're liable to end up someplace else." Clinically, this allegory fits the situation in which we squander our diagnostic resources by ordering banks of

Table 14-2. Self-directed learning skills

1. Formulating clear learning objectives
2. Reading to solve problems
3. Highly selective browsing
4. Establishing and maintaining a personal information system
5. Carrying out self-assessments
6. Executing personal behavior modification

tests without having thought why we are ordering them. Both we and our patient can get swallowed in the end by a false-positive "shark." And in our learning, we play the sea horse every time we let our quest for new knowledge be guided more by whatever journal crosses our desk, or by whatever meeting comes through town, than by tracking down specific learning opportunities on the basis of what we really need to know.

We maintain that your best sources of clear learning objectives in clinical medicine are the problems presented by your own patients. The more that your learning experiences are generated from, and lead to, the resolution of specific patient problems, the more effective (permanent) and relevant (clinically useful) the learning will be. This is, in fact, simply a clinical restatement of a universal educational principle: Learning is best when it takes place in real life; the best learning experience takes place where what is to be learned is also to be applied [24].

From these beginnings you can apply the other self-directed learning skills described in this book. The "critical appraisal guides" will assist both your browsing and selective reading, and as your *Instant Resource Book* develops you will find progressively more of your answers in it. Finally, the self-assessments gained through periodic reviews of your own performance will identify the successes and failures of attempts to modify your clinical behavior.

True to this theme, we will end this chapter and the book.

Here are our answers to the four questions that opened this chapter:

1. *The 27-year-old woman with SLE who is contemplating pregnancy*. In searching for helpful articles on the *prognosis* of SLE we would be concerned about:

a. An inception cohort of not-yet pregnant SLE patients; with
b. The referral pattern described
c. Complete follow-up achieved
d. Objective outcome criteria for the prognostic outcomes and
e. When looking at the effect of pregnancy, control of extraneous prognostic factors such as age, parity, and the initial severity of disease.

One of us went on an information search on this patient, and the results (and the time required for each approach) went like this:

1. Examined the October 1990 version of Scientific American *Medicine* [27], and found a very helpful half page (with several references from 3–5 years old) on the risks of pregnancy to both the mother and the fetus (4 minutes). I would have stopped here if rushed for time, but went on to see whether other approaches would provide more recent information.
2. Examined *Harvey's Principles and Practice of Medicine* (22nd ed.) [9] and found a brief and not-too-helpful paragraph on pregnancy (with references 3 and 10 years old), plus a more informative one on neonatal lupus (3 minutes).
3. Used CD-ROM [Compact Cambridge] for the current year (November 1990), applied the MeSH terms LUPUS ERYTHEMATOSUS, SYSTEMIC, and PREGNANCY, requested a display (of the title, authors, and source), and limited it to HUMAN and ENGLISH. I got 41 citations, and the second one [26] looked like what I wanted. I found it in the stacks and scanned it. It satisfied most of the criteria, was helpful, and included citations for two other "prospective studies" (6 minutes to set up the search, 9 minutes to scan the citations, 4 minutes to find the article).

2. The *likelihood ratios* we calculated looked like this:

		Target disorder				
		Present		Absent		
		Number	Proportion	Number	Proportion	Likelihood ratio
Test result	+ + +	100	0.5495	1	0.0123	45
	+ +	50	0.2747	10	0.1235	2.2
	+	30	0.1648	30	0.3704	0.45
	0	2	0.0110	40	0.4938	0.02
	Total	182	1.0000	81	1.0000	

A cutoff point between + + + and + + would misclassify (50 + 30 + 2 + 1) or 83 patients; a cutoff between + + and + would misclassify (30 + 2 + 1 + 10) or 43 patients; a cutoff between + and 0 would misclassify (2 + 1 + 10 + 30) or 43 patients. Thus either of the latter two would produce the same number of errors, and you could pick the one that did the most good for true positives and true negatives (or produced the least harm among false positives and false negatives). But, given the considerably greater information gained from likelihood ratios, why would you ever want to dichotomize a diagnostic test result such as this one?

3. *Precautions against* AIDS: This search went as follows:

1. Knowing that it was a hot topic in an area with a massive literature, the first look was in the monthly (rather than the annual) *Index Medicus*, and scanned the AIDS headings. Under AIDS SERODIAGNOSIS, an article on risks to surgeons of acquiring HIV [14], published 5 months ago, was cited (2 min-

utes). It was in the stacks (4 minutes to find and scan it), and included a reference to a 1987 set of recommendations for the prevention of HIV transmission in health-care settings published in *MMWR* (Morbidity and Mortality Weekly Reports) [4]. Our library subscribes to that publication, and I went to the current issues, found a recent issue on the management of exposure and the use of zidovudine [7], examined its references, and found a 1989 update on those guidelines [6] (8 minutes). However, the issues containing both the 1987 guidelines and their 1989 update were AWOL,* so the 20 minutes spent looking for them was wasted. An interlibrary loan was requested, but obviously wouldn't arrive in time. I could have called a colleague at another medical school and asked him to fax the latest version, but I went to the next step instead.

2. I looked in Scientific American *Medicine* (October 1990), found an index heading: "epidemiology and transmission, health-care and research workers," and followed it to a nice table summarizing an earlier (1988) update of the precautions (4 minutes) [5]. It wasn't the latest update, but it was there!

4. *Since you began reading this book, how many opportunities have you had to apply its principles in your own clinical practice? Of these, on how many occasions did you actually apply the principles?*

Only you can answer this question!

References

1. Bennett, K. J., Sackett, D.L ., Haynes, R. B., and Neufeld, V. R. A controlled trial of teaching critical appraisal of the clinical literature to medical students. *J.A.M.A.* 257: 2451, 1987.
2. Carnahan, J. E., and Nugent, C. A. The effects of self-monitoring by patients on the control of hypertension. *Am. J. Med. Sci.* 269: 69, 1975.
3. Carveth, S. W., Burnop, T. K., Bechtel, J., et al. Training in advanced cardiac life support. *J.A.M.A.* 235: 2311, 1976.
4. CDC (Centers for Disease Control). Recommendations for prevention of HIV transmission in health-care settings. *M.M.W.R.* 36: No. 2S, 1987.
5. CDC (Centers for Disease Control). Update: Universal precautions for prevention of transmission of human immunodeficiency virus, hepatitis B virus, and other bloodborne pathogens in health-care settings. *M.M.W.R.* 37: 377, 1988.
6. CDC (Centers for Disease Control). Guidelines for prevention of human immunodeficiency virus and hepatitis B virus to health-care and public-safety workers. *M.M.W.R.* 38: No. S-6, 1989.
7. CDC (Centers for Disease Control). Public Health Service statement on management of occupational exposure to human immunodeficiency virus, including considerations regarding zidovudine postexposure use. *M.M.W.R.* 39: No. RR-1, 1990.
8. Covell, D. G., Uman, G. C., and Manning, P. R. Information needs in office practice: are they being met? *Ann. Intern. Med.* 103: 596, 1985.

*Absent With-Out Leave. They weren't on the shelves or tables, and they hadn't been checked out!

9. Harvey, A. McG., Johns, R. J., McKusick, V.A., et al. *The Principles and Practice of Medicine* (22nd ed.) Norwalk, CT: Appleton & Lange, 1988.
10. Harvey, J. T., Neufeld, V. R., and Sackett, D. L. Ranking clinical problems and ocular diseases in ophthalmology: An innovative approach to curriculum design. *Can. J. Ophthalmol.* 23; 6: 255, 1988
11. Haynes, R. B., Gibson, E. S., Taylor, D. W., et al. Process versus outcome in hypertension: A positive result. *Circulation* 65: 28, 1982.
12. Haynes, R. B., Davis, D. A., McKibbon, A., and Tugwell, P. A critical appraisal of the efficacy of continuing medical education. *J.A.M.A.* 251: 61, 1984.
13. Haynes, R. B., McKibbon, K. A., Walker, C. J., et al. Online access to MEDLINE in clinical settings: A study of use and usefulness. *Ann. Intern. Med.* In Press, 1990.
14. Howard, R. J. Human immunodeficiency virus testing and the risk to the surgeon of acquiring HIV. *Surg. Gynecol. Obstet.* 171: 22, 1990.
15. Kitchens, J. M., and Pfeifer, M. P. Teaching residents to read the medical literature: A controlled trial of a curriculum in critical appraisal/clinical epidemiology. *J. Gen. Intern. Med.* 4: 384, 1989.
16. Kitching, A. D., and Guyatt, G. H. The critical appraisal club. *Can. Med. Assoc. J.* 136: 819, 1987.
17. Linn, B. S. Continuing medical education: Impact on emergency room burn care. *J.A.M.A.* 244: 565, 1980.
18. Linzer, M., Brown, J. T., Frazier, L. M., et al. Impact of a medical journal club on house-staff reading habits, knowledge, and critical appraisal skills. *J.A.M.A.* 260: 2537, 1988.
19. Logan, A. S. *Investigation of Toronto General Practitioners' Treatment of Patients with Hypertension.* Toronto: Canadian Facts, 1978.
20. Lomas, J. The role of cesarian section in changing physicians' awareness, attitudes, knowledge, and behavior. Presentation at the 5th Annual Meeting of the International Society of Technology Assessment in Health Care. London, 1989.
21. Mager, R. F. *Preparing Instructional Objectives* (2nd ed.). Belmont, CA: Fearson. 1975.
22. McDonald, C. J., Wilson, G. A., McCabe, G. P., Jr., et al. Physician response to computer reminders. *J.A.M.A.* 244: 1579, 1980.
23. Miller G. E. Personal communication. 1982.
24. Miller, G. E. *Teaching and Learning in Medical School.* Cambridge: Harvard University Press, 1962. P. 70.
25. Neufeld, V. R. Current concepts in continuing medical education: an overview for clinicians. *Ann. Roy. Coll. Phys. Surg. Canad.* 16: 223, 1983.
26. Nossent, H. C., and Swaak, T. J. G. Systemic lupus erythematosus: VI. Analysis of the interrelationship with pregnancy. *J. Rheumatology* 17: 771, 1990.
27. Rubenstein, E., and Federman, D. D. Scientific American *Medicine.* New York: Scientific American. 1978–1983.
28. Sanazaro, P. J., and Worht, M. Concurrent quality assurance in hospital care: Report of a study by private initiative in PSRO. *N. Engl. J. Med.* 298: 1171, 1978.
29. Sibley, J. C., Sackett, D. L., Neufeld, V. R., et al. A randomized trial of continuing medical education. *N. Engl. J. Med.* 302: 511, 1982.
30. Swain, M. A., and Steckel, S. B. Influencing adherence among hypertensives. *Res. Nurs. Health* 4: 213, 1981.
31. Wakefield, J. G., Woodward, C. A., and Neufeld, V. R. Effective self-directed learning in physicians. Final Report to the Ivy Foundation. London, Ontario, 1983.
32. Weaver, F. J., Ramirez, A. G., Dorman, S. B., et al. Trainees' retention of cardiopulmonary resuscitation: How quickly they forget. *J.A.M.A.* 214: 901, 1979.
33. Williamson, J. W., German, P. S., Weiss, R., et al. Health science information management and continuing education of physicians; a survey of U.S. primary care providers and their opinion leaders. *Ann. Intern. Med.* 110: 151,1989.

Index